RADIOLOGY
OF THE NORMAL SKULL

Radiology of the Normal Skull

Robert Shapiro, M.D.

Chairman, Department of Radiology
The Hospital of St. Raphael
Clinical Professor of Radiology
Yale University School of Medicine
New Haven, Connecticut

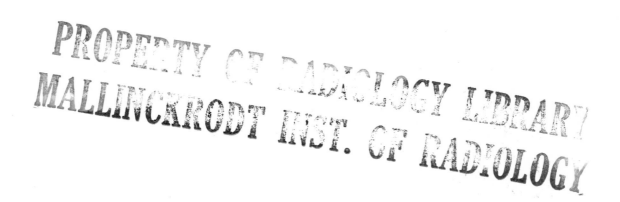

YEAR BOOK MEDICAL PUBLISHERS, INC.

CHICAGO • LONDON

Library of Congress Cataloging in Publication Data

Shapiro, Robert.
    Radiography of the normal skull.

    Bibliography: p.
    Includes index.
    1. Skull—Radiography. I. Title. [DNLM: 1. Skull
—Radiography.   WE705 S5294r]
RC936.S52   617′.5140757   80-23680
ISBN 0-8151-7631-7

*To Pearl, the beloved companion of my life, and
to the cherished, older Ox Bow Four.*

Preface

Some twenty years ago, Arnold Janzen and I wrote a monograph on the normal skull. Since that time, several authors (Taveras and Wood, Newton and Potts) have produced outstanding works on the skull and its contents. Their treatises are multivolume texts which consider the normal skull, the many diseases affecting the skull and its contents, and the specialized techniques for studying these diseases. Until the present book, a single volume devoted exclusively to a detailed radiologic presentation of the normal skull and its variants has not been available.

During the past ten years, I have spent considerable time studying the embryogenesis of the human skull and the comparative anatomy of vertebrate skulls in general. I have also collected data on a large number of normal variants seen in a busy clinical and consulting practice, augmented by contributions from numerous colleagues. A lifetime of teaching reinforces the impression that the identification of many normal variants and the early departure from normalcy still constitutes a significant problem for radiologists, neurologists, neurosurgeons, residents, and medical students. I hope this monograph helps to answer that need.

Although this is a highly personal book, the fruits of discussions with many colleagues over the years have undoubtedly found their way into the manuscript. However, my friends bear no responsibility for the weaver's personal taste nor for any inadvertent errors that may have crept into the warp and woof of the tapestry.

New Haven, 1980   ROBERT SHAPIRO

Acknowledgments

I gratefully acknowledge the opportunity provided by Dr. Edmund S. Crelin to study a large number of human anatomical specimens and by Dr. John Ostrom to study the rich collection of vertebrate skulls at the Peabody Museum. I am particularly beholden to Dr. E. Leon Kier, one of the country's outstanding neuroradiologists, for generously sharing his case material with me. This book might never have been written were it not for the encouragement of Dr. Stephen G. Rothman, who is responsible for chapter 17 on CT scanning of the calvaria, and who collaborated with me on chapter 12, dealing with the sella turcica. I am also indebted to Dr. Robert E. Schaeffer and to Eastman Kodak Company for allowing me to use the tomographic illustrations of the ear in chapter 16.

It is a great pleasure to thank my dear friend and colleague, Dr. Arnold H. Janzen, and Harper & Row, for permitting me to use material from *The Normal Skull*. My thanks also to Drs. Ronald Ablow, Maier B. Ozonoff, John F. Holt, and G. Frank Johnson for lending me some of their case material. A portion of the material in this book has appeared previously in various journals.

I wish to thank Dr. Franklin Robinson, my coauthor for many of the papers, and the editors of *American Journal of Radiology*, *Investigative Radiology*, *Journal of Neurosurgery*, and *Radiology* for granting me permission to use material from these papers. I am especially grateful to the Harvard University Press for permission to use a number of illustrations from the monograph *Embryogenesis of the Human Skull*.

All books like this begin with radiographs, photographs, and artist's illustrations. I am grateful to Nicholas Piscitelli, the masterful chief radiologic technologist at The Hospital of St. Raphael, for his expert radiography of many specimens and for his assistance with the first chapter. I also wish to thank Ovidio Gallo and Doris Barclay for the excellent photography, and Virginia Simon for the superb new drawings. Finally, I must acknowledge, with unbounded gratitude, the invaluable contribution of my secretary, Angela Brunetti, who typed, retyped, and proofread the manuscript. Without her untiring efforts, this book would truly not have been possible.

Contents

1

Technique

Superior radiography of the skull demands meticulous care. This does not necessarily mean the use of expensive, highly sophisticated equipment, although a well-engineered head unit is helpful. It does mean careful positioning of the patient, which requires a good head clamp and a centering device. Adequate work can be done with a standard radiographic unit that includes a Bucky diaphragm with a grid ratio of 10 to 1, a rotating anode tube with a 0.3-mm focal spot, and an anode to film distance in the range of 100 cm. A high-detail screen-film combination is also desirable.

There is no consensus about the technique itself. I like to conduct the examination with the patient sitting, whenever possible. However, satisfactory films can also be obtained with the patient recumbent. Indeed, the latter position is often preferable, particularly for very ill or debilitated patients. The value of stereoscopic films cannot be overemphasized, although an expert can probably do as well with single films. In my opinion, stereoscopy better highlights minor differences and small calcifications, and more clearly delineates the structures at the base of the skull. Ideally, the tube shift (TS) should have the same proportion to the viewer's interpupillary distance (IPD) as the focus to film distance (FFD) has to the viewing distance (VD).

$$\frac{TS}{IPD} = \frac{FFD}{VD}$$

For ordinary radiographic units, a shift equal to 10% of the FFD is usually satisfactory. For isocentric skull devices, a total of a 6-degree shift is adequate.

There are several excellent radiographic atlases with detailed descriptions of the routine and the special views of the skull, as well as methods for obtaining them. No effort will be made to duplicate this material. This chapter will be limited to a brief resume of the standard projections I use. Whenever possible, I routinely take the straight posteroanterior, Caldwell, Towne, submentovertical, and right and left lateral projections. One of the lateral projections is made stereoscopically.

LINES AND PLANES (FIG 1)

1. The anthropological baseline (Reid's or Frankfort baseline) joins the infraorbital point to the superior margin of the external auditory meatus. The anthropological plane passes through both anthropological baselines.

2. The international baseline (orbitomeatal baseline) joins the outer canthus of the eye to the center of the external auditory canal. The international plane passes through both orbitomeatal lines. I prefer this term of reference to that of the anthropological baseline. The anthropological and international baselines meet at an angle of 7 to 10 degrees.

3. The midsagittal plane bisects the skull vertically into two equal halves.

4. The infraorbital line joins both infraorbital points.

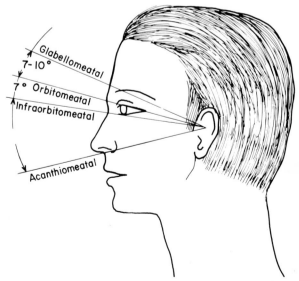

Fig 1.—Common lines and planes used in skull radiography.

1

5. The interorbital (interpupillary) line joins the center of both orbits or pupils.

6. The canthomeatal line joins the outer canthus of the eye to the center of the external auditory canal. This usually, but not always, coincides with the center of the orbit.

PROJECTIONS

1. Straight posteroanterior view (Fig 2). The midsagittal and orbitomeatal planes are perpendicular to the film. The central ray is perpendicular to the film, entering the skull at the external occipital protuberance and exiting at the nasion.

2. Caldwell (inclined posteroanterior) view (Fig 3). The midsagittal and the orbitomeatal planes are perpendicular to the film. The central ray is angled 23 degrees caudad to the orbitomeatal line. The central ray exits at the glabella. In order to visualize fluid levels in the paranasal sinuses, the central ray must be perpendicular to the film and the head tilted so that the international baseline forms an angle of 23 degrees to the central ray.

3. Towne (half-axial anteroposterior) view (Fig 4). The midsagittal and the orbitomeatal planes are perpendicular to the film. The central ray is angled 30 degrees caudad to the orbitomeatal line. The central ray is directed to the center of the film, bisecting a line joining the external auditory meatuses.

4. Base view (Fig 5). I prefer the submentovertical projection whenever possible. The midsagittal plane is perpendicular to the film. The head and neck are hyperextended so that the infraorbitomeatal line is parallel to the film. The central ray is perpendicular to the center of the film, bisecting the midpoint of the infraorbitomeatal plane. I prefer the infraorbitomeatal line of reference for the base view rather than the orbitomeatal line because it projects the mandible more anteriorly.

5. Lateral view (Fig 6). The midsagittal plane of the skull is parallel to the plane of the film. The central ray is perpendicular to the midsagittal plane, directed to the center of the film. It enters the skull 2 cm anterior to, and 2 cm above, the external auditory canal.

Other Views

Occasionally, it is desirable to study the orbit in greater detail. In this case, an optic foramen view should be obtained. Although there are several projections for this purpose, I use the Rhese view, which can be made either anteroposteriorly or posteroanteriorly. I

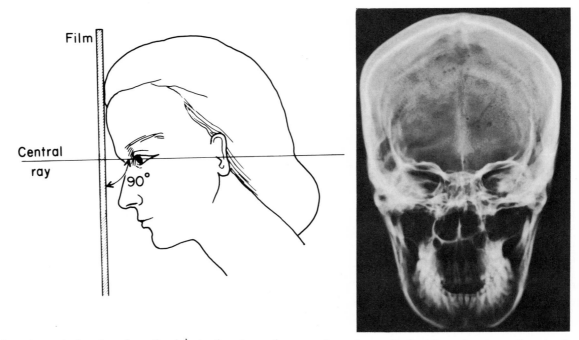

Fig 2.—Straight posteroanterior view. In optimal projection, tops of petrous ridges are slightly below superior margins of orbits. If internal auditory canals are of primary interest, a straight anteroposterior projection may be preferable because of the more posterior location of petrous bone. If clinoids and upper sellar structures are of special interest, a posteroanterior view angled slightly craniad (5 to 8 degrees) will throw the orbital margins and most of the ethmoidal contours downward out of the way.

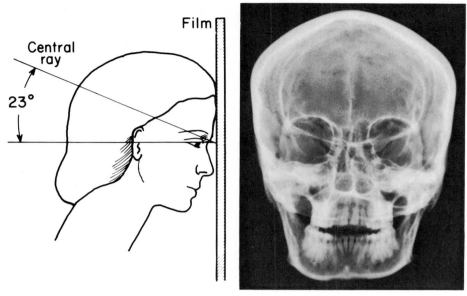

Fig 3.—Caldwell posteroanterior view.

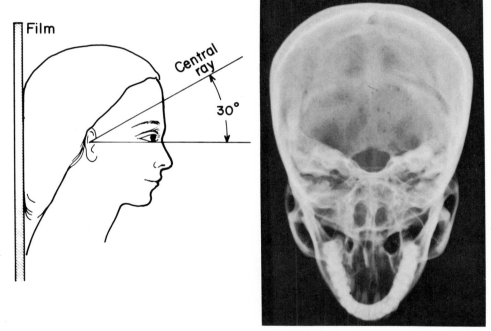

Fig 4.—Towne anteroposterior view. The 30- to 35-degree angle should be used only when Reid's baseline is perpendicular to the tabletop. In patients with thick, short necks and limited cervical flexion, a central ray to tabletop angulation greater than 35 degrees may be necessary. Unfortunately, this results in undesirable distortion and elongation. Under these circumstances, a "reverse" Towne posteroanterior view angled 30 to 35 degrees toward the head is frequently the projection of choice.

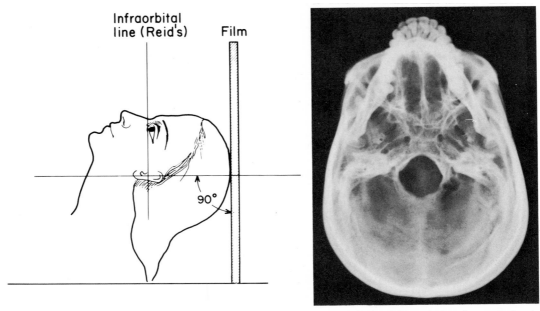

Fig 5.—Base view (submentovertical). Stereoscopic films are particularly helpful in differentiating the complex bony outlines.

prefer the former because it is easier to line up the patient.

6. Rhese view (anteroposterior) (Fig 7). The canthomeatal line is perpendicular to the film. The median sagittal plane is rotated so that it forms an angle of 53 degrees with the plane of the film. The central ray enters the outer third of the orbit perpendicular to the film. In a correctly positioned optic foramen view, the optic foramen is projected into the lower outer quadrant of the orbit.

PARANASAL SINUSES

Whenever possible, I conduct the examination with a horizontal beam and the patient in the sitting position, in order to detect air-fluid levels. A telescopic cone helps to increase definition. I routinely employ the following projections:

1. Caldwell posteroanterior view for visualization of the frontal and ethmoidal sinuses.

2. Waters posteroanterior view for demonstration of the maxillary sinuses (Fig 8). The midsagittal plane and

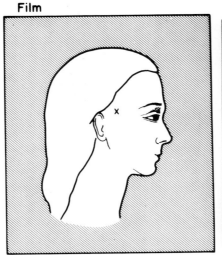
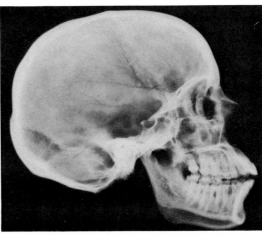

Fig 6.—Lateral view.

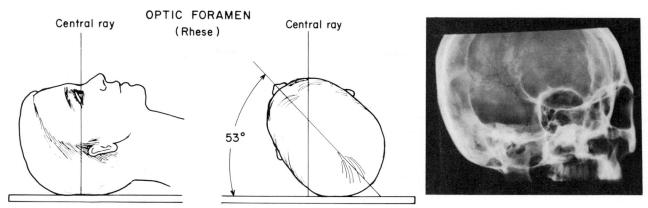

Fig 7.—Rhese view. Rhese projection for the optic foramen.

the central ray are perpendicular to the film. The neck is extended so that the international baseline forms an angle of 37.5 degrees with the central ray. The central ray exits at the nasolabial junction. This view, which is optimal for facial anatomy, projects the temporal petrosa below the maxillary sinuses. In order to demonstrate fluid levels, however, the central ray must be horizontal.

3. Base view for visualization of the ethmoidal and sphenoidal sinuses.

4. Lateral view. The lateral view of the sinuses differs from the lateral projection of the skull in that the central ray is directed more anteriorly in the lateral view, i.e., to the midorbitomeatal line. In addition, the exposure is approximately 10 kvp less. This view provides more information about the paranasal sinuses than any other

single projection. It demonstrates the thickness of the anterior wall of the frontal sinuses, the anteroposterior diameter and depth of the sphenoidal sinuses, and the structure of the ethmoidal cells.

Occasionally, I use the Rhese view for further evaluation of the ethmoidal sinuses, but it is not part of the routine examination.

Mastoids

The examination is carried out with the patient recumbent. As is the case with the skull, there is no unanimity of opinion as to what constitutes an adequate study of the mastoids. I routinely use the following projections:

1. Towne anteroposterior view to compare both petromastoid regions.

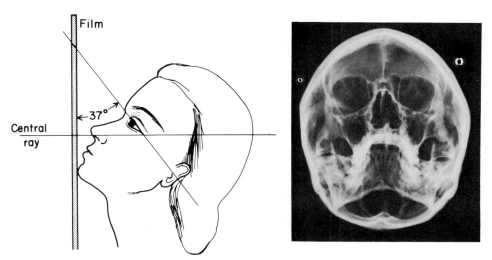

Fig 8.—Waters posteroanterior view. Diagram illustrates a technique with the mouth open. Although correct positioning of the patient is somewhat more difficult, a fine view of the posteroinferior portion of the sphenoidal sinuses is obtained as a dividend.

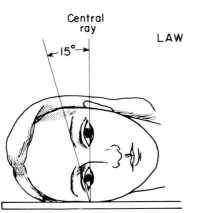
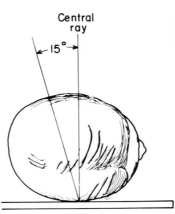
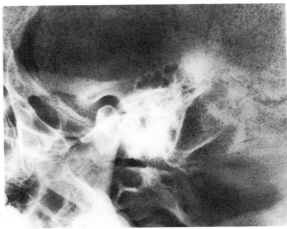

Fig 9.—Law view.

2. Lateral view. I prefer the Law projection (Fig 9), although the Schüller projection is also satisfactory. The head is positioned for a lateral view of the skull. The central ray is angled 15 degrees caudad and 15 degrees anteriorly, exiting through the mastoid closest to the film. It is helpful to tape the appropriate ear lobe forward with adhesive to avoid superimposition.

3. Stenvers view (Fig 10). In this posteroanterior projection the patient is positioned with the orbitomeatal plane perpendicular to the film. The head is rotated so that the midsagittal plane forms an angle of 45 degrees with the plane of the film. The central ray is angled 17 degrees craniad to a point midway between the external auditory meatus and the external occipital protuberance.

4. Owen's modification of the Mayer view (Fig 11). The patient is placed supine on the table. The head is rotated toward the side under study so that the midsag-

ittal plane forms an angle of 30 degrees with the plane of the film. The orbitomeatal plane is perpendicular to the plane of the film. The central ray is angled 30 degrees caudad, entering the head 5 cm above the supraorbital ridge on the side farthest from the film. The central ray exits through the tip of the mastoid nearest the film.

REFERENCES

Camp J. D., Gianturco C. A.: Simplified technique for roentgenographic examination of the optic canals. *Am. J. Roentgenol.* 29:547–549, 1933.

Chaussé C.: Trois incidences pour l'examen du rocher. *Acta Radiol.* 34:274–287, 1950.

Clark K. C.: *Positioning in Radiography.* London, Heinemann, 1938.

Epstein B. S.: Laminagraphy of the sphenoid bone. *Am. J. Roentgenol.* 48:625–631, 1942.

Epstein B. S.: Skull laminagraphy. *Radiology* 38:22–29, 1942.

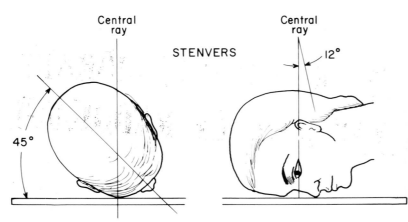
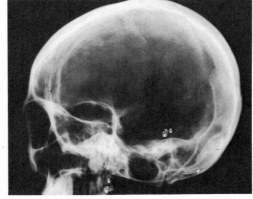

Fig 10.—Stenvers view.

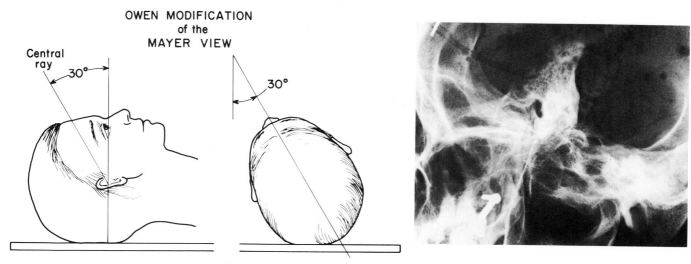

Fig 11.—Owen's modification of the Mayer view.

Etter L. E.: A new method for roentgen anatomic study of the skull. *Radiology* 53:394–402, 1949.

Etter L. E.: *Atlas of Roentgen Anatomy of the Skull.* Springfield, Ill., Charles C Thomas, Publisher, 1964.

Fuchs A. W.: Cranial base. *Radiog. Clin. Photog.* 15:42–50, 1939.

Holvey H. E., Rosenthal L. M., Anson B. J.: Tomography of the skull. *Radiology* 44:425–448, 1945.

Law F. M.: Radiography as an aid in the diagnosis of mastoid disease. *Ann. Otol. Rhinol. Laryngol.* 22:635–637, 1913.

Lazlo P.: Conventional radiography of the temporal bone. *Otolaryngol. Clin. North Am.* 6:323–336, 1973.

Littleton J. T.: *Tomography: Physical Principles and Clinical Applications.* Baltimore, Williams & Wilkins Co., 1976.

Lysholm E.: Apparatus and technique for roentgen examination of the skull. *Acta Radiol.*, suppl. 12, 1931, pp. 67–93.

Mayer E. G.: The technic of the roentgenologic examination of the temporal bone. *Radiology* 7:306–317, 1926.

Merrill V.: *Atlas of Roentgenographic Positions,* ed. 3. St. Louis, C. V. Mosby Co., 1967, vol. 2.

Pfeiffer R. L.: A new technique for roentgenography of the optic canals. *Am. J. Roentgenol.* 29:410–415, 1933.

Stenvers H. W.: Roentgenography of the os petrosum. *Arch. Radiol. Electrother.* 22:97–112, 1947.

Waters C. A.: A modification of the occipitofrontal position in the roentgen examination of the accessory nasal sinuses. *Arch. Radiol. Radiother.* 20:15–17, 1915.

Welin S.: Roentgen ray examination of the paranasal sinuses with particular reference to the frontal sinuses. *Br. J. Radiol.* 21:431–437, 1948.

Zimmer J.: Planigraphy of the temporal bone. *Acta Radiol.* 37:419–430, 1952.

2

Embryology

A working knowledge of the embryology of the skull is essential to understand the broad gamut of normalcy as well as the pathologic.

The entire skull, i.e., base, vault, and facial bones, develops from primitive mesenchyme that encases the cranial end of the notochord and the neural tube in the fifth week of gestation. During the seventh week, cartilaginous centers appear in the mesenchyme of the spheno-occipital region. Similar centers for the nose, periotic capsule, and branchial arches develop by the tenth week. The floor of the skull, the oldest part of the neurocranium from an evolutionary standpoint, is derived from cartilage. The cranial roof, on the other hand, develops from mesenchyme that forms a connective tissue capsule for the forebrain. The bones of the roof ossify from centers that appear in the connective tissue membrane by the eighth to ninth week. These bony foci spread rapidly and undergo varying degrees of fusion.

CALVARIAL BONES DERIVED FROM MEMBRANE

The frontal, parietal, squamosal, and tympanic segments of the temporal bone, the interparietal portion of the occipital bone, the greater wing of the sphenoid and the medial pterygoid lamina (exclusive of the hamulus), the vomer, the lacrimal, the nasal bones, and the zygoma are derived from membrane.

FRONTAL BONE.—The frontal bone develops from paired ossification centers, one on either side of the midline, which appear in the vertical plate by the end of the eighth week of gestation (Fig 12). By 14 weeks, there is substantial bone formation in both the vertical and horizontal (orbital) plates (Fig 13). Further ossification reduces the width of the membrane separating the two centers. As a result, the interfrontal (metopic) suture is relatively narrow at birth. Rarely, it contains a fonticulus (metopic fontanelle).

The frontal sinuses are topographically nasal in origin, arising from the frontal recess in the middle meatus during the fourth fetal month. Development occurs by growth of a series of evaginated folds and furrows along the lateral wall of the recess (Fig 14). At term, the frontal sinuses are still intranasal.

PARIETAL BONES.—Each parietal bone usually develops from a single ossific center during the eighth week of fetal life. Progressive ossification occurs in a radial fashion, extending outward from the original focus to the periphery of the bone (Fig 15). Although both parietal bones are extensively ossified at birth, one or more linear strips of unossified membrane may persist along the margins of the parietal bone. These ossify during the first postnatal year. The sutures adjacent to the parietal

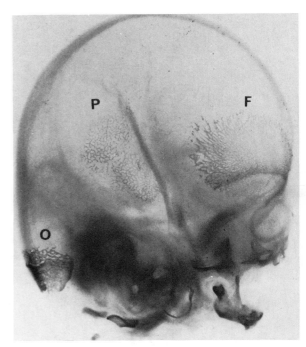

Fig 12.—Lateral aspect of fetal skull at 10 weeks. Spalteholtz preparation. Note frontal ossification center *(F)*, occipital ossification center *(O)*, and parietal ossification center *(P)*. (From Shapiro, R., and Robinson, F.: *Am. J. Roentgenol.* 111:569–577, 1972.)

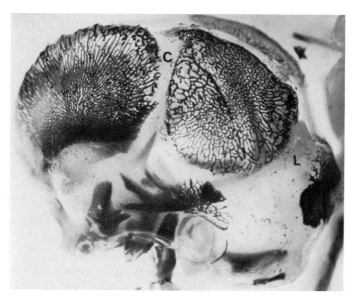

Fig 13.—Lateral aspect of fetal skull at 13 weeks. Spalteholtz preparation. Note sites of future coronal suture (C) and future lambdoidal suture (L). (From Shapiro, R., and Robinson, F.: *Am. J. Roentgenol.* 111:569–577, 1972.)

bones are fairly broad, especially in the parietotemporal area. The anterior fonticulus (fontanelle) is relatively large, but the posterior and lateral fonticuli are small. Occasionally, there is a sagittal fonticulus.

Rarely, the parietal bone ossifies from two centers

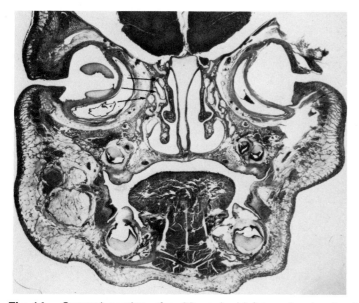

Fig 14.—Coronal section of a 32-week-old fetus showing frontal furrows and anterior ethmoidal cells in the middle meatus (arrows). Frontal anlage and ethmoidal anlage are difficult to differentiate from each other at this stage. (Hematoxylin eosin stain.)

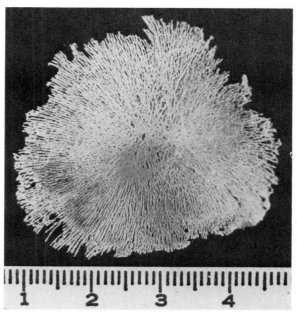

Fig 15.—Inner aspect of isolated parietal bone from 19-week-old fetus. Note radial arrangement of bony trabeculae. (From Shapiro, R., and Robinson, F.: *Am. J. Roentgenol.* 111:569–577, 1972.)

oriented craniocaudally. An anomalous transverse parietal suture is present when these centers fail to fuse.

THE VOMER.—The vomer ossifies from dual centers, one on either side of the midline, which appear during the eighth week of fetal life. By the third month, the centers unite inferiorly to form a groove in which the nasal septal cartilage rests. Progressive ossification results in the formation of two lamellae that fuse superiorly and anteriorly.

LACRIMAL BONES.—Each lacrimal bone arises from a single ossific center that appears at approximately 12 weeks of gestation.

NASAL BONES.—Each nasal bone ossifies from a single center that appears at nine to 12 weeks of gestation.

THE ZYGOMA.—The zygomatic bone ossifies from a single center that appears at about eight weeks of fetal life.

CALVARIAL BONES DERIVED FROM CARTILAGE OR CARTILAGE AND MEMBRANE

TEMPORAL BONE.—The temporal bone at birth is composed of three segments: the squamosal and the tympanic portions derived from membrane, and the petrosa (periotic) derived from cartilage (Fig 16).

The temporal squama ossifies from a single center in

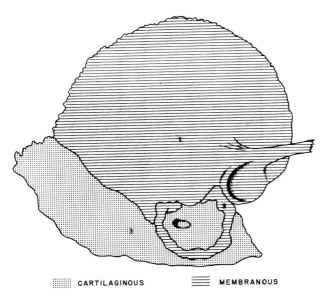

CARTILAGINOUS   MEMBRANOUS

Fig 16.—Temporal bone at birth. Squama *(1)* and tympanic portion *(2)* arise from membrane, whereas petromastoid *(3)* arises in cartilage. Mastoid process has not yet developed.

the inferior half of the bone at approximately the eighth week of fetal life. Ossification progresses superiorly toward the parietal bone, laterally toward the zygoma, and inferiorly to form the postauditory process, which fuses with the tympanic ring. The postauditory process separates the tympanic ring from the petromastoid portion.

The tympanic ring arises from an ossific focus in the outer wall of the tympanic segment during the ninth week of gestation. The ring, which encloses the tympanic membrane, fuses with the squamosa prior to birth.

The cartilaginous petrosa begins to ossify at 16 to 17 weeks of gestation. Ossification proceeds from four principal ossific clusters—opisthotic, pro-otic, pterotic, and epiotic. Progressive fusion of the various bone centers results in almost complete ossification of the otic capsule by the 24th week.

The mastoid antrum is an extension of the epitympanum. It appears during the 22d fetal week and increases in size until term, when it is relatively large and well pneumatized. The mastoid process is not present at birth but develops by the end of the first postnatal year.

The styloid process develops from two centers at the cranial end of the cartilaginous second branchial arch. The proximal tympanohyal center appears before birth and fuses with the petromastoid. The distal stylohyal

center appears in the second postnatal year. Although the two centers usually fuse in the adult, they may occasionally remain separate.

THE ETHMOID.—The ethmoid develops from three primary centers in the cartilaginous nasal septum. The ethmoidal cartilage is composed of two lateral labyrinths and a central portion running from the tip of the nasal process to the sphenoid bone. Ossification of the crista galli occurs by the 12th week. During the fifth fetal month, an ossific focus appears in each lateral mass and develops into the orbital lamina. During the eighth month, ossification extends into the cribriform plate and ethmoturbinates. During the first postnatal year, the perpendicular plate is formed by ossification of the cephalic end of the cartilaginous nasal septum. The unossified distal segment of the central ethmoidal mass gives rise to the cartilaginous nasal septum. The three main components of the ethmoidal bone—the orbital lamina, the cribriform plate, and the perpendicular plate—are not fused at term.

The ethmoidal cells develop by evagination of the nasal mucosa in the superior and middle meatuses. The

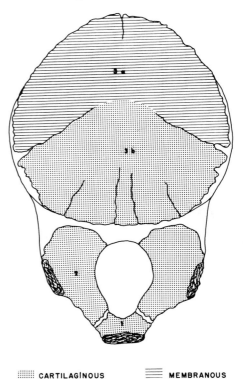

CARTILAGINOUS   MEMBRANOUS

Fig 17.—Occipital bone ossification. Basioccipital *(1)* and paired exoccipital *(2)* centers encircle inferior aspect and sides of foramen magnum. Mendosal sutures separate membranous interparietal *(3a)* segment from cartilaginous supraoccipital *(3b)* portion.

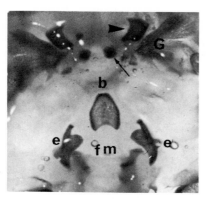

Fig 18.—Base of skull of 14-week-old fetus. Spalteholtz preparation. Basioccipital *(b)* and paired exoccipital centers *(e)* surround foramen magnum *(fm)*. Note also ossification of greater *(G)* and lesser *(arrowhead)* sphenoidal wings and of postsphenoid centers *(arrow)* anterior to basioccipital bone. (From Shapiro, R., and Robinson, F.: *Am. J. Roentgenol.* 126:1063–1068, 1976.)

anterior and posterior ethmoidal cells are pneumatized at birth.

OCCIPITAL BONE.—The occipital bone is derived from both membrane and cartilage (Fig 17). The membranous component is the interparietal segment, i.e., the superior squama, above the mendosal suture. The cartilaginous portion is formed from the union of four principal centers grouped around the foramen magnum: the basioccipital, anterior to the foramen; the paired exoccipitals, one on either side of the foramen; and the supraoccipital, posterior to the foramen, i.e., the inferior squama, below the mendosal suture.

At nine to ten weeks of gestation, a single ossification

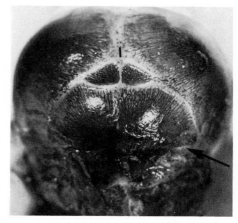

Fig 20.—Occiput of skull of 14-week-old fetus. Spalteholtz preparation. Note bipartite os incae below lambda *(1)*. The rest of interparietal segment is separated from supraoccipital segment by mendosal suture *(arrow)*. (From Shapiro, R., and Robinson, F.: *Am. J. Roentgenol.* 126:1063–1068, 1976.)

center in the tectum synoticum (the chondrocranial roof connecting the auditory bullae) gives rise to the supraoccipital segment. At the same time, there is a single ossific focus in each lateral occipital condyle, in the midline basiocciput, and in the membranous interparietal segment (Fig 18). By 12 weeks, the interparietal and supraoccipital segments are fused in the midline but separated laterally by the mendosal sutures (Fig 19). Progressive ossification reduces the mendosal sutures to narrow slits. Not infrequently, there is a vertical midline linear strip of unossified membrane at the superior margin of the interparietal segment. Similar unossified

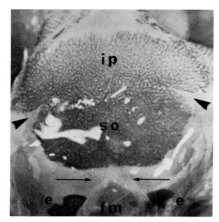

Fig 19.—Posterior aspect of fetal skull at 12 weeks. Spalteholtz preparation. Note interparietal segment *(ip)*, supraoccipital segment *(so)*, exoccipitals *(e)*, foramen magnum *(fm)*, mendosal sutures *(arrowheads)*, and innominate synchondrosis *(arrows)*. (From Shapiro, R., and Robinson, F.: *Am. J. Roentgenol.* 126:1063–1068, 1976.)

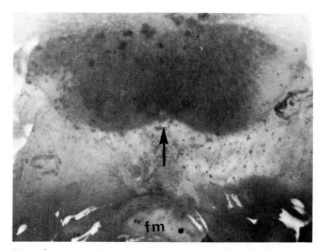

Fig 21.—Occiput of fetal skull at 4 months. Spalteholtz preparation. Note cleft in midportion of inferior margin of supraoccipital segment *(arrow)*, and foramen magnum *(fm)*. (From Shapiro, R., and Robinson, F.: *Am. J. Roentgenol.* 126:1063–1068, 1976.)

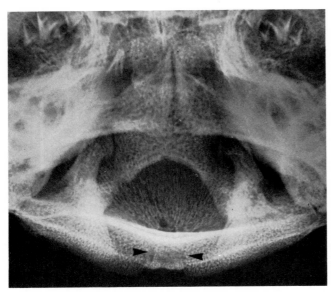

Fig 22.—Exaggerated Waters view of dry skull of full-term stillborn fetus showing Kerckring's bone *(arrowheads)* almost completely fused to supraoccipital segment. (From Shapiro, R., and Robinson, F.: *Am. J. Roentgenol.* 126:1063–1068, 1976.)

strips may be present anywhere along the margins of the interparietal bone. These membranous remnants usually ossify during the first postnatal year. Rarely, the interparietal segment arises from two or more centers which fail to unite (os incae) (Fig 20).

Occasionally, there is a midline cleft in the inferior margin of the cartilaginous supraoccipital segment (Fig 21). The cleft may persist or subsequently ossify. Infrequently also, there is a small median bony projection arising from the inferior margin of the supraoccipital segment (Kerckring's bone). Rarely, Kerckring's bone is separate and lies in a broad midline cleft (Figs 22 and

23). One or more supernumerary ossicles may be present in the innominate synchondrosis between the supraoccipital and exoccipital segments.

The ventral portion of each occipital condyle is formed by ossification extending laterally from the basiocciput. The dorsal portion of the condyles develops from the exoccipital bones. At term, a prominent synchondrosis separates the basioccipital and exoccipital segments on either side (Fig 24). Progressive narrowing of the synchondroses results in their complete obliteration at age 2 to 4. The supraoccipital is separated from the exoccipital segments by the broad innominate synchondrosis, which becomes obliterated at the same time.

SPHENOID BONE.—The sphenoid bone is derived from cartilage, with the exception of the greater wing and the medial pterygoid lamina (exclusive of the hamulus), which have a membranous origin.

As early as 6½ weeks of gestation, there are chondral centers in the region of the sella turcica. Shortly thereafter, there is chondrification of the lesser wings (orbitosphenoids), which are unfused and isolated from the prehypophyseal portion of the body of the sphenoid. Both the prepituitary and postpituitary segments of the body of the sphenoid are chondrified. At about the same time, the greater wings (alisphenoids) can be identified joined to the posterolateral aspect of the body by the alar processes. The aperture for the optic foramen is wide open anteriorly. There is also a wide aperture between the lesser and greater wings for the future superior orbital fissure. By nine weeks, there is progressive chondrification of the lesser wings both medially and laterally (Fig 25). There is also chondrification of the

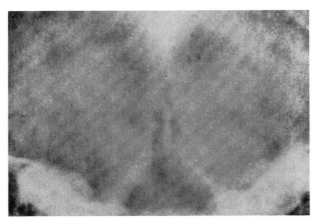

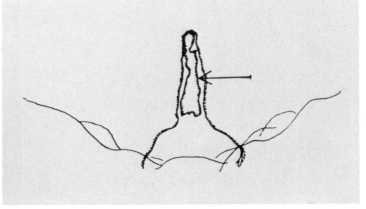

Fig 23.—Towne projection showing ununited Kerckring's bone in skull of adult.
(From Shapiro, R., and Robinson, F.: *Am. J. Roentgenol.* 126:1063–1068, 1976.)

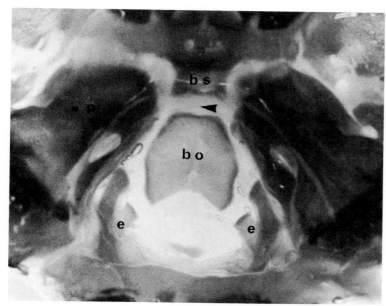

Fig 24.—Base of skull of 22-week-old fetus. Spalteholtz preparation. Note prominent spheno-occipital synchondrosis *(arrowhead)* separating basisphenoid *(bs)* from basioccipital bone *(bo)*; petrous bones *(p)*; and exoccipitals *(e)*. (From Shapiro, R., and Robinson, F.: *Am. J. Roentgenol.* 126:1063–1068, 1976.)

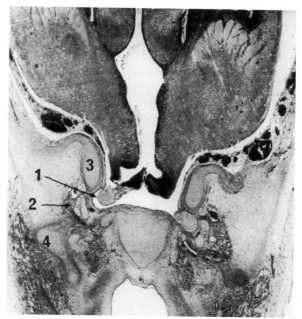

Fig 25.—Section through plane of forebrain and sphenoid in 9-week-old fetus showing embryonal cartilaginous matrix surrounding vascular and neural structures within anlage of sphenoidal fissure. At this age, bone formation has not yet occurred. Note optic nerve *(1)*; neurovascular structures within sphenoidal fissure *(2)*; embryonal cartilaginous matrix of lesser sphenoidal wing *(3)*; and embryonal cartilaginous matrix of greater sphenoidal wing *(4)*. Paraffin-embedded section; modified Masson stain. (From Shapiro, R., and Robinson, F.: *Am. J. Roentgenol.* 101:814–827, 1967.)

lateral pterygoid plate and of the hamular process of the medial pterygoid plate. In fact, cartilage can be seen in the hamulus at eight weeks. At nine weeks, the craniopharyngeal canal is usually filled in with cartilage. By ten weeks, ossification has spread to the membranous medial pterygoid plate and to the anterior aspect of the alar process, lateral and inferior to the foramen rotundum. By 11 weeks, one can recognize ossification in the lesser wing and in the lateral pterygoid plate. Lesser wing ossification progresses to form the shape of a C, open medially by 13 weeks. At 15 weeks, there is ossification of the posterior part of the alar process and also, to a limited degree, of the foramen rotundum. By 18 to 19 weeks, the greater and lesser wings are diffusely ossified (Figs 26 and 27). The medial and lateral pterygoid plates fuse with each other at approximately 20 weeks and with the lingula shortly thereafter. At this time, the margins of the foramen rotundum are fully ossified, and the pterygoid canal is partially ossified (Fig 28). The latter is almost completely ossified at 36 weeks (Fig 29).

Ossification of the cartilaginous optic foramen begins along its anterolateral margin in the lesser sphenoidal wing at 12 weeks. By this time, there is also ossification of the principal presphenoid center that forms the me-

dial border of the optic foramen. Simultaneously, ossification appears in the anteroinferior portion of the optic strut and continues until it fuses with the presphenoid at 17 to 18 weeks to form a large, keyhole-shaped foramen. Ossification of the posterosuperior portion of the optic strut begins either from a spur on the medial aspect of the lesser wing or from dual spurs on the lesser wing and lateral margin of the presphenoid. In either case, a thin bridge of bone ultimately extends from the lesser wing to the presphenoid. The anteroinferior and posterosuperior segments of the optic strut fuse into a single structure by 38 weeks (Fig 30).

The body of the sphenoid consists of two major components—the presphenoid and the basisphenoid—and a third minor contribution anteriorly from the greater wing. The presphenoid develops from multiple ossific centers. The principal pair of presphenoid centers are close to the posterior portion of the lesser wing. Additional paired accessory centers are located anterior, posterior, and medial to the primary major presphenoid centers. The basisphenoid ossifies from paired medial

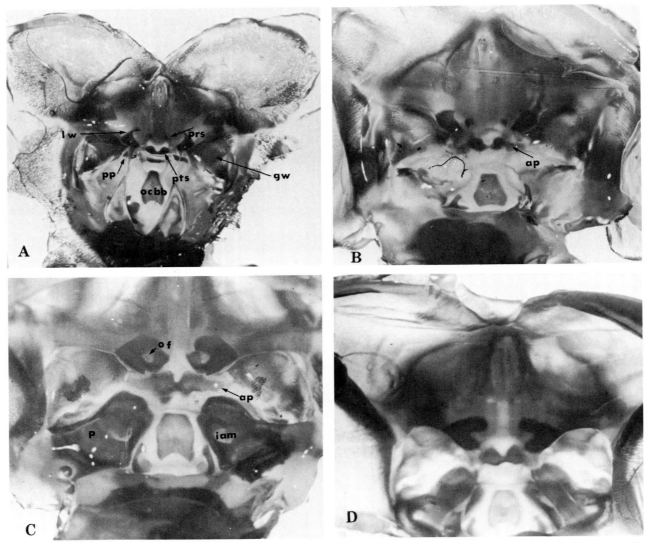

Fig 26.—Inner aspect of base of transilluminated fetal skull at 14 weeks **(A)**, 16 weeks **(B)**, 18 weeks **(C)**, and 20 weeks **(D)** showing progressive ossification of sphenoid bone. The more complete formation of the optic foramen in **C** (18 weeks) compared with **D** (20 weeks) illustrates the variable growth and development in biology. Spalteholtz preparation. Note alar process *(ap)*; greater wing *(gw)*; lesser wing *(lw)*; internal auditory meatus *(iam)*; optic foramen *(of)*; petrous bone *(p)*; pterygoid plate *(pp)*; presphenoid center *(prs)*; postsphenoid center *(pts)*; and basioccipital center *(ocbb)*. (From Shapiro, R., and Robinson, F.: *Embryogenesis of the Human Skull* [Cambridge, Mass.: Harvard University Press, 1980].)

and lateral centers that begin to ossify at approximately 13 weeks of gestation. Fusion of the basisphenoid centers can be seen at 20 weeks. Ossific union of the presphenoid and basisphenoid centers occurs during the seventh fetal month. This is preceded by fusion of the various presphenoid foci during the fifth to sixth fetal month.

The postsphenoid develops from two pairs of centers: a medial pair and a lateral pair. At 16 weeks, ossifica-

tion of these centers is evident. By 20 weeks, the ossific postsphenoid centers are contiguous in the midline but not completely fused. Complete union does not occur until the seventh to eighth fetal month. The postsphenoid usually fuses with the presphenoid during the seventh fetal month and with the greater wing shortly thereafter. The postsphenoid unites with the lesser wing during the ninth month of gestation.

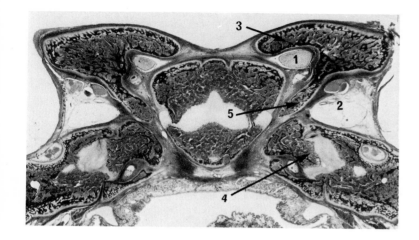

Fig 27.—Coronal section through plane of optic foramen in 20-week-old fetus showing optic nerve (1) and neurovascular bundle (2) within sphenoidal fissure. Note well-defined ossification of lesser (3) and greater (4) sphenoidal wings, and optic strut (5). Darker areas represent more advanced ossification. Celloidin-embedded section; modified Masson stain. (From Shapiro, R., and Robinson, F.: *Am. J. Roentgenol.* 101:814–827, 1967.)

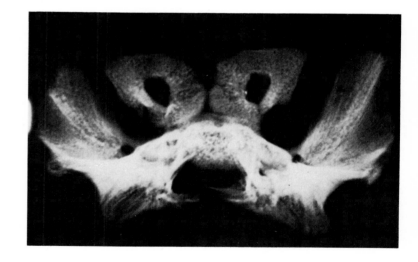

Fig 28.—Radiograph of dry sphenoid bone from stillborn fetus at approximately 20 weeks' gestation.

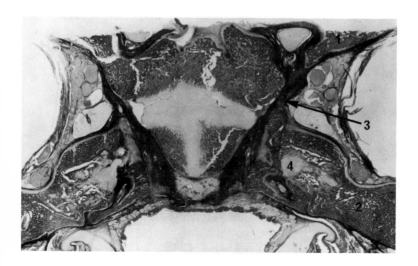

Fig 29.—Coronal section through plane of optic foramen and sphenoidal fissure in 36-week-old fetus. Note relatively complete ossification of lesser (1) and greater (2) sphenoidal wings, and optic strut (3). A few islands of unossified cartilage remain in greater wings (4). Celloidin-embedded section; modified Masson stain. (From Shapiro, R., and Robinson, F.: *Am. J. Roentgenol.* 101:814–827, 1967.)

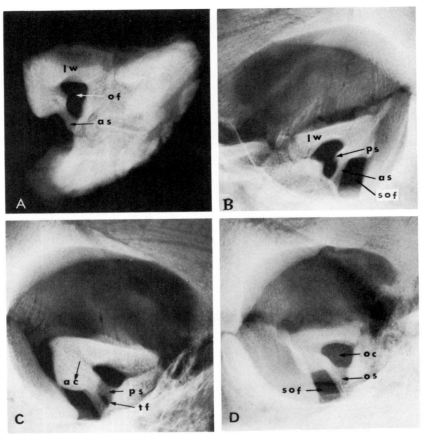

Fig 30.—Radiographs of dissected, dry fetal sphenoid bones showing formation of optic canal; ×3. **A,** 28-week-old fetus. A large keyhole-shaped optic foramen *(of)* is still present. **B,** 31-week-old fetus. Posterior optic strut segment *(ps)* is beginning to form. Anterior optic strut segment *(as)* separates optic foramen from superior orbital fissure *(sof)*. **C,** 35-week-old fetus. Posterior strut segment *(ps)* is fully formed and separated from anterior segment by a temporary foramen *(tf)*. **D,** 38-week-old fetus. Two strut segments are fused into single optic strut *(os)*. An optic canal *(oc)* with cranial and orbital openings has formed. (From Kier, E. L.: *Invest. Radiol.* 1:346–362, 1966.)

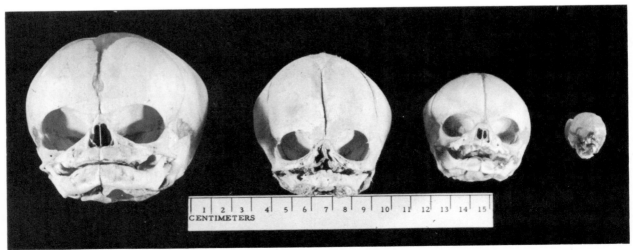

Fig 31.—Frontal view of fetal skulls at 10, 20, 30, and 40 weeks, showing progressive growth. (From Shapiro, R., and Robinson, F.: *Embryogenesis of the Human Skull* [Cambridge, Mass.: Harvard University Press, 1980].)

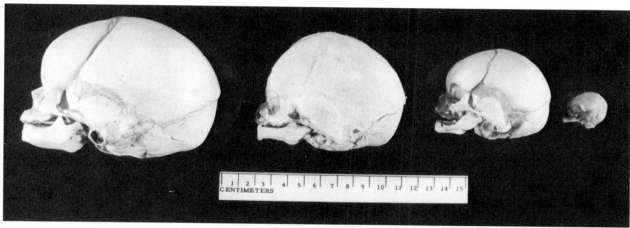

Fig 32.—Lateral view of fetal skulls at 10, 20, 30, and 40 weeks showing progressive growth of calvaria. Note comparatively slow growth of facial skeleton. (From Shapiro, R., and Robinson, F.: *Embryogenesis of the Human Skull* [Cambridge, Mass.: Harvard University Press, 1980].)

REFERENCES

Arey L. B.: *Development Anatomy: A Textbook and Laboratory Manual of Embryology,* ed. 5., Philadelphia, W. B. Saunders Co., 1946.

Augier M.: Squelette cephalique, in Poirier P., Charpy A. (eds.): *Traite d'anatomié humaine,* ed. 4. Paris, Masson & Cie, 1931, vol 1.

Bast T. H., Anson B. J.: *The Temporal Bone and the Ear.* Springfield, Ill., Charles C Thomas, Publisher, 1949.

Berkvens T.: Radiography of the fetal skull. *Acta Radiol.* 34:250–252, 1950.

Caffey J.: On the accessory ossicles of the supraoccipital bone: Some newly recognized roentgen features of the normal infantile skull. *Am. J. Roentgenol.* 70:401–412, 1953.

Crelin E. S.: *Anatomy of the Newborn: An Atlas.* Philadelphia, Lea & Febiger, 1969.

Debeer G. R.: *The Development of the Vertebrate Skull.* Oxford, London, Clarendon Press, 1937.

Fawcett E.: Notes on development of human sphenoid. *J. Anat.* 44:207–222, 1910.

Franken E. A.: The midline occipital fissure: Diagnosis of fracture versus anatomic variants. *Radiology* 93:1043–1046, 1969.

Gasser R. F.: Early formation of the basicranium in man, in Bosma J. F. (ed.): *Development of the Basicranium.* NIH 76–989. U.S. Dept. of Health, Education, and Welfare, 1976, pp. 29–43.

Henderson S. G., Sherman L. S.: Roentgen anatomy of the skull in the newborn infant, in Etter L. (ed.): *Atlas of Roentgen Anatomy of the Skull.* Springfield, Ill., Charles C Thomas, Publisher, 1964.

Inman V. T., Saunders J. B.: Ossification of the human frontal bone with specific references to its presumed pre- and postfrontal elements. *J. Anat.* 71:383–394, 1937.

Kier E. L.: Embryology of the normal optic canal and its anomalies: An anatomic and roentgenographic study. *Invest. Radiol.* 1:346–362, 1966.

Kier E. L.: The infantile sella turcica: New radiologic and anatomic concepts based on a developmental study of the sphenoid bone. *Am. J. Roentgenol.* 102:747–767, 1968.

Kodama G.: Developmental studies of the presphenoid of the human sphenoid bone, in Bosma J. F. (ed.): *Development of the Basicranium.* NIH 76–989. U.S. Dept. of Health, Education, and Welfare, 1976, pp. 141–155.

Kodama G.: Developmental studies on the body of the human sphenoid bone, ibid, pp. 156–165.

Kodama G.: Developmental studies on the orbito-sphenoid of the human sphenoid bone, ibid, pp. 166–1976.

Lowman R. M., Robinson F., McAllister W. B.: Craniopharyngeal canal. *Acta Radiol.* (Diag.) 5:41–54, 1966.

Mall F. P.: On ossification centers in human embryos less than one hundred days old. *Am. J. Anat.* 5:433–458, 1905–1906.

Patton B. M.: *Human Embryology.* Philadelphia, Blakiston Co., 1946.

Pierce R. H., Mainen M. W., Bosma J. F.: *The Cranium of the Newborn Infant: An Atlas of Tomography and Anatomical Sections.* Bethesda, Md., U.S. Dept. of Health, Education, and Welfare, 1978.

Sasaki H., Kodama G.: Developmental studies on the postsphenoid of the human sphenoid bone, in Bosma, J. F. (ed.): *Development of the Basicranium.* NIH 76–989. U.S. Dept. of Health, Education, and Welfare, 1976, pp. 177–190.

Scammon R. E., Calkins L. A.: *The Development and Growth of the External Dimensions of the Human Body in the Fetal Period.* Minneapolis, University of Minnesota Press, 1929.

Scammon R. E.: in Morris' *Human Anatomy,* ed. 10. Philadelphia, The Blakiston Co., 1942.

Shapiro R., Robinson F.: *Embryogenesis of the Human Skull: An Anatomic and Radiographic Atlas.* Cambridge, Mass., Harvard University Press, 1980.

3

The Neonatal Skull

CONFIGURATION AND RELATIONSHIPS

There are a number of important external differences between the neonatal and the adult skull. The newborn skull is characterized by prominent frontal and parietal eminences, large orbits, wide nasal apertures, rudimentary development of the paranasal sinuses and mastoids, and a relatively flat base. The ratio of head size to total body length is greater in the newborn than in the adult. There is also a distinct difference in the relative size of the skull and face. The ratio of the area of the neonatal skull to that of the facial bones is 4 to 1 because of the relatively large size of the brain and the slower development of the maxilla, mandible, and frontal and maxillary sinuses. This difference gradually diminishes with age (3 to 1 at two years, 2.5 to 1 at three years) until the adult proportion of 1.5 to 1 is reached (Fig 33). The average circumference of the skull

is approximately 35 cm at birth, 44 cm at six months, and 47 cm at one year. (±2 standard deviations). The size of the skull vault is intimately related to brain growth. A reduction of the normal ratio between vault and face should suggest microcephaly (Fig 34). In microcephaly, brain growth stops prematurely, and early sutural closure ensues. The shape of the skull is significantly influenced by heredity after the effects of molding have disappeared (Fig 35). On the other hand, the size of the chondrocranium is not significantly influenced by brain growth. Rather, it appears to be controlled by the genetic information inherent in the primitive prechondral mesenchyme. Since the chondrocranium constitutes the roof of the face as well as the floor of the skull, its dimensions govern the width and protrusion of the face.

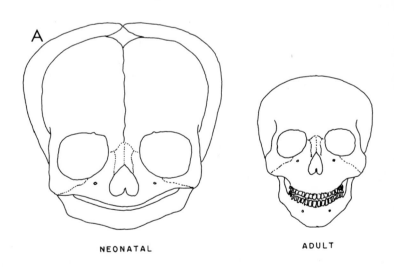

NEONATAL   ADULT

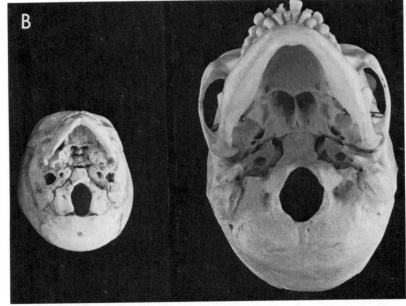

Fig 33.—A, relative size of face and cranium in neonatal and adult skull. Facial bones are drawn to same size, with cranial vault of each in proportion. This demonstrates relatively greater height of vault and width of base in infantile skull. **B,** base view of neonatal skull *(left)* and adult skull *(right)* showing striking differences in craniofacial proportions.

18

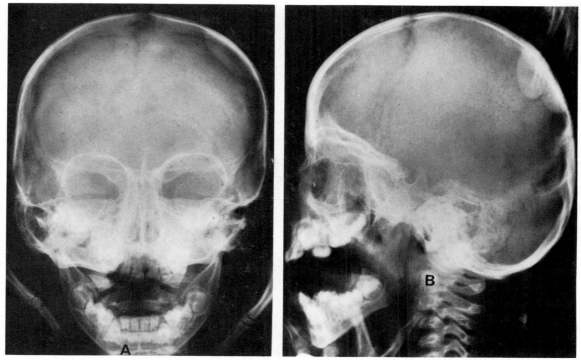

Fig 34.—Posteroanterior **(A)** and lateral **(B)** views of skull of a 4-year-old microcephalic boy with adult craniofacial proportions recognized during first year of life.

GENERAL APPEARANCE

The thin bones of the skull show no differentiation into the various tables. The overall appearance is one of fairly uniform density. This is due to the rudimentary

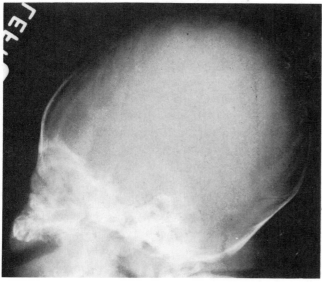

Fig 35.—Typical molding of parietal bones in neonate. (Courtesy of Dr. R. Ablow.)

development of the vascular grooves and ridges and the absence of convolutional markings. Occasionally, a few, unimpressive convolutional markings may be present. A striking contrast is presented by the infant with craniolacunia (lückenschädel), which is a developmental defect in ossification of the membranous vault. Radiography demonstrates prominent oval-shaped radiolucencies (the nonossified membrane) ringed by a denser periphery (ossified membrane) (Fig 36). Craniolacunia is always associated with some form of spinal dysraphism and tends to disappear by the end of the first year of life. Premature infants tend to have a poorly ossified vault and a lax skin. The redundant skin folds frequently produce radiolucent streaks on the roentgenogram that should not be confused with fractures or suture lines (Fig 37). Forward folding of the ear may also create an erroneous impression of a mass on the lateral film. Occasionally, a sliver of air is trapped in the fossa of the ear. This should not be mistaken for an osteolytic lesion or pneumocephalus.

The standard views of the newborn skull in Figures 38 to 50 are labeled in some detail to facilitate the recognition of various important features and landmarks discussed in the following text.

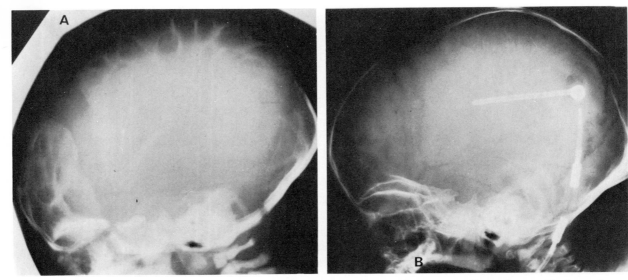

Fig 36.—A, craniolacunia in neonate. Abnormality involves only membranous vault, sparing cartilaginous base. **B,** complete return to normalcy one year after shunting for hydrocephalus.

The cranial fossae in the neonate are shorter and have a steeper declivity than in the adult. This is particularly true of the anterior fossa, where the roofs of the orbits slope sharply. The posterior fossa varies in depth and height. Because the neonatal skull is relatively soft, it is susceptible to deformation by extrinsic pressure. Thus, the dependent portion of the skull is flattened in infants who constantly lie in one position. Postural flattening is most common posteriorly, particularly in neonates with motor retardation. Occasionally, there is a prominent posterior bulge of the interparietal portion of the occipital bone, i.e., bathrocephaly. This has no significance and generally disappears during the first year of life. Rarely, it may be more pronounced and persist into adult life.

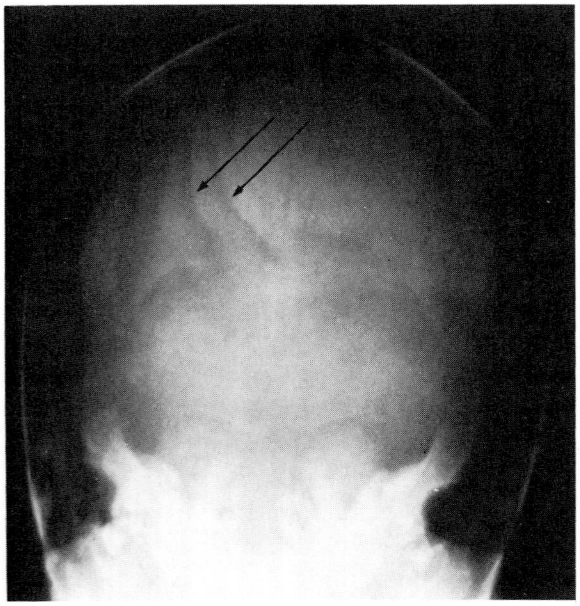

SYNCHONDROSES, SUTURES, AND FONTICULI (FONTANELLES)

The enchondral bones at the base of the skull are separated by cartilaginous bars called synchondroses (considered in detail in chapter 2). The membranous bones of the vault are separated by broad, radiolucent bands of fibrous tissue in the region of the sutures and fonticuli (Fig 51).

There are six constant fonticuli: (1) The broad, diamond-shaped anterior fonticulus between the anteromedial margins of the parietal bones and the frontal bones is the largest. It usually closes by age 2, although it may disappear considerably earlier. Rarely, the anterior fonticulus may contain a separate ossicle, the anterior fonticulus bone (Fig 52). (2) The posterior fonticulus between the posterior parietal and occipital bones is considerably smaller. It may disappear in utero; if present at birth, it usually closes after several months. (3) and (4) The paired anterolateral (sphenoidal) fonticuli

Fig 37.—Prominent scalp folds *(arrows)* in an infant. These may vary in appearance on different films because of mobility of loose scalp in relationship to underlying calvaria.

are bounded by the frontal, temporal, and parietal bones and the greater sphenoidal wing; they usually close by the third or fourth postnatal month. (5) and (6) The paired posterolateral (mastoid) fonticuli are bounded by the temporal, parietal, and occipital bones; they have a variable closure date and may remain open until the latter part of the second year.

In addition to the major fonticuli, there may rarely be accessory fonticuli: the metopic fonticulus within the metopic suture (Fig 53), and the glabellar fonticulus in the nasofrontal suture. Terrafranca and Zellis have reported three cases of persistent metopic fonticulus in two generations of the same family, suggesting that this trait may be hereditary.

Sutures are considered in greater detail in chapter 10. However, a few pertinent remarks concerning sutures in the neonate are in order here. In the first 24 hours after birth, the sutures may overlap due to molding. This recedes rapidly so that there is only minimal overlapping at the end of three or four days. If sutural overlapping persists beyond the first week of life, one should be concerned about the possibility of retarded brain growth. Because the sutures are broad, the determination of early sutural widening is extremely difficult. Unfortunately, there are no objective criteria, and even the experienced radiologist may have considerable trouble in recognizing early subtle pathologic widening. If available, a baseline film for comparison is most helpful. Bulging of the soft tissues through the anterior fonticulus during the first postnatal year is also helpful in establishing the diagnosis of increased intracranial pressure when sutural widening is suspected. One should not be misled by spurious widening due to some obliquity on the lateral roentgenogram. Wormian bones may be present in any suture but are more common in the lambdoidal suture and, to a lesser extent, in the posterior sagittal and squamosal sutures. The sutural bone occasionally found in the region of the anterolateral fonticulus is called the epipteric bone (Fig 54). Sutural bones are commonly found in large numbers in osteogenesis imperfecta, cleidocranial dysostosis, and pyknodysostosis.

FRONTAL BONE.—The frontal bone is divided into halves by the metopic (interfrontal) suture, which extends from the anterior fonticulus to nasion.

Although the newborn skull is generally devoid of vascular markings, there is one important exception—the frontal diploic vein (Fig 55). This structure runs vertically upward from the supraorbital region and may be unilateral or bilateral. The radiolucency it produces is gray rather than black. When unilateral, it should not be confused with a fracture, particularly when it is branched or serpiginous.

The nasal bones are usually mineralized at birth. Absence of normal ossification occurs in mongolism as well as in the premature infant.

PARIETAL BONES.—The parietal bones are separated from the frontal bones by the coronal suture, from one another by the midline sagittal suture, from the occipital bone by the lambdoidal suture, and from the temporal squamosa by the squamosal suture. There may be one or more unossified strips of membrane along any margin of the parietal bone that should not be mistaken for fractures (Figs 56 to 58). In the absence of known trauma and localized soft tissue swelling, such linear radiolucencies should be regarded as normal variants. The strips usually ossify completely by the end of the first year.

OCCIPITAL BONE.—The occipital bone consists of four bony masses around the foramen magnum separated by synchondroses—the basioccipital, the paired exoccipitals, and the occipital squamosa. The occipital squamosa is in turn separated by the mendosal sutures into the supraoccipital segment inferiorly (derived from cartilage) and the interparietal segment superiorly (derived from membrane). At its superior central margin, the interparietal segment often contains a thin, linear strip of unossified membrane, the superior longitudinal fissure (Fig 59). Similar fissures may occur along any margin of the interparietal segment. These fissures usually ossify by the end of the first year and should not be confused with fractures. Rarely, the interparietal segment ossifies from two or more centers which may not fuse. In this case, various forms of os incae result (Fig 60). Since the supraoccipital portion is normally derived from a single ossific focus in cartilage, any vertical linear radiolucency in this area should be regarded as a fracture (Fig 61). I have never seen a bona fide midline cerebellar suture or synchondrosis in the supraoccipital portion of the newborn occipital bone.

One or more supernumerary ossicles may be present in the innominate synchondrosis between the exoccipitals and the supraoccipital segment (Fig 62). According to Caffey, these usually unite by the end of the first

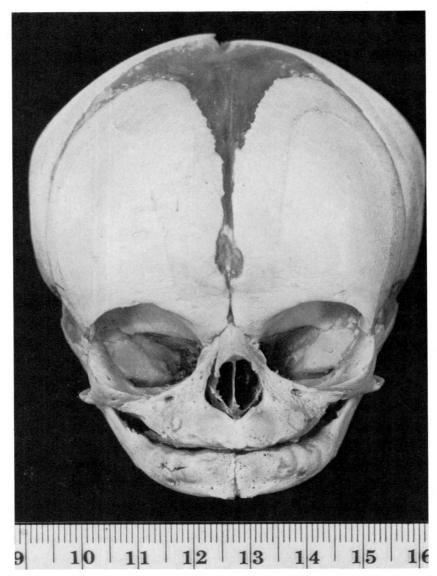

Fig 38.—Frontal photograph of skull of full-term stillborn fetus. (From Shapiro, R., and Robinson, F.: *Embryogenesis of the Human Skull* [Cambridge, Mass.: Harvard University Press, 1980].)

ABBREVIATIONS FOR FIGURES 38–50

acp	anterior clinoid process
af	anterior fonticulus
alf	anterolateral fonticulus
beocsy	basiexoccipital synchondrosis
carc	carotid canal
cc	condyloid canal
cpc	craniopharyngeal canal
cs	coronal suture
ds	dorsum sellae
dv	diploic vein
ebcp	cribriform plate
ebop	orbital plate of ethmoid bone
ec	ethmoid cells
fb	frontal bone
fbhp	horizontal (orbital) plate of frontal bone
fbvp	vertical plate of frontal bone
fes	frontoethmoidal suture
fla	foramen lacerum
fm	foramen magnum
fmf	floor middle fossa
fmxs	frontomaxillary suture
fns	frontonasal suture
fo	foramen ovale
fr	foramen rotundum
iam	internal acoustic meatus
imxs	intermaxillary suture
ins	internasal suture
insy	innominate synchondrosis
iof	infraorbital foramen
iofs	inferior orbital fissure
issy	intersphenoid synchondrosis
l	labyrinth
lb	lacrimal bone
ls	lambdoidal suture
m	mandible
mc	condylar process of mandible
mcr	coronoid process of mandible
mef	mental foramen
mf	metopic fonticulus
mns	mendosal suture
mps	median palatine suture
ms	metopic (frontal) suture
msa	mastoid antrum
msy	mandibular synchondrosis
mx	maxilla
mxans	anterior nasal spine of maxilla
mxfp	frontal process of maxilla
mxpp	palatine process of maxilla
mxsi	maxillary sinus
mxzp	zygomatic process of maxilla
nb	nasal bone
nc	nasal cavity
nfs	nasofrontal suture
nmxs	nasomaxillary suture
ns	nasal septum
o	ossicles
ocb	occipital bone
ocbb	basioccipital bone
ocbex	exoccipital portion of occipital bone
ocbip	interparietal portion of occipital squama
ocbso	supraoccipital portion of occipital squama
ocbsq	squamous portion of occipital bone
occ	occipital condyle
of	optic foramen
orb	orbit
pab	palatine bone
pamxs	palatomaxillary suture
pb	parietal bone
pc	pterygoid canal
pf	posterior fonticulus
pfo	pterygoid fossa
plf	posterolateral fonticulus
psqs	petrosquamosal suture
sbb	basisphenoid
sbbo	body of sphenoid bone
sbgw	greater sphenoidal wing
sblpp	lateral pterygoid plate
sblw	lesser sphenoidal wing
sbmpp	medial pterygoid plate
sbpp	pterygoid plate
sf	sphenoidal fissure
sfs	sphenofrontal suture
smf	superior median fissure
socsy	sphenooccipital synchondrosis
sor	superior orbital rim
sqs	squamosal suture
ss	sagittal suture
ssc	superior semicircular canal
ssqs	sphenosquamosal suture
st	sella turcica
stmf	stylomastoid foramen
szs	sphenozygomatic suture
tbm	mastoid portion of temporal bone
tboc	otic capsule of temporal bone
tbp	petrous portion of temporal bone
tbsq	squamous portion of temporal bone
tbt	tympanic portion of temporal bone
tbzp	zygomatic process of temporal bone
tc	tympanic cavity
tus	tuberculum sellae
vb	vomer bone
zb	zygomatic bone
zfs	zygomaticofrontal suture
zmxs	zygomaticomaxillary suture
zts	zygomaticotemporal suture

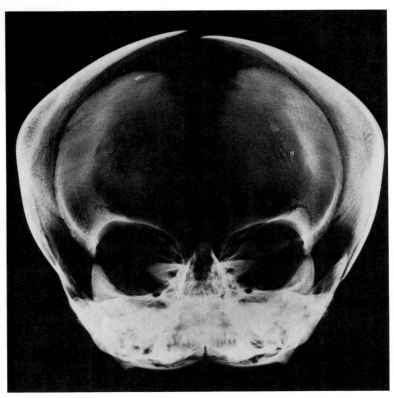

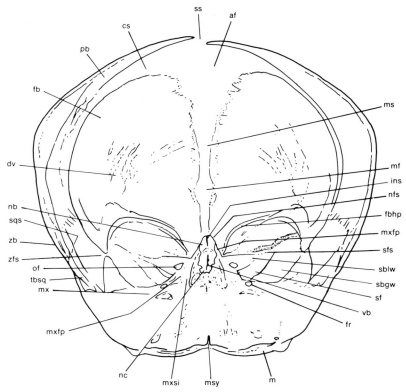

Fig 39.—Radiograph in Caldwell projection of dry skull of full-term stillborn fetus. (From Shapiro, R., and Robinson, F.: *Embryogenesis* *of the Human Skull* [Cambridge, Mass.: Harvard University Press, 1980].)

year. The foramen magnum is normally symmetric but varies somewhat in size and shape. The common configuration is ovoid or a rounded triangle but not a perfect circle. Occasionally, the normal foramen is asymmetric because of asymmetric closure of the adjacent synchondroses. A Kerckring's bone is sometimes found at the superior aspect of the foramen magnum (Fig 63).

SPHENOID BONE.—At term, the intersphenoid synchondrosis is usually obliterated. However, it may be open and manifest itself as a narrow, linear radiolucent streak that ossifies completely during the first year. There may also be residual unossified cartilaginous foci within the body of the sphenoid and the dorsum sellae that ossify after birth. The synchondrosis between the basisphenoid and basiocciput is prominent. The ossified lesser wings are unfused medially since the planum sphenoidale is as yet unossified. The planum sphenoidale undergoes ossification during the first three postnatal years.

The clivus is relatively short compared to the rest of the skull. The craniopharyngeal canal is normally obliterated, although a primitive vascular channel passing from the sellar floor through the body of the sphenoid bone may be patent. This channel follows the general course of the stalk of Rathke's pouch but contains no epithelial elements. At term, the rudimentary sphenoidal sinus is still in the posterior nasal capsule. Hence, there is no pneumatization of the sphenoid bone. Pneumatization of the sphenoid bone commences during the third or fourth postnatal year.

TEMPORAL BONE AND PARANASAL SINUSES.—The mastoid process is nonexistent at birth. Only the tympanic cavity and mastoid antrum are pneumatized at this time. The paranasal sinuses are also inconspicuous. The frontal sinuses lie in the nasal fossa, while the maxillary sinuses consist of a single small cell on either side of the lateral nasal wall. However, the ethmoidal sinuses are sufficiently pneumatized to be recognizable on the lateral roentgenogram (Fig 64). The structures of the internal ear are well developed (Figs 65 and 66). Occasionally, there is a tiny intradural ossicle close to the medial

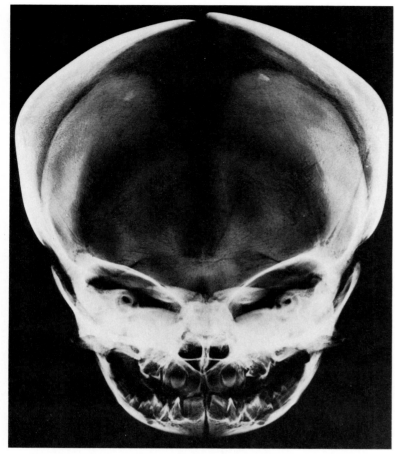

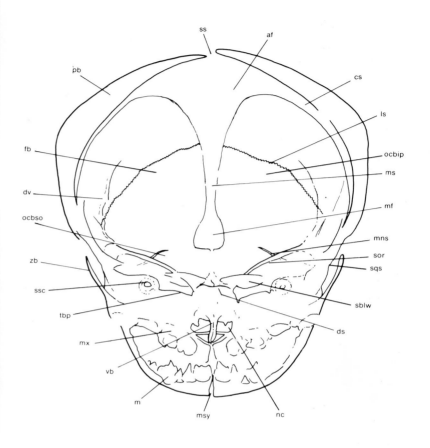

Fig 40.—Radiograph in straight posteroanterior projection of dry skull of full-term stillborn fetus. (From Shapiro, R., and Robinson, F.: *Embryogenesis of the Human Skull* [Cambridge, Mass.: Harvard University Press, 1980].)

aspect of the petrous tip. It is usually bilateral and has no clinical significance (Fig 67).

MANDIBLE.—The mandible is divided into two lateral halves by a midline bar of cartilage. The rami are broad and relatively large. The body contains multiple radiolucent dental crypts within which the denser crowns of the deciduous teeth can be seen.

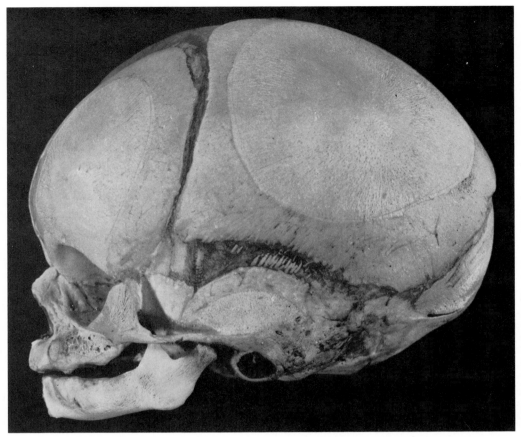

Fig 41.—Lateral photograph of skull of full-term stillborn fetus. (From Shapiro, R., and Robinson, F.: *Embryogenesis of the Human Skull* [Cambridge, Mass.: Harvard University Press, 1980].)

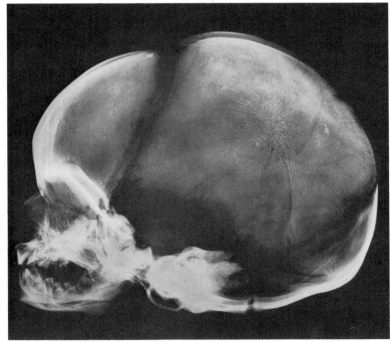

Fig 42.—Radiograph in lateral projection of dry skull of full-term stillborn fetus. (From Shapiro, R., and Robinson, F.: *Embryogenesis of the Human Skull* [Cambridge, Mass.: Harvard University Press, 1980].)

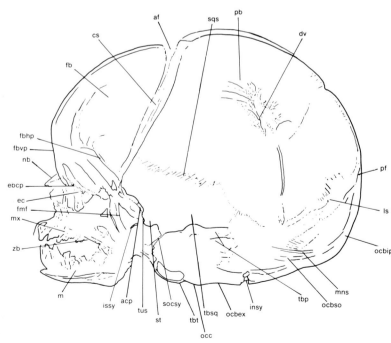

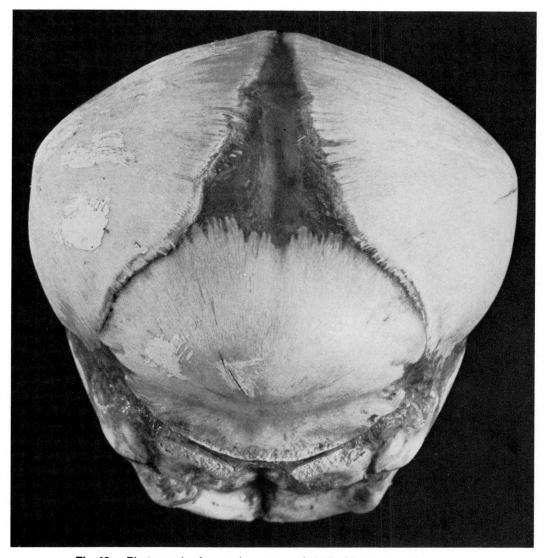

Fig 43.—Photograph of posterior aspect of skull of full-term stillborn fetus.

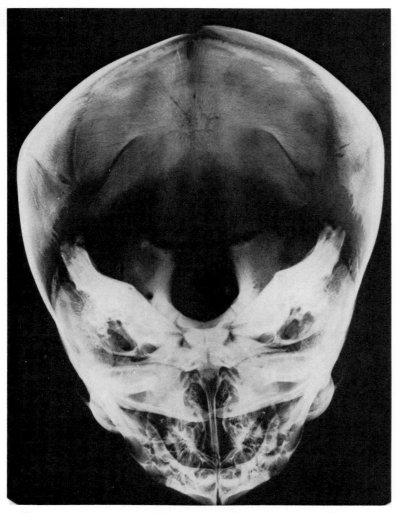

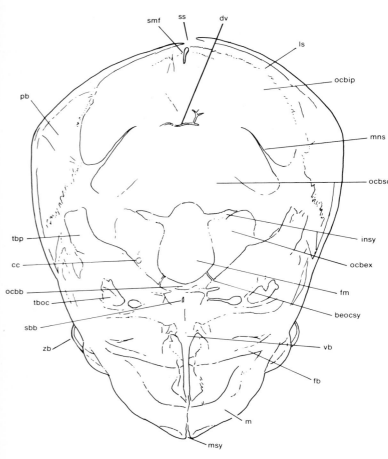

Fig 44.—Radiograph in Towne projection of dry skull of full-term stillborn fetus. (From Shapiro, R., and Robinson, F.: *Embryogenesis* *of the Human Skull* [Cambridge, Mass.: Harvard University Press, 1980].)

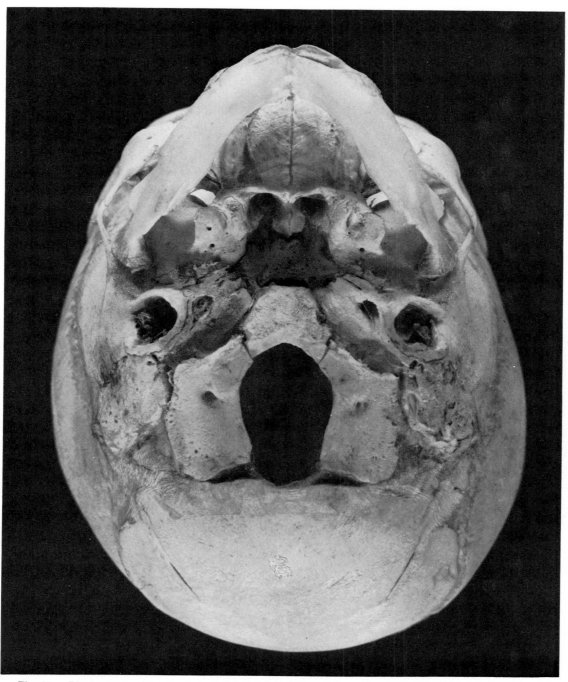

Fig 45.—Photograph of base of skull of full-term stillborn fetus. (From Shapiro, R., and Robinson, F.: *Embryogenesis of the Human Skull* [Cambridge, Mass.: Harvard University Press, 1980].)

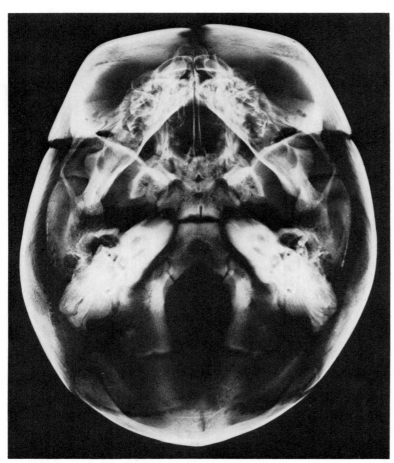

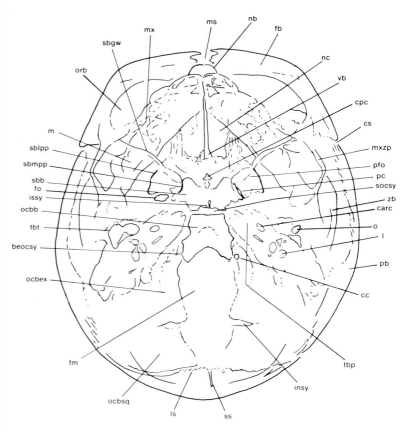

Fig 46.—Radiograph in submentovertical projection of dry skull of full-term stillborn fetus. (From Shapiro, R., and Robinson, F.: *Embry-* *ogenesis of the Human Skull* [Cambridge, Mass.: Harvard University Press, 1980].)

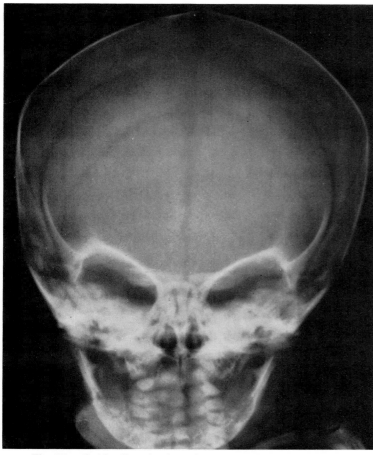

Fig 47.—Caldwell projection of neonatal skull of live infant.

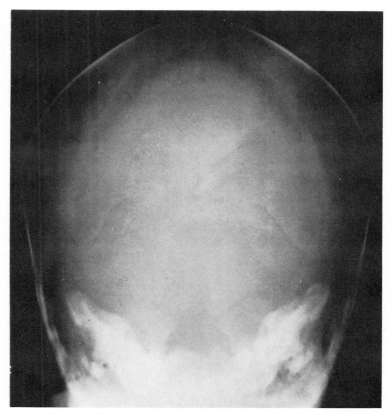

Fig 49.—Towne projection of neonatal skull of live infant.

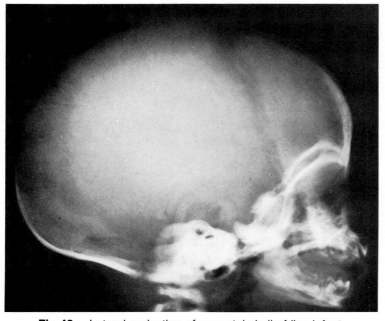

Fig 48.—Lateral projection of neonatal skull of live infant.

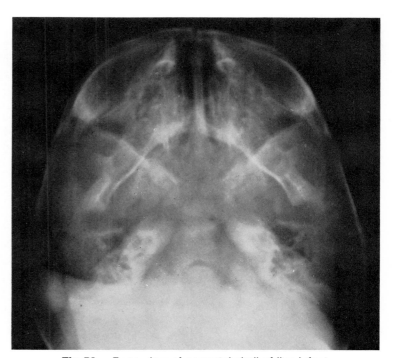

Fig 50.—Base view of neonatal skull of live infant.

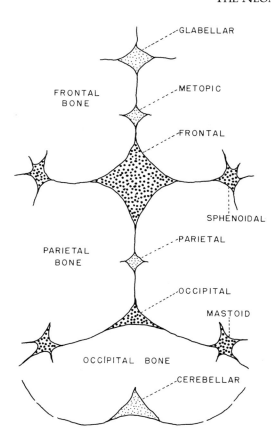

Fig 51.—Fonticuli at birth. Constant fonticuli are identified by heavy stippling and accessory fonticuli by light stippling.

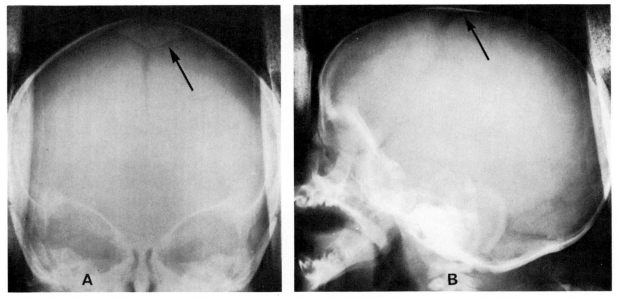

Fig 52.—Frontal **(A)** and lateral **(B)** projections of infant skull showing a large anterior fonticulus bone *(arrow)*. (Courtesy of Dr. J. F. Holt.)

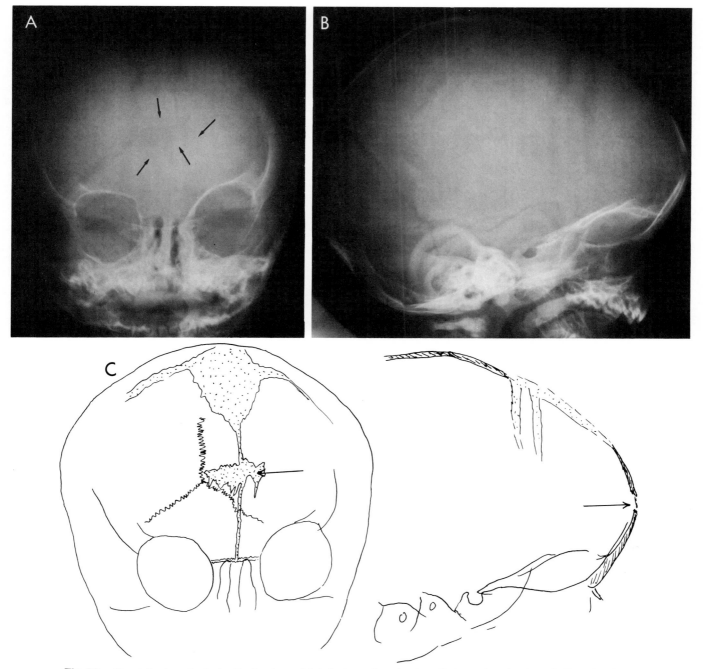

Fig 53.—Persistent metopic fonticulus in a child. **A,** frontal projection. **B,** lateral projection. **C,** line drawing.

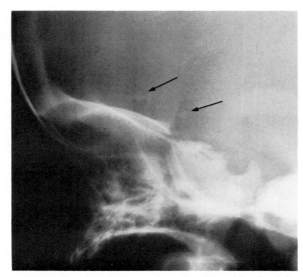

Fig 54.—Bilateral epipteric bones in anterolateral fonticuli *(arrows).*

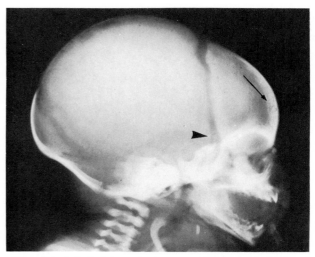

Fig 55.—Frontal diploic vein in neonate *(arrow).* Note also the epipteric bone *(arrowhead).*

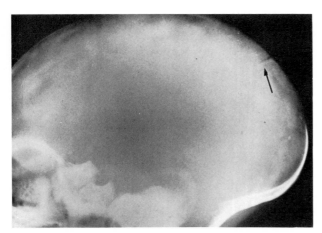

Fig 56.—Unossified parietal strip *(arrow)* in relationship to sagittal suture in newborn. (From Shapiro, R., and Robinson, F.: *Am. J. Roentgenol.* 115:569–577, 1972.)

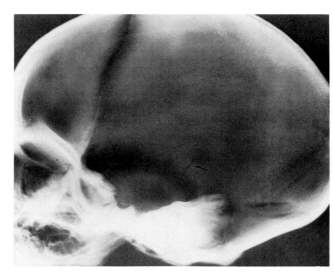

Fig 57.—Roentgenogram of dry skull of full-term stillborn fetus showing parietal strip *(arrow)* in relationship to squamosal suture. (From Shapiro, R., and Robinson, F.: *Am. J. Roentgenol.* 115:569–577, 1972.)

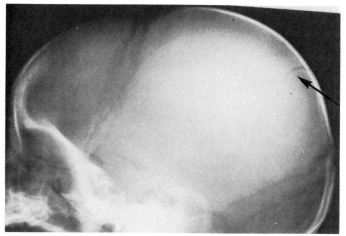

Fig 58.—Fracture of parietal bone *(arrow)* in 4-month-old child who fell out of the crib. There was a palpable local hematoma. Differential diagnosis from an unossified membranous strip may at times be difficult or impossible. (From Shapiro, R., and Robinson F.: *Am. J. Roentgenol.* 115:569–577, 1972.)

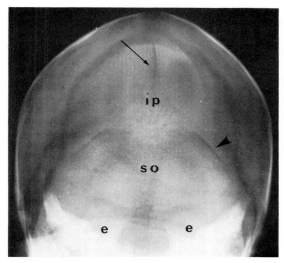

Fig 59.—Towne projection of neonatal skull. Note midline unossified membranous strip *(arrow)* in interparietal segment of the occipital bone *(ip)*. The latter is separated by mendosal suture *(arrowhead)* from supraoccipital segment *(so)*. Paired exoccipital segments *(e)* are on either side of foramen magnum. (From Shapiro, R., and Robinson, F.: *Am. J. Roentgenol.* 126:1063–1068, 1976.)

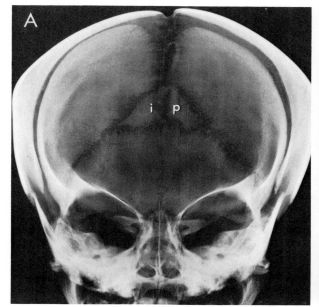
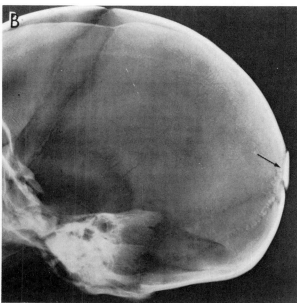

Fig 60.—Frontal **(A)** and lateral **(B)** projections of skull of full-term infant showing a classic triangular os incae *(ip)*. Note sclerotic appearance in lateral projection *(arrow)*. (From Shapiro, R., and Robinson, F.: *Am. J. Roentgenol.* 127:469–471, 1976.)

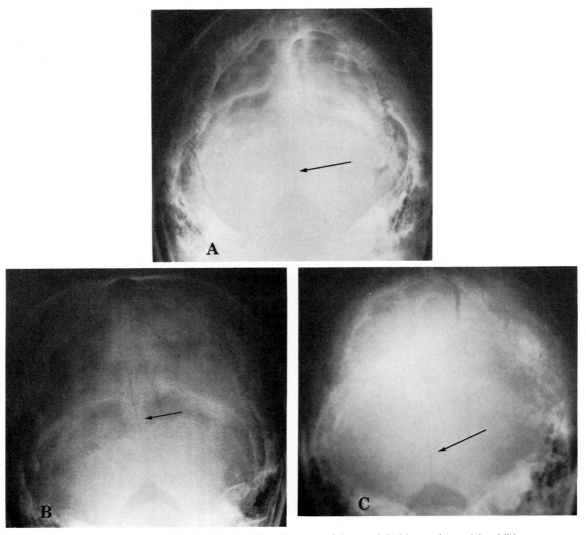

Fig 61.—Three cases **(A, B, C)** of midline fracture of the occipital bone *(arrow)* in children.

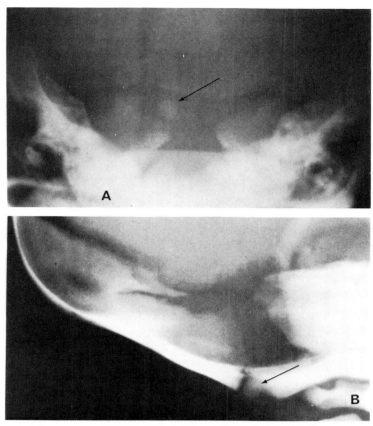

Fig 62.—Towne projection **(A)** and lateral projection **(B)** of infant skull showing a supernumerary bone in the innominate synchondrosis *(arrow)*.

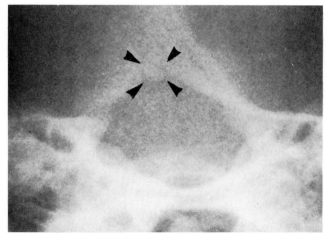

Fig 63.—Kerckring's bone *(arrowheads)* in a child.

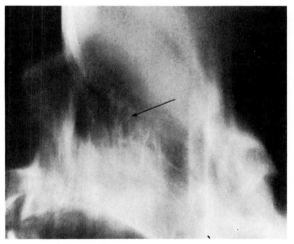

Fig 64.—Lateral radiograph of dry skull of full-term stillborn fetus showing pneumatized ethmoidal cells *(arrow)*.

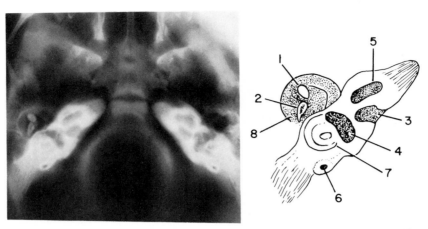

Fig 65.—Body-section radiograph *(left)* and line drawing *(right)* of full-term neonatal skull in submentovertical projection at the plane of the cochlea. Drawing portrays findings in right temporal bone. The stapes is missing. Note the malleus *(1);* incus *(2);* internal auditory canal *(3);* vestibule *(4);* cochlea *(5);* posterior semicircular canal *(6);* horizontal semicircular canal *(7);* and epitympanic cavity *(8).*

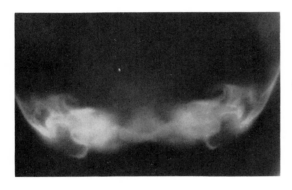
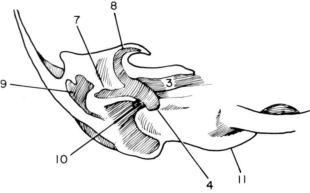

Fig 66.—Body-section radiograph *(left)* and line drawing *(right)* of skull of full-term neonate in anteroposterior projection at the plane of the vestibule. Drawing portrays findings in right temporal bone. Note the internal auditory canal *(3);* vestibule *(4);* horizontal semicircular canal *(7);* superior semicircular canal *(8);* antrum *(9);* oval window *(10);* and occipital bone *(11).*

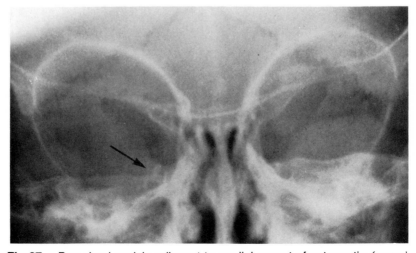

Fig 67.—Pea-sized ossicle adjacent to medial aspect of petrous tip *(arrow).*

REFERENCES

Caffey J.: On the accessory ossicles of the supraoccipital bone. *Am. J. Roentgenol.* 70:401–412, 1953.

Caffey J.: *Pediatric x-ray diagnosis,* ed. 7. Chicago, Year Book Medical Publishers, 1972.

Chasler C. N.: *Atlas of Roentgen Anatomy of the Newborn and Infant Skull.* St. Louis, Warren H. Greene, 1972.

Currarino G., Weinberg A.: Os supra petrosum of Meckel. *Am. J. Roentgenol.* 121:139–142, 1974.

Dedick A. P., Caffey J.: Roentgen findings in the skull and chest in 1,030 newborn infants. *Radiology* 61:13–20, 1953.

Girdany B. R., Blank E.: Anterior fontanel bones. *Am. J. Roentgenol.* 95:148–153, 1965.

Henderson S. G., Sherman L. S.: The roentgen anatomy of the skull in the newborn infant. *Radiology* 46:107–118, 1946.

Henderson S. G., Sherman L. S.: Roentgen anatomy of the skull in the newborn infant, in Etter L. (ed.): *Atlas of Roentgen Anatomy of the Skull.* Springfield, Ill., Charles C Thomas, Publisher, 1964.

Kruff E.: Occipital dysplasia in infancy. *Radiology* 85:501–506, 1965.

LeWald L. T.: Congenital absence of superior orbital wall associated with pulsating exophthalmos. *Am. J. Roentgenol.* 30:756–764, 1933.

Nellhaus G.: Head circumference from birth to eighteen years: Practical composite international and interracial graphs. *Pediatrics* 41:106–114, 1968.

Robertson E. G.: Pulsating exophthalmos due to defective development of the sphenoid bone. *Am. J. Roentgenol.* 62:44–51, 1949.

Shopfner C. E., Wolfe T. W., O'Kell R. T.: The intersphenoid synchondrosis. *Am. J. Roentgenol.* 104:184–193, 1968.

Silver H. K., Deamer W. C.: Graphs of the head circumference of the normal infant. *J. Pediatr.* 33:167–171, 1948.

Terrafranca R. J., Zellis A.: Congenital hereditary cranium bifidum occultum frontalis with a review of anatomical variations in lower mid sagittal region of frontal bones. *Radiology* 61:60–66, 1953.

4

The Skull in Childhood

According to Watson and Lowery, 80% of brain growth is completed by the end of the third year and 95% by the end of the eighth year of life. Since skull growth and development parallel brain growth, it is not remarkable that the appearance of the skull at the end of the third year resembles that of the adult. Further development at a slow rate continues so long as there is general somatic growth.

TABLES

As the skull matures, it increases in thickness and differentiates into three more or less distinct tables. In addition to the appositional new bone laid down at the margins of the membranous calvarial components, new bone is also deposited on their endocranial and exocranial surfaces. As in long-bone modeling, there is simultaneous bone resorption. This involves the diploic surfaces of the inner and outer tables, thereby widening the diploe.

VASCULAR MARKINGS AND SUTURES

Vascular markings in the diploe and inner table make their appearance to a varying degree. The fonticuli become obliterated, and the sutures decrease markedly in width. The metopic suture usually becomes obliterated by the end of the second year, although it may occasionally persist into adult life. It should not be mistaken for a fracture of the frontal bone, particularly when slightly asymmetric or when the straight endocranial aspect of the suture is projected as a vertical radiolucent line (Fig 68).

The mendosal sutures usually disappear during the latter half of the first year. Rarely, a single mendosal suture remains open and should not be confused with a fracture. Similarly, the innominate synchondrosis between the supraoccipital and the exoccipital segments, and the synchondroses between the basioccipital and

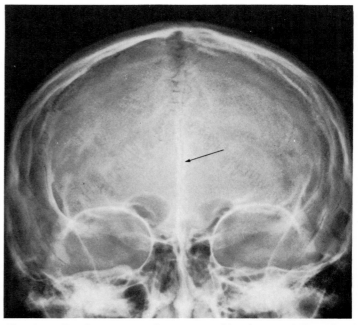

Fig 68.—Persistent metopic suture with characteristic sclerotic margins *(arrow)* in 12-year-old boy. Suture begins at bregma and usually extends to nasion. It is generally, though not always, midline in position.

exoccipital segments of the occipital bone are usually obliterated by age 2 to 4. Occasionally, these synchondroses may not close simultaneously on both sides.

Knowledge of the location and direction of the normal sutures and synchondroses is helpful in avoiding an erroneous diagnosis of a fracture based on an asymmetric linear radiolucency. Ossification of the spheno-occipital synchondrosis begins at age 12 to 13 in girls and 14 to 15 in boys. However, the synchondrosis does not completely fuse until age 16 to 20. Occasionally, the spheno-occipital synchondrosis persists into adult life. The coronal, lambdoidal, and sagittal sutures persist throughout childhood and adolescence. Physiologic sutural diastasis may occur following rapid recovery from nutritional deprivation in infancy and childhood.

CONVOLUTIONAL MARKINGS

The terms "convolutional markings," "digital markings," and "brain markings" are used interchangeably. They designate the impressions made on the inner table of the skull by the gyri of the brain. During the first year of life, there are few digital markings. They increase progressively in number and prominence up to the sixth year, maintain a plateau until age 10, and then regress (Fig 69). This regression usually continues during adolescence, although it is not unusual to find prominent convolutional markings in young adults (Fig 70). The convolutional markings tend to be equally prominent in the vault and base, although they may occasionally be limited to the occipital bone. When they are absent, retardation or arrest of brain growth should be suspected, and checked by periodic measurement of the internal diameters of the skull. On the other hand, increased prominence of the convolutional markings may accompany the rapid brain growth that follows successful treatment of severe nutritional deficiency.

INDICATIONS OF INCREASED INTRACRANIAL PRESSURE

In the absence of sutural spreading or sellar changes, prominent convolutional markings per se are an unreliable index of increased intracranial pressure. In infants, sutural diastasis may be the only radiographic sign of generalized increased intracranial pressure. However, resorption of the inner aspect of the base of the dorsum sellae may also be present, particularly later in childhood. Sellar erosion with normal sutures in children is usually due to local disease, e.g., craniopharyngioma. Specific sellar changes are discussed in chapter 12, dealing with the sella turcica. Although sutural diastasis may develop rapidly in infants and young children (two to four weeks after the onset of symptoms) (Fig 71), in older children it is often indicative of a more chronic process. In these patients, the sella turcica is usually also abnormal.

PITUITARY FOSSA

The pituitary fossa in the child tends to be small and round. Although the chiasmatic sulcus varies, it is usu-

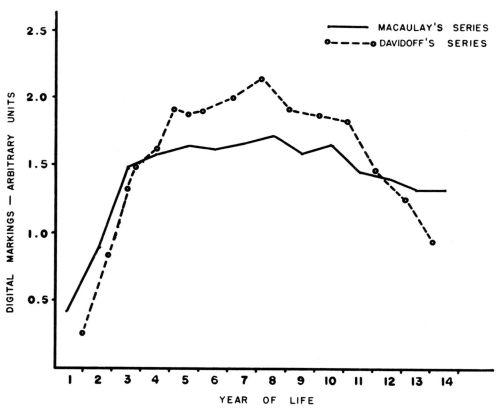

Fig 69.—Incidence of convolutional markings in childhood. (After Macaulay, *Br. J. Radiol.* 24:647–652, 1951.)

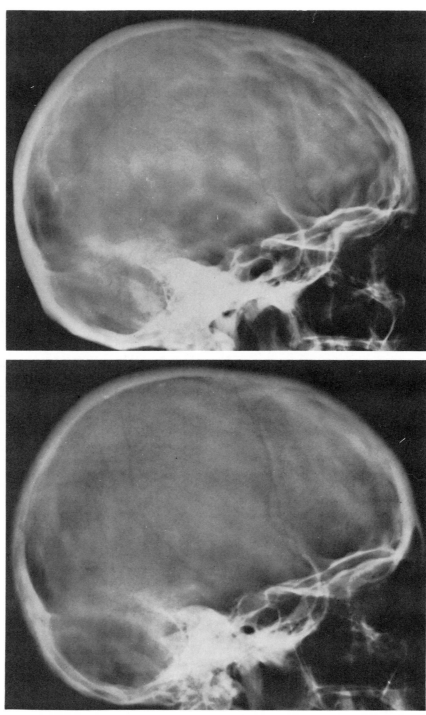

Fig 70.—Prominent convolutional markings of inner table of skull in 22-year-old woman with headaches *(top).* Same patient at age 30 *(bottom)* shows considerable diminution in prominence of convolu-tional markings. It is interesting that the headaches persisted with no apparent organic basis for the complaint.

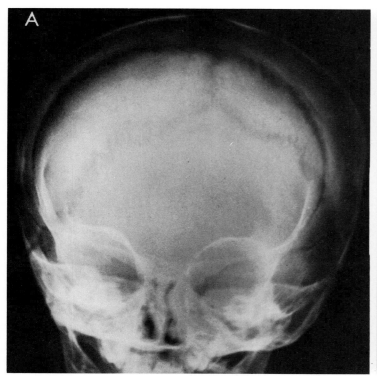

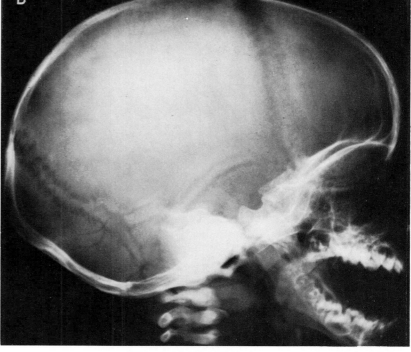

Fig 71.—Frontal **(A)** and lateral **(B)** radiographs showing obvious sutural diastasis in a two-year-old girl with medulloblastoma of cere-bellar vermis. Clinical and radiologic signs of increased intracranial pressure developed within a period of one month.

ally prominent. The so-called J-shaped sella due to a large chiasmatic sulcus and a small tuberculum sellae is normal in infancy and childhood. The planum sphenoidale, which is not present at birth, develops during the first postnatal year and grows posteriorly during the first two or three years to cover the cranial end of the roof of the optic canal. The notch separating the limbus sphenoidale from the presphenoid normally may be seen during the first five to six years. This notch is obliterated after the limbus fuses with the presphenoid, usually by the end of the sixth year. Occasionally, it remains open in adult life. According to Silverman, the pituitary fossa in males tends to be larger than the sella in females until age 13. At that time, the fossa in the female catches up with, and surpasses, the fossa in the male in size. Silverman's data suggest that the area of the pituitary fossa may be more closely related to body height than to age (Figs 72 to 76).

PARANASAL SINUSES

Pneumatization of the vertical plate of the frontal bone begins during the latter half of the second post-natal year and progresses slowly to reach the level of nasion by the fourth year. By six to eight years, the frontal sinuses are usually readily visable in the vertical plate as a result of further growth. Continued pneumatization occurs throughout childhood but is quite variable (Fig 77).

Pneumatization of the sphenoid bone commences at age 4 and continues throughout childhood and adolescence with considerable variability. The maxillary sinuses also undergo variable growth and development during the same period. On the lateral roentgenogram, the adenoids behind the pharyngeal airway produce a density of varying size that may be very prominent in some children. Prior to age 1 month, however, a soft tissue mass in this region should be considered abnormal, according to Capitanio and Kirkpatrick. The absence of lymphoid tissue in the posterior nasopharynx in childhood should raise the question of an immune deficiency state.

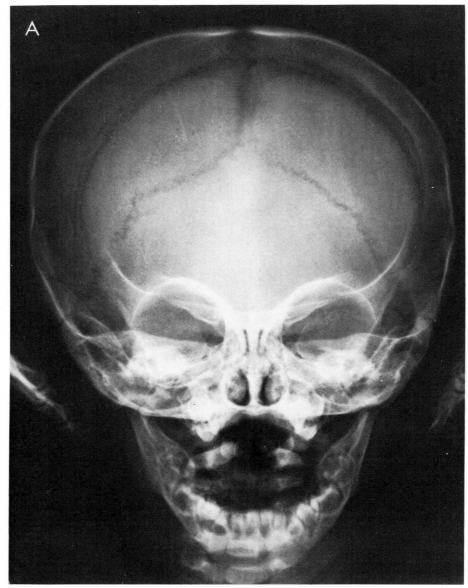

Fig 72.—Normal skull at one year. **A,** posteroanterior view. Anterior fontanelle is normally widely patent, but posterior fontanelle is closed. Sutures are open and well defined. **B,** lateral view. *(Continued)*

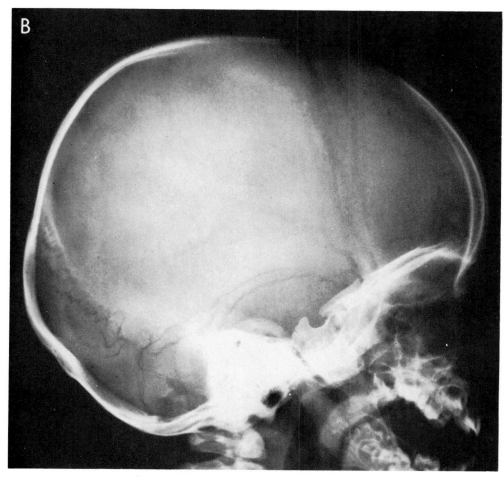

Fig 72 (cont.).—See legend on facing page.

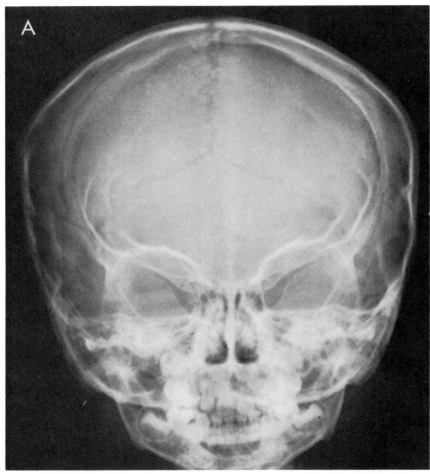

Fig 73.—Normal skull at two years. **A,** posteroanterior view. Fonticuli are closed, and vault has begun to differentiate into inner and outer tables and diploë. Convolutional margins are usually present at this age. **B,** lateral view. *(Continued)*

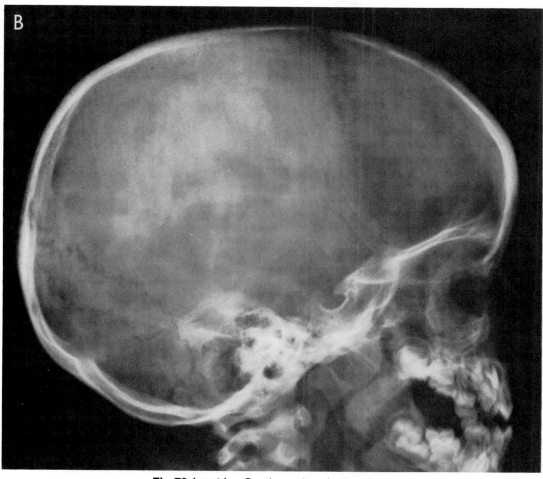

Fig 73 (cont.).—See legend on facing page.

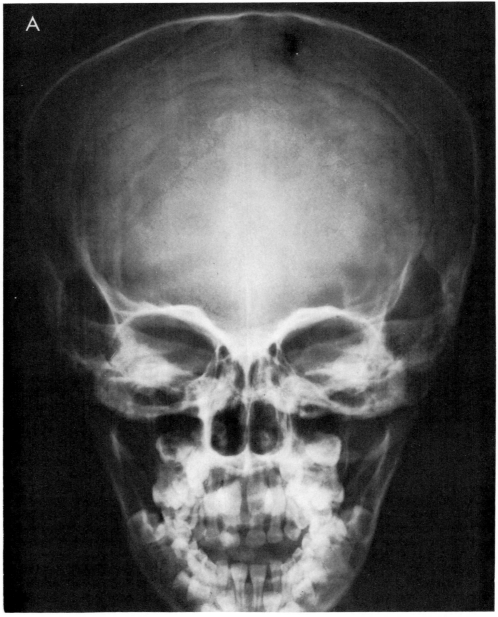

Fig 74.—Normal skull at five years. **A,** posteroanterior view. **B,** lateral view. Nasopharyngeal lymphoid tissue presents as a smoothly marginated soft tissue density. *(Continued)*

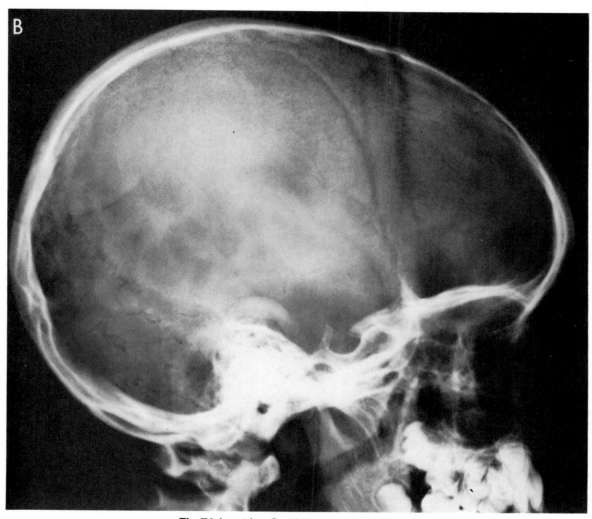

Fig 74 (cont.).—See legend on facing page.

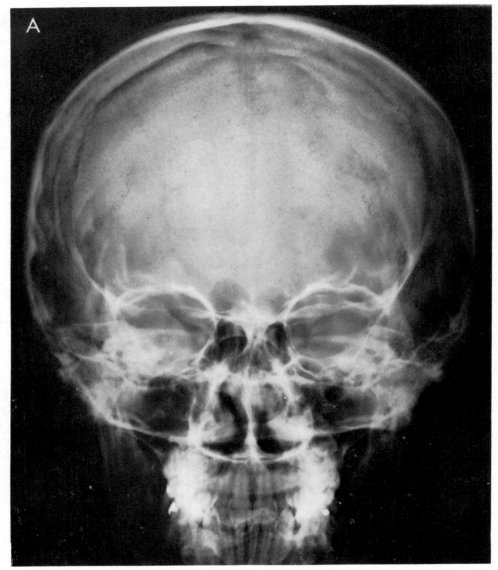

Fig 75.—Normal skull at 12 years. **A,** posteroanterior view. **B,** lateral view. *(Continued)*

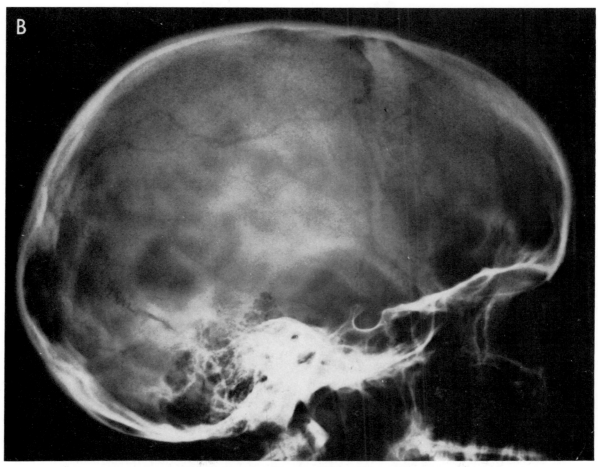

Fig 75 (cont.).—See legend on facing page.

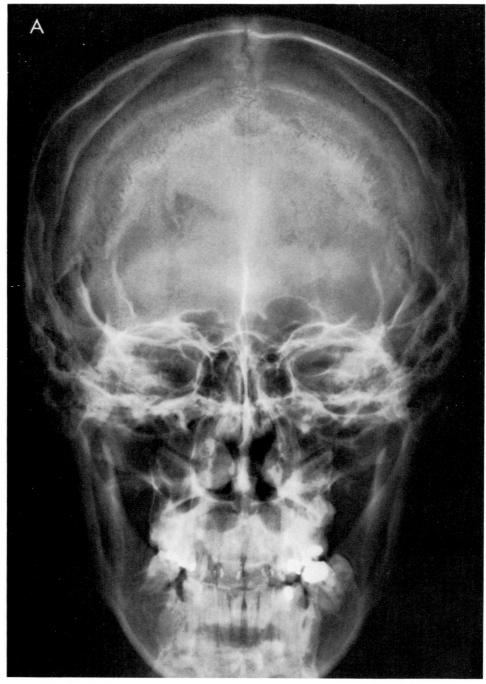

Fig 76.—Normal skull at 18 years. **A,** posteroanterior view. **B,** lateral view. *(Continued)*

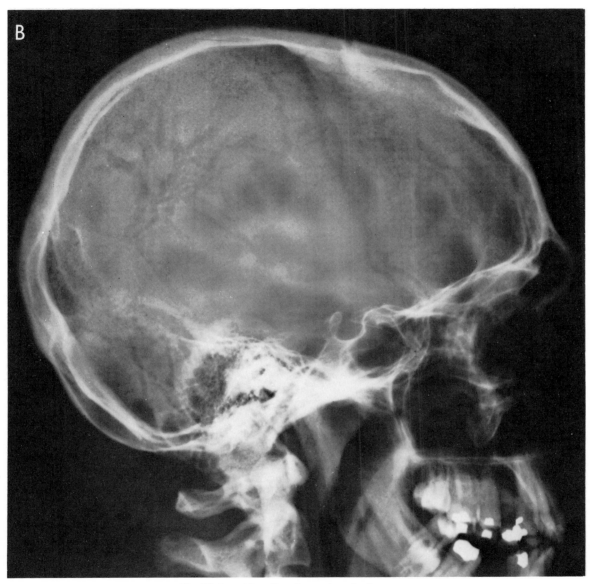

Fig 76 (cont.).—See legend on facing page.

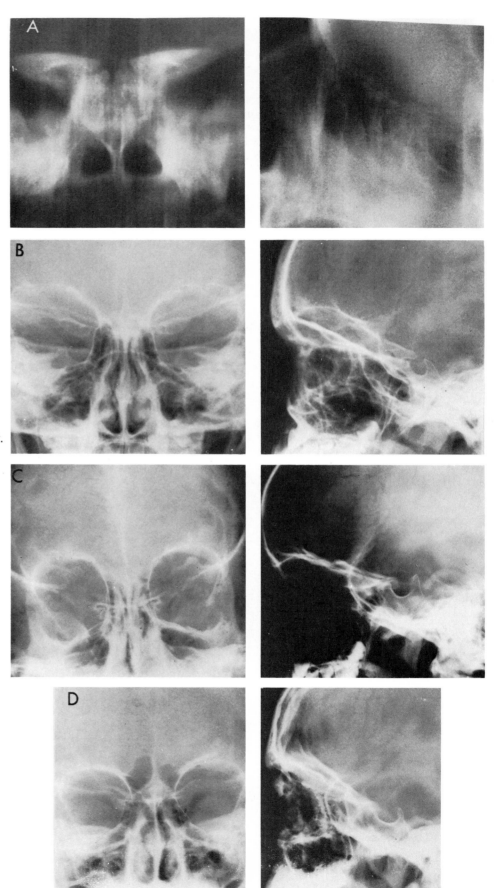

Fig 77.—Normal paranasal sinus development. **A,** full-term stillborn neonate. **B,** age 3 years. **C,** age 5 years. **D,** age 10 years.

REFERENCES

Abraham J. M., Snodgrass G. J. A. I.: Sotos' syndrome of cerebral gigantism. *Arch. Dis. Child.* 44:203–210, 1969.

Allen W. E. III, Kier E. L., Rothman L. G.: Pitfalls in the evaluation of skull trauma: A review. *Radiol. Clin. North Am.* 11:479–503, 1973.

Anderson H., Gomes S. P.: Craniosynostosis: Review of the literature and indications for surgery. *Acta Paediatr. Scand.* 57:47–54, 1968.

Austin J. H. M., Gooding C. A.: Roentgenographic measurement of skull size in children. *Radiology* 99:641–646, 1971.

Campbell J. A.: Roentgen aspect of cranial configuration. *Radiol. Clin. North Am.* 4:11–31, 1966.

Christensen J. B., Lachman E., Brues A. M.: A study of the roentgen appearance of cranial vault sutures: Correlation with their anatomy. *Am. J. Roentgenol.* 83:615–627, 1960.

Cronqvist S.: Roentgenologic evaluation of cranial size in children. *Acta Radiol.* 7:97–111, 1968.

Davidoff L. M.: Convolutional digitations seen in the roentgenogram of immature human skulls. *Bull. Neurol. Inst. New York* 5:61–71, 1936.

Dorst J. P.: Functional craniology: An aid in interpreting roentgenograms of the skull. *Radiol. Clin. North Am.* 2:347–366, 1964.

Dorst J. P.: Changes of the skull during childhood, in Newton T. H., Potts D. G. (eds.): *The Skull.* Book 1: *Radiology of the Skull and Brain,* vol. 1. St. Louis, C. V. Mosby Co., 1971.

DuBoulay G.: The significance of digital impressions in children's skulls. *Acta Radiol.* 46:112–122, 1956.

Enlow D. H.: *The Human Face: An Account of the Postnatal Growth and Development of the Craniofacial Skeleton.* New York, Harper & Row, 1968.

Epstein J. A., Epstein B. S.: Deformities of the skull surfaces in infancy and childhood. *J. Pediatr.* 70:636–647, 1967.

Francis C. C.: Growth of the human pituitary fossa. *Hum. Biol.* 20:1–20, 1948.

Gerald B. E., Silverman F. N.: Normal and abnormal interorbital distances with special reference to mongolism. *Am. J. Roentgenol.* 95:154–161, 1965.

Gooding C. A.: Skull vault: Size and shape, in Newton T. H., Potts D. G. (eds.): *The Skull.* Book 1: *Radiology of the Skull and Brain,* vol. 1. St. Louis, C. V. Mosby Co., 1971.

Gooding C. A.: Cranial sutures and fontanelles, ibid.

Gordon I. R. S.: Measurement of cranial capacity in children. *Br. J. Radiol.* 39:377–381, 1966.

Gordon I. R. S.: Microcephaly and craniostenosis. *Clin. Radiol.* 21:19–31, 1970.

Haas L. L.: Roentgenological skull measurements and their diagnostic applications. *Am. J. Roentgenol.* 67:197–209, 1952.

Harwood-Nash D. C., Fitz C. R.: *Neuroradiology in Infants and Children.* St. Louis, C. V. Mosby Co., 1976, vol. 1.

Macaulay D.: Digital markings in radiographs of the skull in children. *Br. J. Radiol.* 24:647–652, 1951.

McRae D. L.: Observations on craniolacunia. *Acta Radiol.* 5:55–64, 1966.

Robinson R. G.: Congenital perforations of the skull in relation to the parietal bone. *J. Neurosurg.* 19:153–158, 1962.

Shapiro R., Janzen A. H.: *The Normal Skull: A Roentgen Study.* New York, P. B. Hoeber, 1960.

Silverman F. N.: Roentgen standards for size of the pituitary fossa from infancy thru adolescence. *Am. J. Roentgenol.* 78:451–460, 1957.

Watson E. H., Lowery G. H.: *Growth and Development of Children,* ed. 5. Chicago, Year Book Medical Publishers, 1967.

5

Functional Craniology

BASIC STRUCTURAL-FUNCTIONAL RELATIONSHIPS

Well into the present century the skull was viewed as an isolated structural unit. In the 1940s, Weidenreich, van der Klaauw, Moss, and Young emphasized the importance of function through a variety of embryologic, comparative anatomical, anthropological, and experimental studies. Nonetheless, in the following two decades, only a few radiologists exhibited an interest in the effect of various pathologic processes upon skull growth and development. In 1964, Dorst's classic paper focused attention on the importance of the functional approach to the analysis of skull roentgenograms. Time has proven the validity of this concept.

Van der Klaauw first pointed out that the skull should "be regarded as a complex of relatively separate functional components, sometimes detached, sometimes united in a morphological whole, but even in this case to a certain extent independent in size, relative position, and grouping." In general, the function of bones (and therefore of the bony skull) is to support and protect the contiguous soft tissues. The form of the skull is, therefore, determined by the soft tissues it encloses. Hence, significant abnormalities of the brain and its investments early in life are always associated with abnormalities of the overlying skull.

The skull can be conveniently divided into two main functional units: (1) neural, and (2) facial. The neural component can in turn be subdivided into (a) the cerebral capsule or brain case, and (b) the sensory capsule investing the organs of smell, vision, and hearing. For practical purposes, it is simpler to consider the internal ear as a neural component, and the orbit and nose as a facial component. The facial component can likewise be divided into two parts: (a) the nasomaxillary complex, and (b) the mandible.

The major functional components should not be confused with morphological units such as individual bones of the skull. Although a single bone or segment thereof may form a functional unit, the latter may also consist of several different bones. Thus, the vertical plate of the frontal bone is a functional component of the brain case, whereas the horizontal plate is a functional unit of the orbit. Moreover, every skull bone has three separate functional components: the inner table, the diploë, and the outer table.

The cartilaginous base of the human skull is the most primitive portion phylogenetically. It is not surprising, therefore, that the chondrocranium of the eight-week human fetus resembles that of the elasmobranch shark. Since the genetic information governing growth of the primitive chondrocranium is probably inherent in the prechondral mesenchyme, development of the chondrocranium is limited and not significantly influenced by the surrounding soft tissues. Diseases characterized by defective enchondral bone formation, i.e., achondroplasia, demonstrate abnormalities of the skull base, i.e., short cranial base, small foramen magnum, and sunken root of nose (Fig 78).

The cranial vault, on the other hand, is derived from membrane that appears to have no inherent growth limitation. Hence, the membranous bones of the vault are able to respond to the dramatic growth of the contiguous soft tissues, i.e., the neural mass. The neural mass consists of the brain, the leptomeninges, and the cerebrospinal fluid. If the neural mass is abnormally small or large, the cerebral capsule is likewise abnormally small or large. If the neural mass is abnormal in shape, the calvaria tends to be abnormally shaped. Since major cerebral growth occurs during gestation and the first three postnatal years, gross disease of the brain in this period is likely to be reflected by corresponding changes in the size and shape of the overlying calvaria. Clinically, this is evidenced in a variety of pathologic conditions that are associated with asymmetry of the calvaria. Thus, Childe showed that subdural collections

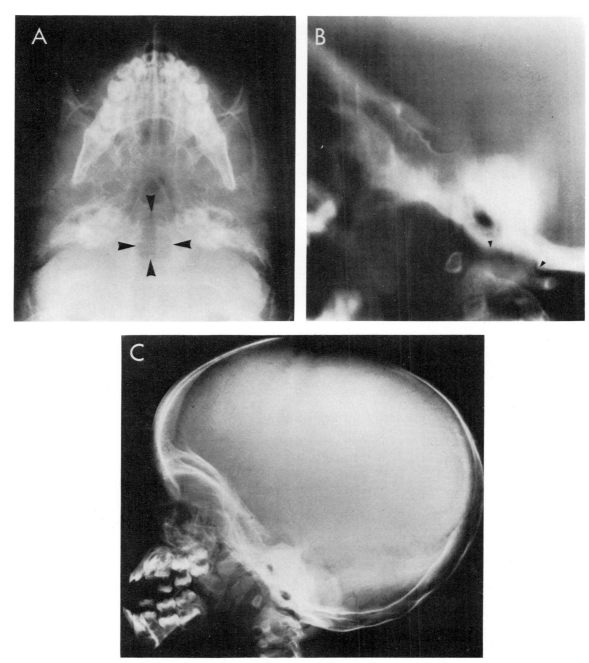

Fig 78.—Submentovertical radiograph **(A)** and lateral tomogram **(B)** in 16-month-old child with achondroplasia. Note small size of foramen magnum *(arrowheads)* due to inherent defect in enchondral bone formation. Conventional lateral film **(C)** shows the short base, sunken nose, and prominent vault.

of fluid—chronic hematoma or hygroma, cerebral agenesis or atrophy associated with arachnoidal cysts or ventricular enlargement, slow-growing temporal lobe astrocytomas, giant aneurysms of the internal carotid artery in the middle fossa, and neurofibromatosis—commonly produce localized changes in the ipsilateral hemicranium. These changes include elevation of the lesser sphenoidal wing, lateral bulging of the greater wing, and anterior bulging of the middle fossa (Figs 79 to 81).

Similarly, Davidoff and co-workers described the bony changes associated with unilateral cerebral atrophy: diminution in size and thickening of the ipsilateral

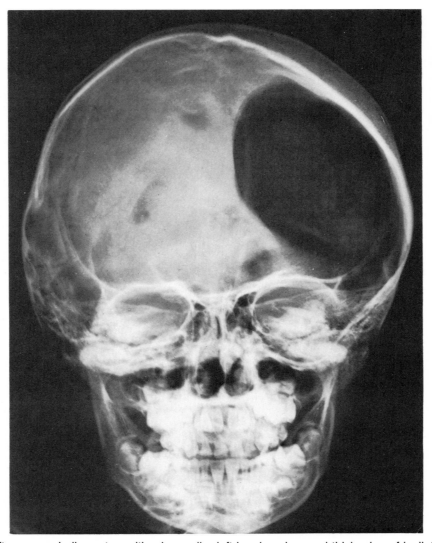

Fig 79.—Large left porencephalic cyst resulting in smaller left hemicranium and thickening of ipsilateral parietal bone.

hemicranium, elevation of the ipsilateral orbit and pet-rous bone, and hypertrophy of the ipsilateral paranasal sinuses. To these signs McCrae added displacement of the crista galli and of the groove for the superior sagittal sinus toward the involved side. The thickening of the inner table is a response to the falling away of the atrophic brain in the absence of an abnormal localized fluid collection (Figs 82 to 84).

The posterior fossa may also fail to develop normally and remain small in various congenital abnormalities of the hindbrain, e.g., cerebellar hypoplasia (Fig 85). Con-trariwise, the posterior fossa may be enlarged in various disease processes which increase the neural mass,

i.e., arachnoid cyst, Dandy-Walker syndrome, and slow-growing tumors (Fig 86).

Any part of a pathologically thin bony calvaria (due to osteogenesis imperfecta, severe chronic hydrocepha-lus) is responsive to abnormal stress and may become deformed. Similar deformities can also develop in the brain case of normal infants who persistently lie in one position (Fig 87).

Moss and Young have pointed out that the frontal bone is not a single functional unit. The inner table is an intrinsic part of the cerebral capsule, since its peri-osteum is the outer layer of the dura. Hence, the size and shape of the inner table are primarily determined

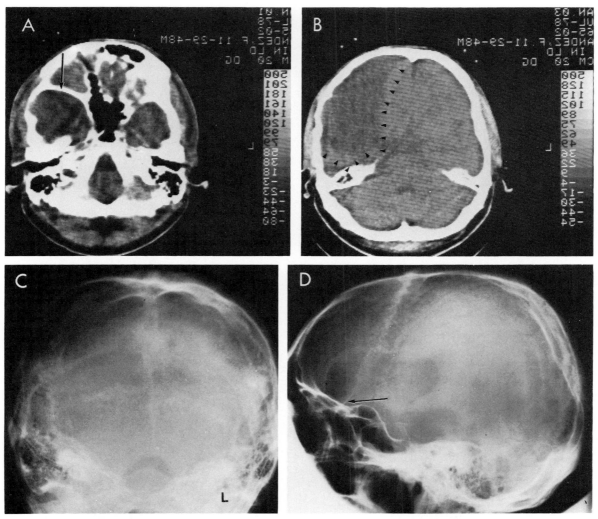

Fig 80.—Agenesis of right temporal lobe associated with arachnoid cyst filling ipsilateral middle fossa. Note thinning of right temporal bone and expansion of ipsilateral middle fossa, as well as anterior displacement of involved sphenoidal wing *(arrow)* on the CT scan **(A).** The CT scan also clearly demonstrates the arachnoid cyst *(arrowheads,* **B**). Conventional Towne view **(C)** shows expanded right hemicranium. Lateral view **(D)** shows anterior displacement of right sphenoidal wing *(arrow).*

by the configuration of the frontal lobes. On the other hand, the outer table is not part of the cerebral capsule and, therefore, is functionally independent of the latter. During the first few years of life, the inner table drifts anteriorly in response to the stimulus of the growing frontal lobes. Because the diploe is relatively undeveloped at this time, the inner table passively carries the outer table with it. When the rapid growth of the frontal lobes is diminished at age 6 to 7, growth of the frontal inner table also becomes arrested. However, the functionally independent outer table continues to drift anteriorly in response to growth of the nasomaxillary facial complex. This results in progressive separation of the inner and outer tables of the frontal bone. The intervening spacial gap is filled by the frontal sinuses (Fig 88).

The relative size of the cerebral capsule compared to that of the face is a significant biologic relationship. In aquatic animals, e.g., the hippopotamus, a large head and skull may accompany a large body because the buoyant effect of water helps support a large head. In most terrestrial animals, however, a large body is apt to be associated with a small head and skull because the head must be carried in the air. In general, cranial en-

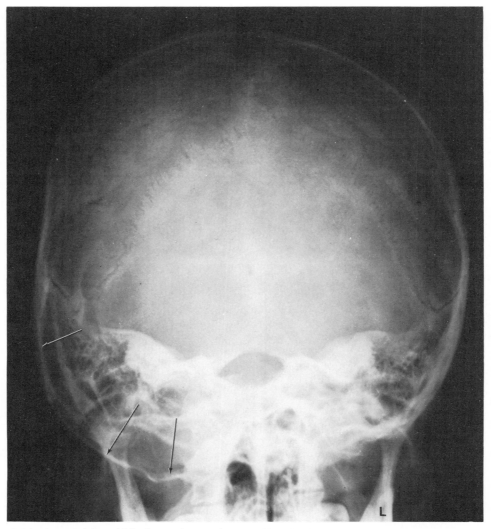

Fig 81.—Bulging and thinning of right middle fossa *(arrows)* caused by slowly growing cystic astrocytoma of right temporal lobe.

largement due to increased brain growth is associated with a reduction in facial size and, hence, relatively weak muscles of mastication.

The skull of the normal adult human tends to have a concordant craniofacial relationship. It is important to remember that the size of the skull depends upon the size of the neural mass, while the size of the face is related to general somatic growth. The diagnosis of microcephaly or macrocrania depends upon recognition of an abnormal craniofacial ratio. This observation can best be made on the lateral skull roentgenogram. The normal craniofacial area ratio is 4 to 1 in the neonate (Fig 89). Growth of the facial skeletal complex begins after birth and continues into puberty, when the adult craniofacial area ratio of 1.5 to 1 is reached.

The orbit, composed of cerebral and facial elements, functionally behaves as part of the face. The interorbital distance is normally fairly wide at birth, and reaches adult size by age 12. When the interorbital distance is excessive, the condition is termed hypertelorism. This may be a normal familial trait. However, it may also be associated with mental retardation and a variety of developmental anomalies and systemic diseases, e.g., midline facial defects, trisomy 13–15, and infantile hypercalcemia. In the newborn, approximately half of the globe lies anterior to the orbit, whereas the adult globe is almost entirely recessed within the orbit (Fig 90).

A prominent supraorbital ridge in the adult human with microcephaly represents the summation of two separate growth processes. The vertical plate of the

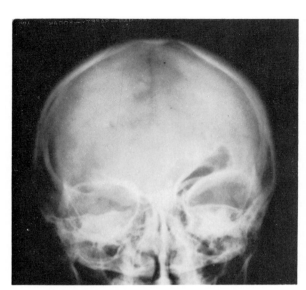

Fig 82.—Davidoff-Dyke-Masson syndrome. Left cerebral hemiatrophy with homolateral hypertrophy of left frontal sinus. Elevation of orbital roof, lesser sphenoidal wing, and petrous ridge on left side. (From Collins, L. M., and Schwartz, C. W.: *The Skull and Brain Roentgenologically Considered* [Springfield, Ill., Charles C Thomas, Publisher, 1951].)

frontal bone adapts to the reduced frontal lobe mass by slowing its growth, thereby producing a sloping forehead. On the other hand, the horizontal plate of the frontal bone functionally related to the orbit continues to envelop the normal soft tissue contents and grows over the globe as usual. The conspicuous protuberant supraorbital ridge is reminiscent of that seen in the gorilla (Fig 91). Enlargement of the orbital cavity is a re-

sponse to stimulation from augmented soft tissue contents, e.g., tumors and meningocele secondary to bony defect (Fig 92). A small orbit is usually associated with microphthalmos or enucleation of the eye in early childhood. A small orbit associated with exophthalmos may be present in craniosynostosis involving the periorbital sutures (Fig 93).

The mandible at birth is also relatively small, with short rami and poorly developed condyles. However, these structures steadily increase in size throughout childhood. Defective intrauterine development of the first branchial arch results in agenesis or hypoplasia of the condyles. Hypoplasia of the mandible occurs in a variety of developmental and chromosomal abnormalities as well as in systemic diseases, e.g., mandibular dysostosis, trisomy 13–15 and 17–18, cri du chat syndrome, infantile hypercalcemia, and arthrogryposis (Fig 94).

The maxilla is also small at birth. It begins to increase in size anteriorly and inferiorly concomitantly with the growth of the nasal septum. The growth of the maxilla continues in response to eruption of the maxillary teeth and enlargement of the maxillary sinus. Hypoplasia of the maxilla is not uncommon in achondroplasia and various dysplasias, e.g., mandibulofacial dysostosis (Treacher Collins syndrome), craniofacial dysostosis (Crouzon's disease), and acrocephalosyndactyly (Apert's disease) (Fig 95). It is important to remember that the width of the midface is determined by the width of the floor of the skull. The midface cannot be wider than the floor as it would have nothing with which to articulate. The proxi-

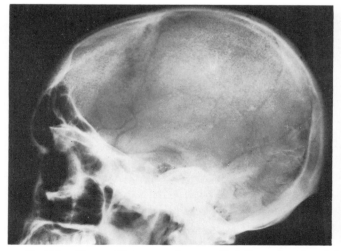
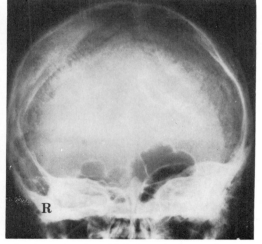

Fig 83.—Sturge-Weber syndrome with left cerebral hemiatrophy, hypertrophy of left frontal sinus, elevation of left petrous bone, and thickening of left hemicranium.

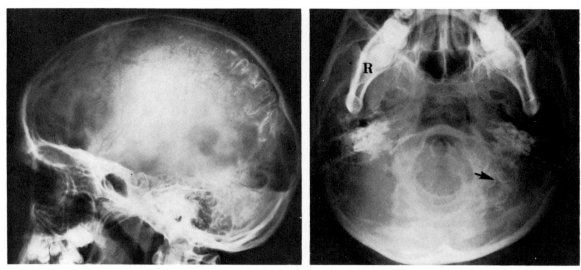

Fig 84.—Sturge-Weber syndrome with small left posterior fossa on side of calcification *(arrow)*.

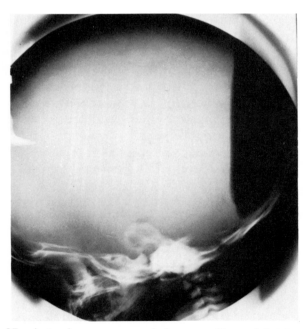

Fig 85.—Lateral pneumoencephalogram with occipital horns up. Note markedly dilated symmetric occipital horns and small posterior fossa with a low position of inion.

mal half of the nasal complex is well developed in early childhood, but the distal portion continues to grow throughout childhood.

It is worthwhile repeating that the form of the inner table is determined by the size and shape of the neural mass. On the other hand, the structure of the outer table is quite variable phylogenetically because it is biologically independent. In various thick-skulled animals, e.g., the pig, the form of the outer table has little re-

semblance to that of the inner table (Fig 96). Indeed, the outer table may have migrated so far from the inner table that the external form of the skull bears little relationship to the size of the brain. Obviously, in these circumstances, the term "brain case" is inappropriate. The outer table in such animals is responsive to other needs, i.e., the need to provide thick bony ridges for attachment of powerful trunk and masticatory muscles.

In man, with a relatively thin calvaria, the outer and inner tables tend to be more or less concordant. Hence, the shape of the outer table is similar to that of the inner table. The discordant areas in man include the frontal sinuses and mastoids; the temporal lines, where the temporal muscles attach; and the external occipital protuberance, where the neck and trunk muscles attach. Since the temporal muscles that close the jaws are facial components, they are governed by facial growth. Hence, the temporal line has an abnormally low position in hydrocephalus, while the reverse is true in microcephaly. Dwarf dogs have a craniofacial relationship and frontal sinus development similar to that in man, while large dogs exhibit craniofacial discordance (Fig 97).

The diploë has at least two functions: (1) the reduction of total bone weight by increasing the amount of trabecular bone at the expense of compact bone, and (2) hematopoiesis. The hematopoietic function does not appear to be a seminal one in the normal person. However, significant changes in the diploë are recognizable on the skull film in a variety of conditions characterized by excessive hematopoiesis, e.g., severe chronic he-

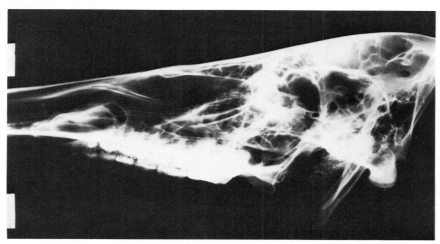

Fig 96.—Lateral radiograph of skull of pig showing exuberant frontal sinuses and wide diploë. Note discordance between cranial cavity and large facial structures. (From Shapiro, R., and Schorr, S.: *Invest. Radiol.* 15:191–202, 1980.

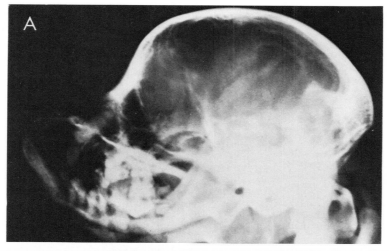

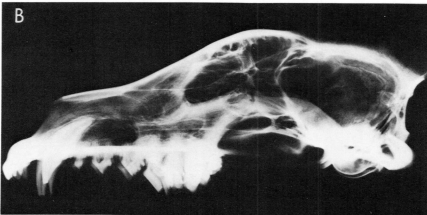

Fig 97.—Lateral radiographs of skull of a Shi-tsu dwarf-dog **(A)** and a large dog, i.e., wolf **(B).** Note concordant craniofacial relationship with small frontal sinuses similar to man in the former, and a discordant craniofacial relationship with large frontal sinuses in the latter. (From Shapiro, R., and Schorr, S.: *Invest. Radiol.* 15:191–202, 1980.

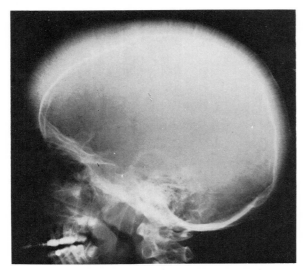

Fig 98.—Lateral radiograph of skull of 11-year-old girl with severe thalassemia major showing wide diploë as reflection of excessive hematopoiesis.

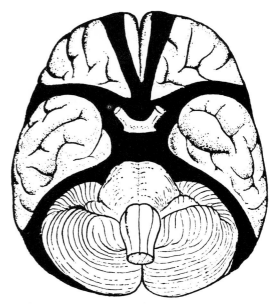

Fig 99.—Undersurface of adult human brain. Principal dural fiber tracts (black) arise from their attachments to skull base in region of the sella. Anterior, middle, and posterior tracts underlie sagittal, coronal, and lambdoidal sutural areas, respectively. (After Young and Moss.)

expands in the direction of the sagittal, lambdoidal, and squamosal sutures, resulting in a brachycephalic configuration (Fig 100). Contrariwise, premature fusion of the sagittal suture interferes with lateral enlargement of the cerebral capsule. The growing neural mass expands in the anteroposterior direction, resulting in a dolichocephalic skull (Fig 101).

In the presence of premature closure of both the transverse and the sagittal sutures, the neural mass cannot expand either in width or length. This produces an oxycephalic or turricephalic configuration because the direction of least resistance is superior. Premature fusion of the metopic suture produces trigonocephaly, narrowing of the anterior portion of the skull. Plagiocephaly is the asymmetry due to premature closure of one

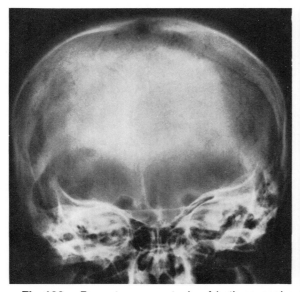
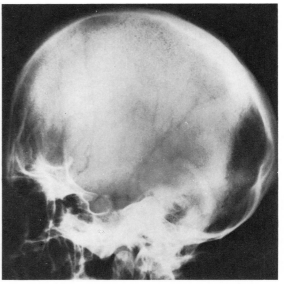

Fig 100.—Premature synostosis of both coronal sutures and sagittal suture resulting in brachycephaly (short head) and turricephaly (high head). Note also the hypertelorism.

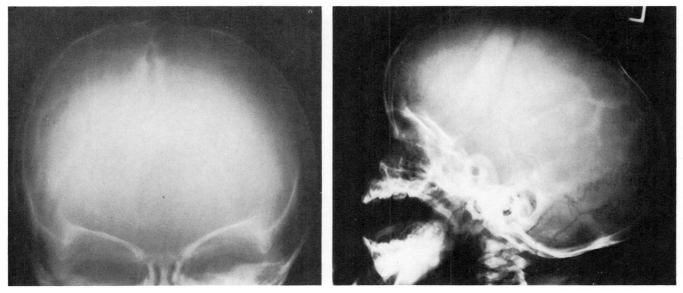

Fig 101.—Posteroanterior *(left)* and lateral *(right)* skull radiographs showing premature closure of sagittal suture producing scaphocephaly in 7-month-old infant.

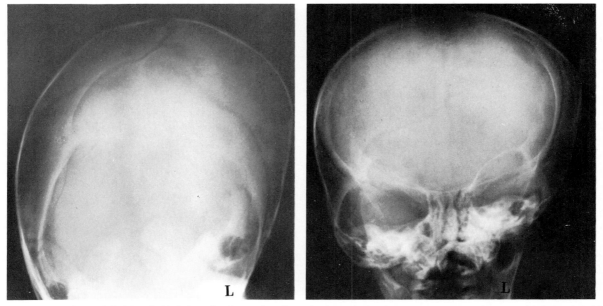

Fig 102.—Towne *(left)* and Caldwell *(right)* projections showing plagiocephaly due to premature closure of left lambdoidal suture.

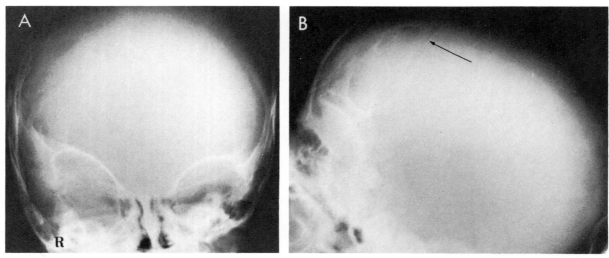

Fig 103.—Plagiocephaly due to premature synostosis of right coronal suture. Note smaller harlequin right orbit **(A)**. On the lateral view **(B)** only the left coronal suture is open *(arrow)*.

coronal or lambdoidal suture (Figs 102 and 103). The ipsilateral anterior fossa, and sometimes hemicranium, tends to be smaller. This is associated with elevation of the involved orbital roof and lesser sphenoidal wing. The degree of skull deformity varies directly with the number of sutures involved and the time of onset of the premature fusion—the earlier the synostosis, the greater the deformity.

REFERENCES

Anderson E., Kieffer S. A., Wolfson J. J., et al.: Thickening of the skull in surgically treated hydrocephalus. *Am. J. Roentgenol.* 110:96–101, 1970.

Baer M. J.: Patterns of growth of the skull as revealed by vital staining. *Hum. Biol.* 26:80–126, 1954.

Burrows E. H.: Bone changes in orbital neurofibromatosis. *Br. J. Radiol.* 36:549–561, 1963.

Campbell J. A.: Roentgen aspect of cranial configurations. *Radiol. Clin. North Am.* 4:11–31, 1966.

Capitanio M. A., Kirkpatrick J. A.: Widening of the cranial sutures. *Radiology* 92:53–59, 1969.

Childe A. E.: Localized thinning and enlargement of the cranium with special reference to the middle fossa. *Am. J. Roentgenol.* 70:1–22, 1953.

DeBeer G. R.: *The Development of the Vertebrate Skull.* London, Oxford University Press, 1937.

Dorst J. P.: Functional craniology: An aid in interpreting roentgenograms of the skull. *Radiol. Clin. North Am.* 2:347–366, 1964.

DuBoulay G.: The significance of digital impressions in children's skulls. *Acta Radiol.* 46:112–122, 1956.

Duggan C. H., Keener E., Gay B. B.: Secondary craniostenosis. *Am. J. Roentgenol.* 109:277–292, 1970.

Dyke C. G., Davidoff L. M., Masson C. B.: Cerebral hemiat-

rophy with homolateral hypertrophy of the skull and sinuses. *Surg. Gynecol. Obstet.* 58:588–600, 1933.

Faber H. K., Towne E. B.: Early operation in premature cranial synostosis for the prevention of blindness and other sequelae. *J. Pediatr.* 22:286–307, 1943.

Freeman J. M., Borkowf S.: Craniostenosis: Review of the literature and report of 34 cases. *Pediatrics* 30:57–70, 1962.

Giblin N., Alley A.: Studies in skull growth: Coronal suture fixation. *Anat. Rec.* 88:143–153, 1944.

Greene D.: Asymmetry of the head and face in infants and children. *Am. J. Dis. Child.* 41:1317–1326, 1931.

Griscom T., Oh K.: The contracting skull. *Am. J. Roentgenol.* 11:106–110, 1970.

Hardman J.: Asymmetry of the skull in relation to subdural collections of fluid. *Br. J. Radiol.* 12:455–461, 1939.

Jackson H.: Asymmetry and growth of the skull. *Br. J. Radiol.* 29:521–535, 1956.

Jupe M. H.: The reaction of the bones of the skull to intracranial lesions. *Br. J. Radiol.* 11:146–164, 1938.

Kruyff E. R.: Occipital dysplasia in infancy: The early recognition of craniovertebral abnormalities. *Radiology* 85:501–507, 1965.

Kruyff E. R., Jeffs R.: Skull abnormalities associated with Arnold-Chiari malformation. *Acta Radiol.* 5:9–24, 1966.

Lachman E.: The life history of cranial vault sutures as revealed in the roentgenogram. *Am. J. Roentgenol.* 79:721–725, 1958.

LeWald L. T.: Congenital absence of superior orbital wall associated with pulsating exophthalmos. *Am. J. Roentgenol.* 30:756–764, 1933.

Macaulay D.: Digital markings in radiographs of skull in children. *Br. J. Radiol.* 24:645–652, 1951.

Massler M., Schour I.: The growth pattern of the cranial vault in the albino rat as measured by vital staining with alizarine red "S". *Anat. Rec.* 110:83–101, 1951.

Mednick L. W., Washburn S. L.: The role of the sutures in

the growth of the brain case of the infant pig. *Am. J. Phys. Anthropol.* 14:175–192, 1956.

Momose K. J.: Developmental approach in the analysis of roentgenograms of the pediatric skull. *Radiol. Clin. North Am.* 9:99–116, 1971.

Moore A. E.: Neurofibromatosis associated with proptosis and defect of orbital wall. *Aust. N.Z. J. Surg.* 5:314–318, 1936.

Moss M. L.: Growth of the calvaria in the rat: The determination of osseous morphology. *Am. J. Anat.* 94:333–362, 1954.

Moss M. L.: Experimental alteration of sutural area morphology. *Anat. Rec.* 127:569–589, 1957.

Moss M. L.: Fusion of the frontal suture in the rat. *Am. J. Anat.* 102:141–160, 1958.

Moss M. L.: The pathogenesis of premature cranial synostosis in man. *Acta Anat.* 37:351–370, 1959.

Moss M. L., Young R. W.: A functional approach to craniology. *Am. J. Phys. Anthropol.* 18:281–292, 1960.

Neuhauser E. B. D.: The contour of the skull in the presence of increased or diminished intracranial pressure. *Assoc. Res. Neurol. Mental Dis.*, Research Public. 34:351–359, 1954.

Riesenfeld A.: The variability of the temporal lines: Its causes and effects. *Am. J. Phys. Anthropol.* 13:599–620, 1955.

Robertson E. G.: Pulsating exophthalmos due to defective development of the sphenoid bone. *Am. J. Roentgenol.* 62:44–51, 1949.

Robinson R. G.: Local bulging of the skull and external hydrocephalus due to cerebral agenesis. *Br. J. Radiol.* 31:691–700, 1958.

Rockliffe W. C., Parsons J. H.: Plexiform neuroma of orbit. *Tr. Path. Soc. London* 55:27–38, 1904.

Schwartz A., Lavy S.: Evolution of roentgenographic skull changes with unilateral loss of brain substance in children. *Neurology* 12:133–139, 1962.

Scott J. H.: The growth of the human face. *R. Soc. Med.* 47:91–100, 1954.

Scott J. H.: Dento-facial development and growth. Oxford, England, Pergamon Press, 1967.

Seaman W. B., Furlow L. T.: Anomalies of the bony orbit. *Am. J. Roentgenol.* 71:51–59, 1954.

Sear H. R.: Some notes on craniostenosis. *Br. J. Radiol.* 10:445–487, 1937.

Silverman F. N.: Premature synostosis of the cranial sutures: A review. *Ohio Med. J.* 50:131–137, 1954.

Sondheimer F. K., Grossman H., Winchester P.: Suture diastasis following rapid brain weight gain. *Arch. Neurol.* 23:314–318, 1970.

Van der Klaauw C. J.: Size and position of the functional components of the skull: A contribution to the knowledge of skull structure. *Arch. Neederl. Zool.* 7:16–37, 1946.

Watson E. H., Lowery G. H.: *Growth and Development of Children*, ed. 4. Chicago, Year Book Medical Publishers, 1962.

Weidenreich F.: The brain and its role in the phylogenetic transformation of the human skull. *Trans. Am. Philosoph. Soc.* 31:321–442, 1941.

Wheeler J. M.: Pulsation of eyeball associated with defects in wall of orbit. *Bull. Neurol. Inst. New York* 5:476–484, 1936.

Young R. W.: The influence of cranial contents on postnatal growth of the skull in the rat. *Am. J. Anat.* 105:383–410, 1959.

6

General Appearance of the Adult Skull

ASYMMETRY

The normal skull is not always perfectly symmetric (Fig 104). This slight asymmetry per se is usually not significant, in contrast to the more marked asymmetry produced by a variety of pathologic processes. Underdevelopment of a cerebral hemisphere is commonly associated with displacement of the crista galli and the groove for the superior longitudinal sinus toward the side of the lesion, elevation of the homolateral petrous pyramid, extensive pneumatization of the homolateral paranasal sinuses, and thickening of the homolateral calvaria (see Figs 82 and 83). The calvarial thickening is a compensatory mechanism for the underdeveloped cerebral hemisphere. Likewise, slow-growing brain tumors, neurofibromatosis, subdural collections in childhood, porencephaly, and the rare giant cisterna magna may produce localized thinning or bulging of the overlying calvaria (see Figs 79 to 81). The erosion usually involves the inner table but may also be associated with bulging of the diploe and outer table. The smooth margins and the benign character of the erosion indicate remodeling, which means that the underlying pathologic process has been present for a significant period. A so-called leptomeningeal cyst, resulting from a fracture associated with a dural tear, initially produces erosion of the inner table but may eventually involve all three tables. The pulsating brain and its leptomeningeal envelope herniate through the dural tear to erode the margins of the fracture.

Occasionally, an asymmetric skull may pose a problem in interpretation, even for the experienced observer. At times it may be difficult to decide whether a relatively flat hemicranium is the normal or abnormal side. The same holds true for an unusually rounded hemicranium. Under these circumstances, the following findings help point to the abnormal side: (1) thinning or thickening of the calvaria associated with diminished or

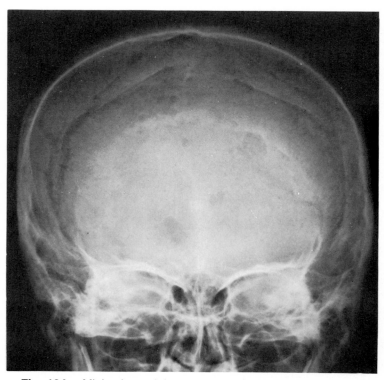

Fig 104.—Minimal cranial asymmetry (normal variant). Median sagittal plane seems bowed instead of straight. However, convolutional markings of inner table are symmetric, and diploë is also symmetric in thickness.

absent convolutional markings; (2) elevation of the lesser sphenoidal wing, orbit, and petrous pyramid, singly or in combination; and (3) abnormal sutural closure or widening.

THE TABLES

The individuality of the three tables varies considerably from person to person, as does the total thickness of the calvaria. In some skulls each table is sharply demarcated, while in others one can barely discern the outlines of the individual tables (Fig 105). The inner and outer tables are composed of compact bone; the diploë consists of cancellous bone filled with vascular spaces. The thickness of the inner and the outer tables varies only slightly. The great variability in overall thickness of the calvaria is due to substantial differences in the thickness of the diploë. In the past, it has been said that the skull of the Negro tends to be thicker and denser than that of the Caucasian. According to Mosely, this is incorrect.

The character and the thickness of the diploë greatly influence the textural appearance of the skull. Some skulls have a fairly uniform granular appearance, while others are coarsely mottled and porous (Fig 106). The areas of honeycomb-like porosity are usually most prominent in the superior parietal and, to a lesser extent, in the frontal region (Fig 107). The impression of porosity is produced by diploic vascular channels coursing at right angles to the tables of the skull. Occasionally, the outer table appears striated along the vertex in the lateral view, due to silhouetting of the sagittal suture (Fig 108).

The smooth outer table is frequently thinner along the parietal eminences. It tends to be thicker in the vertical portion of the frontal bone in persons with poorly pneumatized frontal sinuses. The inner table is normally eroded by pulsations of the brain and blood vessels. The inner table may be equal in thickness to the outer table or thinner or thicker. In any given skull, the thickness of the bones of the vault varies in different regions. The temporal squamosa and the occipital bones in the region of the occipital fossae tend to be thinner than the rest of the vault. Similar thinning may also be present in the inferolateral aspect of the frontal bone (Figs 109 and 110). Occasionally, this normal thinning may be so marked that it is mistaken for a pathologic process.

Marked symmetric bilateral thinning of the parietal bones has long been a familiar entity to anatomists. The thinned areas, which may be flat or grooved, involve the parietal eminences lateral to the sagittal suture. The thinning is primarily due to decreased thickness or actual disappearance of the outer table (Fig 111). Progression of the atrophic process results in thinning of the diploë as well. The inner table remains intact. This striking change may occur in either sex and is more common in elderly men. However, Nash and Camp reported it in approximately 10% of all patients under age 31. The posterior half of the adult parietal bone at any age may also exhibit a midline depression. This intraparietal

thinning likewise takes place at the expense of the outer table.

Steinbach and Obata suggest that symmetric biparietal thinning may be due to decreased osteoblastic activity at a site where there is little stress or strain. They call attention to the fact that the galea aponeurotica, which is not attached to the parietal bone, exerts its greatest force upon the superior parasagittal area. Interestingly, the latter is usually least affected in symmetric biparietal thinning. The preservation of the inner table is attributed to the osteoblastic activity resulting from the pulsations of the underlying brain.

In the lateral view, the biparietal thinning is visualized as an oval or quadrilateral area of decreased density. In the frontal projection, the condition can be overlooked unless the film is examined under a bright light or is underexposed (Fig 112). This interesting variant can readily be differentiated from osteoporosis circumscripta by the sharp linear demarcation from normal bone and the preservation of the diploë in osteoporosis circumscripta.

The occipital bone may seem to be thinned out and bulging on lateral skull radiographs that are slightly rotated (Fig 113). This spurious thinning should not be misinterpreted as an abnormal finding. The correct interpretation can readily be made by comparing the findings on the lateral film with those in Caldwell view and the base view. If the latter views are normal, the finding on the lateral skull film is due either to rotation or to normal slight asymmetry, which is not uncommon. Uncommonly, symmetric or asymmetric thinning and bulging of the midportion of the occipital bone may be due to congenital enlargement of the cisterna magna (Fig 114).

Rarely, in old age, especially in women, the entire calvaria may exhibit pronounced senile osteoporosis. This is particularly striking in the presence of sutural sclerosis.

HYPEROSTOSIS

Hyperostosis of the inner table is usually most prominent in the frontal bone (hyperostosis frontalis interna). However, it may involve any portion of the skull and occasionally the entire vault (hyperostosis diffusa) (Fig 115). The process is found in both sexes but is much more frequent in women over age 40. Some authors have attempted to link this condition with various clin-

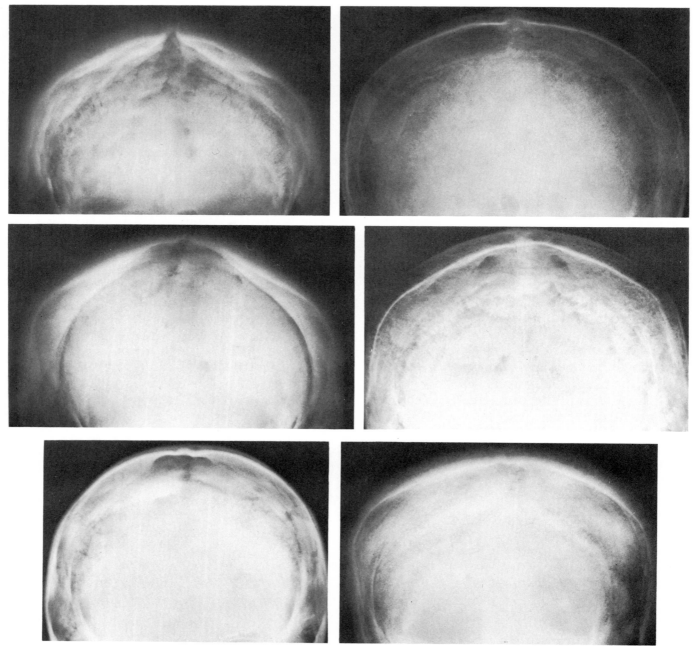

Fig 105.—Variations in thickness and identity of tables of calvaria in normal skulls. Although outer table may be thicker, inner table is usually projected on films with greater prominence. This may be due to undulating contour of inner table *(top left)*. When diploë has a fine, spongy appearance, inner and outer tables may be seen despite a wide range in thickness of bone *(top right, middle left,* and *bottom right)*. Tables are best defined in skulls with a coarse, spongy texture containing numerous vessels *(middle right)*. Many thin calvaria exhibit fusion of inner and outer tables or only scanty diploic structure *(bottom left)*. *(Continued)*

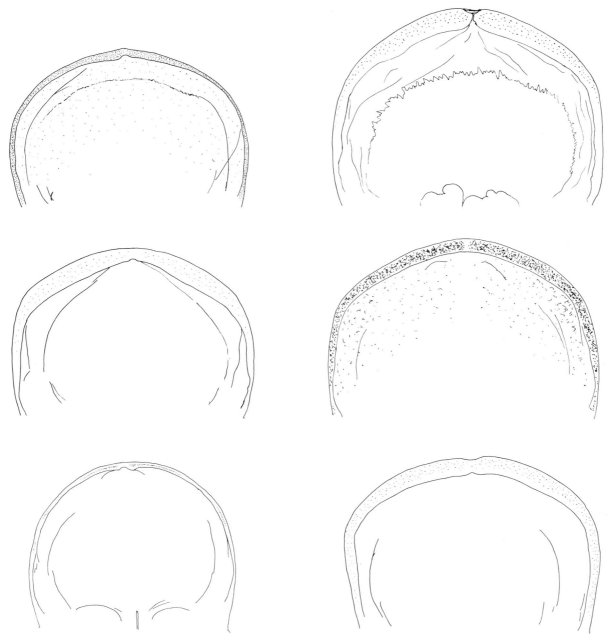

Fig 105 (cont.).—Diagrams of radiographs on facing page.

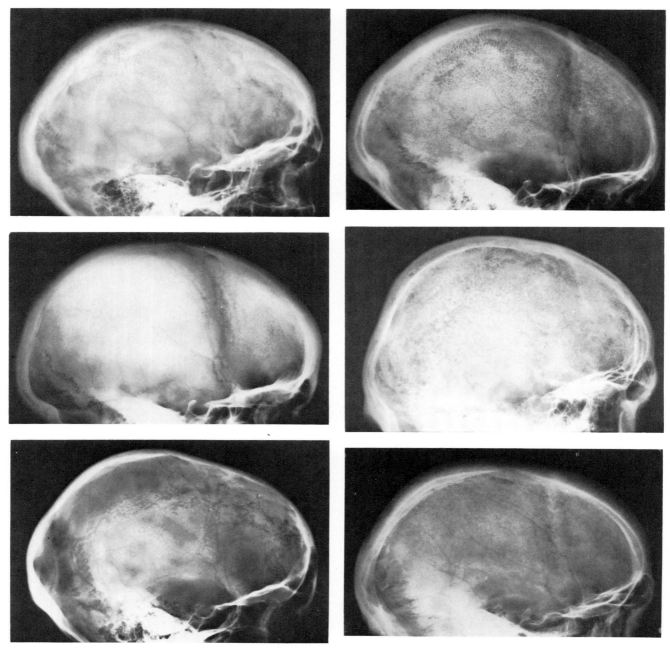

Fig 106.—Variation in appearance of texture and vascular architecture of diploë in normal skulls. *(Continued)*

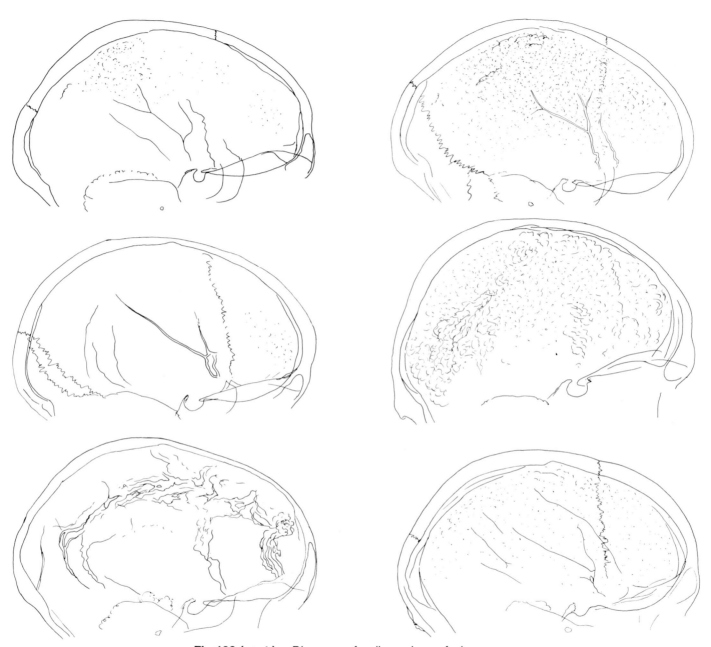

Fig 106 (cont.).—Diagrams of radiographs on facing page.

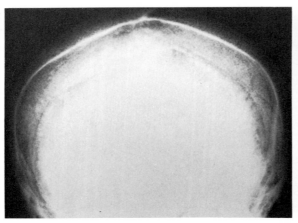 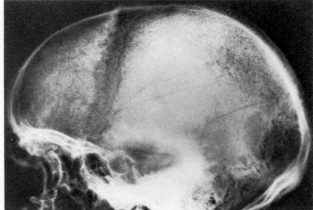

Fig 107.—Normal skull with thick diploë presenting porous granular appearance in lateral projection.

ical findings (the so-called Morgagni-Stewart-Morel-Moore syndrome, consisting of frontal hyperostosis, headache, obesity, hypertension, and vague endocrine disorders). In my experience, hyperostosis of the inner table commonly occurs as an isolated finding without any clinical significance.

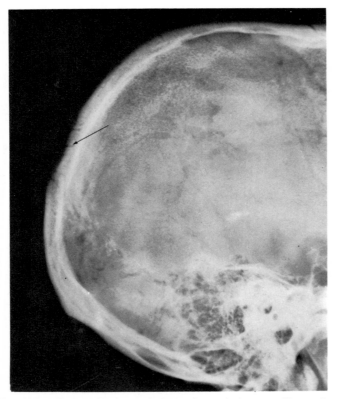

Fig 108.—Perpendicular striations *(arrow)* due to silhouetting of sagittal suture along outer table. This is produced by serrated external surface of the suture.

Roentgenologically, hyperostosis interna manifests itself by irregular, dense, osseous excrescences projecting from the inner table. The hyperostosis may be nodular, flat, or appear as a broad sheet. It frequently has a scalloped appearance, symmetrically distributed on both sides of, but not reaching, the midline. This bilateral symmetric undercutting of the thickened inner table by pulsating venous channels draining into the superior sagittal sinus is typical of the condition (Figs 116 to 118). These characteristics serve to differentiate this benign form of hyperostosis from the hyperostosis produced by a bilateral frontal meningioma. In the latter instance, the bony sclerosis crosses the midline, and there is no undercutting of the thickened inner table.

Unilateral or bilateral focal bony thickening in the region of the pterion is a common normal finding. A diagnosis of meningioma should not be entertained on the basis of the unilateral variant unless there are other convincing roentgenographic or clinical changes of meningioma. Occasionally, a small single hyperostosis is noted on the inner table of the temporal bone, most commonly in the squamosa anterior to the petrous pyramid (Fig 119). This normal finding can be difficult to distinguish from a small meningioma en plaque. The identification of prominent vascular grooves directed toward such a localized hyperostosis is helpful in establishing a diagnosis of meningioma. Frontal projections that are slightly rotated may result in one sphenoidal wing appearing denser than its mate. A similar spurious thinning of one sphenoidal wing may also be produced by rotation. These changes should generally be disregarded in the absence of any other findings. An effort should be made to get perfectly centered stereoscopic

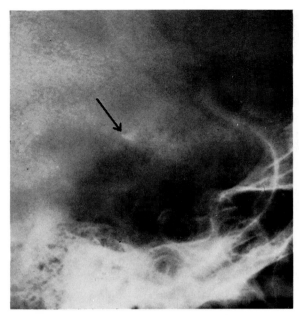

Fig 119.—Solitary enostosis of temporal bone. Patient was referred for suspected calcifying intracranial neoplasm. Stereoscopy readily showed that sharp spicule of bone arose from inner table.

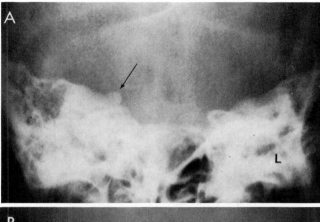

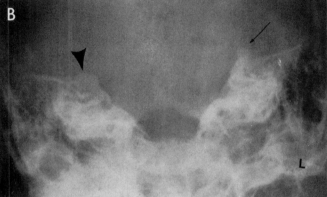

Fig 121.—Towne projection **(A)** showing rounded bony knob on superior aspect of right petrous ridge *(arrow)* in 32-year-old asymptomatic woman. (From Shapiro, R.: *Radiology* 128:354, 1978.) **B,** asymmetric bilateral bony excrescences on petrous ridge. On the right, knob is relatively flat *(arrowhead);* left knob is larger and more rounded *(arrow).*

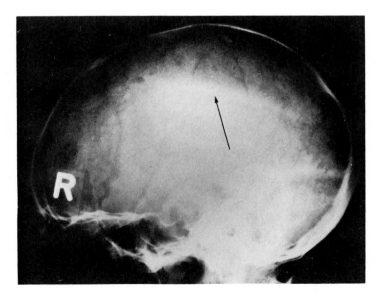

Fig 120.—Prominent temporal line for attachment of temporalis muscle and fascia muscle *(arrow).*

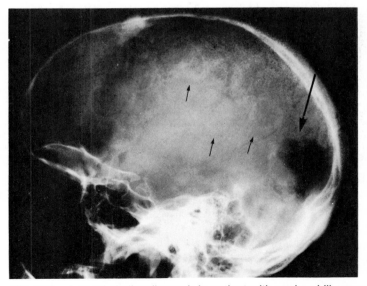

Fig 122.—Lateral skull radiograph in patient with eosinophilic granuloma *(large arrow).* Note multiple annular shadows with dense rim *(small arrows)* due to radiopaque hair dressing.

facts which mimic intracranial calcification are pigtails, radiopaque hair dressings (Fig 122), and the opaque paste used in electroencephalography to fasten the electrodes to the scalp.

REFERENCES

Arendt J.: Bone rarefaction after skull injuries. *Radiology* 45:608–613, 1945.

Bull J. W. D.: Diagnosis of chronic subdural haematomata in children and adolescents. *Br. J. Radiol.* 22:68–80, 1949.

Burrows E. H.: Bone changes in orbital neurofibromatosis. *Br. J. Radiol.* 36:549–561, 1963.

Camp J. D., Nash L. A.: Developmental thinness of the parietal bones. *Radiology* 42:42–47, 1944.

Childe A. E.: Localized thinning and enlargement of the cranium. *Am. J. Roentgenol.* 70:1–22, 1954.

Davidoff L. M., Dyke C. G.: Relapsing juvenile subdural hematoma. *Bull. Neurol. Inst. New York* 7:95–111, 1938.

Davidoff L. M., Gass H.: Convolutional markings in the skull roentgenograms of patients with headache. *Am. J. Roentgenol.* 61:317–323, 1949.

Denstad T.: Hyperostosis cranii. *Acta Radiol.* 28:129–138, 1947.

Dyke C. G., Davidoff L. M., Masson C. B.: Cerebral hemiatrophy with homolateral hypertrophy of the skull and sinuses. *Surg. Gynecol. Obstet.* 58:588–600, 1933.

Eckstein H. B., Chir M., Hoare R. D.: Congenital parietal "foramina" associated with faulty ossification of the clavicles. *Br. J. Radiol.* 36:220–221, 1963.

Epstein B. S.: The concurrence of parietal thinness with postmenopausal, senile, or idiopathic osteoporosis. *Radiology* 60:29–35, 1953.

Ethier R.: Skull vault: Thickness and texture, in Newton T. H., Potts D. G. (eds.): *The Skull.* Book 1: *Radiology of the Skull and Brain,* vol. 1. St. Louis, C. V. Mosby Co., 1971.

Greig D. M.: On symmetrical thinness of parietal bones. *Edinburgh Med. J.* 33:645–671, 1926.

Hardman J.: Asymmetry of the skull in relation to subdural collections of fluid. *Br. J. Radiol.* 12:455–461, 1939.

Hare H. F.: Roentgen changes in vault accompanying diseases resulting from metabolic disturbances. *Radiology* 36:706–711, 1941.

Jackson H.: Asymmetry and growth of the skull. *Br. J. Radiol.* 29:521–535, 1956.

Jupe M. H.: The reaction of the bones of the skull to intracranial lesions. *Br. J. Radiol.* 11:146–164, 1938.

Just N. W. M., Goldenberg M.: Computed tomography of the enlarged cisterna magna. *Radiology* 131:385–391, 1979.

Kasabach H. H., Dyke C. G.: Osteoporosis circumscripta of the skull as a form of osteitis deformans. *Am. J. Roentgenol.* 28:192–203, 1932.

McRae D. L.: Focal epilepsy: Correlation of the pathological and radiological findings. *Radiology* 50:439–457, 1948.

Moore M. T.: Morgagni-Stewart-Morel syndrome. *Arch. Intern. Med.* 73:7–12, 1944.

Moore S.: Hyperostosis cranii. Springfield, Ill., Charles C Thomas, Publisher, 1955.

Moore S.: Hyperostosis frontalis interna. *Surg. Gynecol. Obstet.* 61:345–362, 1935.

Moore S.: Metabolic craniopathy. *Am. J. Roentgenol.* 35:30–39, 1936.

Moore S.: Acromegaly and contrasting conditions: Notes on roentgenography of the skull. *Am. J. Roentgenol.* 68:565–569, 1952.

Pedersen J.: Hyperostosis cranialis interna: Morgagni and Stewart-Morel syndrome. *Arch. Med. Scandinav.* 128:71–102, 1947.

Pendergrass E. P., Perryman C. P.: Porencephaly. *Am. J. Roentgenol.* 56:441–463, 1946.

Pendergrass E. P., Schaeffer, J. P., Hodes, P. J.: *The Head and Neck in Roentgen Diagnosis,* ed. 2. Springfield, Ill., Charles C Thomas, Publisher, 1956.

Penfield W.: Cranial clues to intracranial abnormality. *Am. J. Roentgenol.* 67:535–550, 1952.

Salmi A., Voutilainen A., Holsti L. R., et al.: Hyperostosis cranii in a normal population. *Am. J. Roentgenol.* 87:1032–1040, 1962.

Schwartz C. W.: The normal skull from a roentgenologic viewpoint. *Am. J. Roentgenol.* 39:22–42, 1938.

Schwartz C. W.: Anomalies and variations in the normal skull. *Am. J. Roentgenol.* 42:367–373, 1939.

Schwartz, C. W.: Pitfalls to be avoided in the roentgen diagnosis of intracranial disease. *Radiology* 42:34–41, 1944.

Smith S., Hemphill R. C.: Hyperostosis frontalis interna. *J. Neurol. Neurosurg. Psychiatry* 19:42–45, 1956.

Steinbach H. L., Obata, W. G.: The significance of thinning of the parietal bones. *Am. J. Roentgenol.* 78:39–45, 1957.

Stenhouse D.: Plain radiography of the skull in the diagnosis of intracranial tumors. *Br. J. Radiol.* 21:287–300, 1948.

Taveras J. M., Wood E. H.: *Diagnostic Neuroradiology,* ed. 2. Baltimore, Williams & Wilkins Co., 1976.

Wilson A. K.: Roentgenological findings in bilateral symmetrical thinness of the parietal bones (senile atrophy). *Am. J. Roentgenol.* 51:685–695, 1944.

7

Anatomy of the Adult Skull

There is a good deal of confusion about the meaning of the terms "skull," "cranium," and "calvaria." "Skull" and "cranium" are often used synonymously to denote the skeleton of the head exclusive of the mandible. Originally, however, "cranion" (Gr. *kranos*, helmet) referred to that part of the head covered with hair. Similarly, "calvaria" or "calvarium" (L. *calvus*, hairless, smooth) meant skullcap or top of the skull.

In spite of these original meanings, some anthropologists have made the following arbitrary distinctions: skull—the entire skeleton of the head and face including the mandible; cranium—the skull exclusive of the mandible; calvaria—the skull exclusive of the facial bones. However, the Basle nomenclature uses the terms "skull" and "cranium" interchangeably to refer to the entire skeleton of the head. In this system, the maxillae, palatine bones, zygomatic bones, mandible, and hyoid bone constitute the facial bones, and "cranial bones" include all the others. The cranium is further subdivided into the cerebral cranium (facial, ethmoid, sphenoid, occipital, vomer, and the paired nasals, lacrimals, and inferior turbinates) and the visceral cranium (mandible, maxillae, zygomatics, and palatines). These divisions are artificial and not universally accepted. For practical purposes in this text, the skull is divided into (1) the calvaria, or cranium, encasing the brain, consisting of eight bones (frontal, ethmoid, sphenoid, occipital, and the paired parietal and temporal bones); and (2) the 14 facial bones (the paired nasals, lacrimals, maxillae, zygomatics, palatines and inferior nasal conchae (inferior turbinates), and the unpaired vomer and mandible).

ANATOMY OF THE BONES

Frontal Bone

The frontal bone consists of a vertical portion (frontal plate or squama) and a horizontal (orbital) portion that forms the roofs of the orbits and part of the roof of the nasal cavity (Figs 123 to 125). The frontal plate articulates with both parietal bones along the coronal sutures and with the greater sphenoidal wings along the sphenofrontal sutures. Inferiorly, the frontal plate ends in the supraorbital arch, which continues laterally as the zygomatic process to articulate with the zygomatic bone. Medially, the supraorbital arch ends in the internal angular process that articulates with the lacrimal bone and the frontal process of the maxilla. The supraorbital foramen, or notch, pierces the inner third of the arch. Between the internal angular processes, the nasal notch of the frontal bone articulates with the nasal bones and the frontal process of the maxilla. The frontal (nasal) spine projects down from the center of the nasal notch.

The anterior outer surface of the frontal plate is usually smooth and convex, but the bosses may vary considerably, particularly in children. Occasionally, the frontal bosses are asymmetric, and the halves of the frontal bone appear to lie at different levels on the lateral roentgenogram. The concave cerebral surface has convolutional markings for the frontal lobes, depressions for the pacchionian bodies, and vascular grooves (Fig 124). The edges of the groove for the superior sagittal sinus unite inferiorly to form a ridge (frontal crest) to which the falx cerebri is attached. This ridge ends in the foramen caecum. The cribriform plate of the ethmoid that fits into the ethmoidal notch separates both orbital plates inferiorly. Posteriorly, the orbital plates articulate with the greater sphenoidal wings.

The frontal sinuses are located between the two tables of the frontal plate on either side of the midline. They may extend superiorly, laterally, and posteriorly to a varying degree.

The vertical portion of the frontal bone is seen to best advantage on the straight posteroanterior roentgenogram. The orbital portion, however, is better demonstrated in the lateral and Caldwell projections.

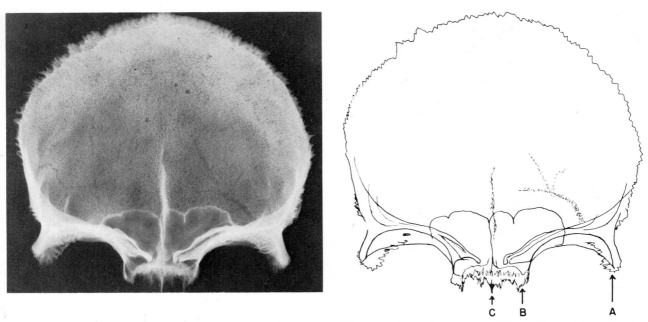

Fig 123.—Radiograph of frontal bone. Note the zygomatic process *(A)*, internal angular process *(B)*, and frontal (nasal) spine *(C)*.

Ethmoid Bone

The ethmoid is a small, irregular, cuboid bone consisting of a median portion and the two lateral labyrinths (Figs 126 to 129). Lying between the orbits, the ethmoid contributes to the formation of the floor of the anterior cranial fossa and to the nasal and orbital walls.

The median portion consists of the vertical perpendic-

ular plate and the horizontal cribriform plate that fills the ethmoidal notch of the frontal bone. The cribriform plate is perforated by many foramina that transmit the branches of the olfactory nerves. Projecting up from its anterior surface in the midline is the crista galli. The perpendicular plate is a thin, flat bone that hangs down from the inferior surface of the cribriform plate to form the upper part of the bony nasal septum. It is attached

Fig 124.—Photograph of internal aspect of frontal bone. Note pacchionian depressions *(arrowheads)* and vascular grooves *(arrow)*.

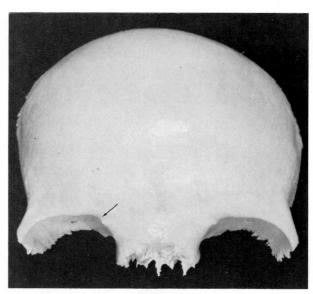

Fig 125.—Photograph of external aspect of frontal bone. This specimen does not have a supraorbital foramen but shows a broad supraorbital notch *(arrow)*.

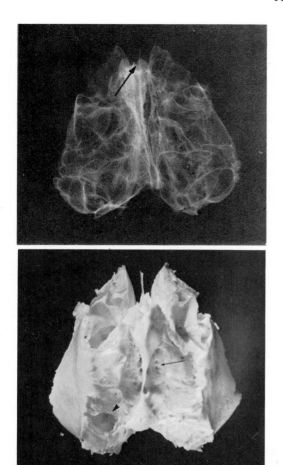

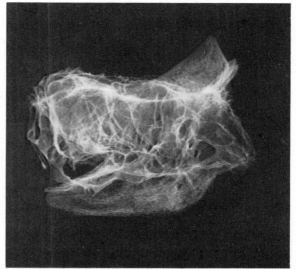

Fig 126.—Radiograph *(top)* and photograph *(bottom)* of ethmoid bone in vertical projection from its orbital surface. Anterior end of perpendicular plate is seen at top of photograph. Openings in cribriform plate *(arrow)* are more clearly visible in photograph than in radiograph. A left posterior ethmoid cell is unroofed *(arrowhead)*.

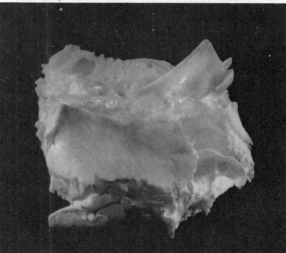

Fig 128.—Radiograph *(top)* and photograph *(bottom)* of ethmoid bone in lateral projection. Photograph is obliqued slightly to show more of superior aspect.

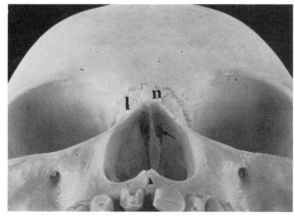

Fig 127.—Photograph of skull showing external surface of cribriform plate of ethmoid *(arrow)*. Note also the nasal bone *(n)*, lachrymal bone *(l)*, and nasal process of maxilla *(arrowhead)*.

to the frontal spine anterosuperiorly, to the cribriform plate at its upper border, to the sphenoidal crest posteriorly, and to the vomer and cartilaginous nasal septum inferiorly.

The paired lateral masses (ethmoidal labyrinths), which contain the ethmoidal cells, hang down from the lateral margin of the cribriform plate. The lateral wall of the ethmoidal labyrinth (lamina papyracea) forms part of the medial wall of the orbit, while the medial wall of the labyrinth forms the greater part of the lateral wall of the nasal cavity. Projecting down from the medial wall of each ethmoidal labyrinth are the scroll-shaped superior and middle turbinate bones.

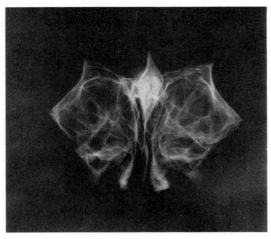

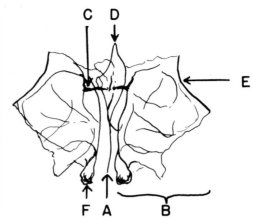

Fig 129.—Posteroanterior view of ethmoid. This is view commonly seen in Caldwell projection of paranasal sinuses. Note the perpendicular plate *(A)*, lateral mass of ethmoidal labyrinth *(B)*, cribriform plate *(C)* and crista galli *(D)*, which are seen with varying clarity, depending partly on size of crista galli. Also shown are lamina papyracea *(E)* and middle turbinate *(F)*.

The ethmoidal labyrinths are rather poorly seen in the posteroanterior projection, owing to superimposition. They are well demonstrated in the submentovertical, lateral, and optic foramen views. The cribriform plate can be visualized in the lateral roentgenograms as the most inferior depression of the floor of the anterior fossa just behind the crista galli.

Parietal Bones

The parietal bones are paired quadrilateral bones with a concave cerebral surface and a convex outer surface. The outer surface is crossed by the temporal ridge about a third or more of the way up. In the posteroanterior projection, the squamosal suture should not be mis-

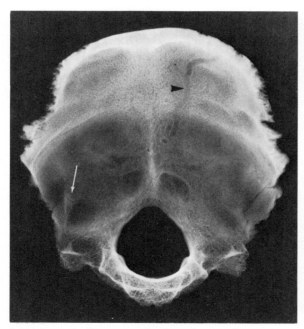

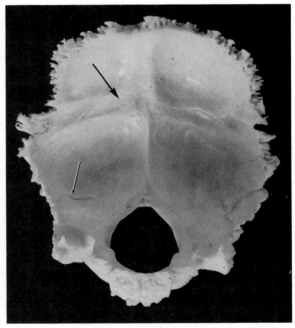

Fig 130.—Occipital bone in Towne projection. A vascular groove *(arrowhead)* is visible on the radiograph *(left)*. Radiograph and photograph also show remnant of suture between exoccipital and su- praoccipital centers *(small arrow)*. Confluence of sinuses is seen in photograph *(large arrow)*.

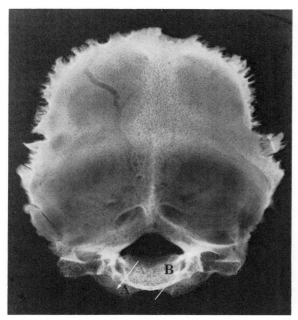 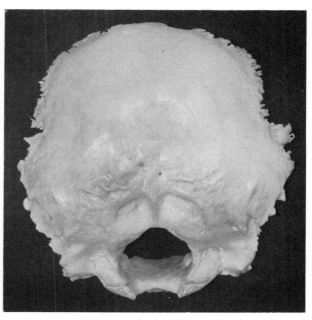

Fig 131.—Radiograph *(left)* and photograph *(right)* of occipital bone. This corresponds to anteroposterior view with angulation of 20 degrees rather than conventional 30 to 35 degrees. Note the occipital condyle *(A)* and hypoglossal canal *(B)*.

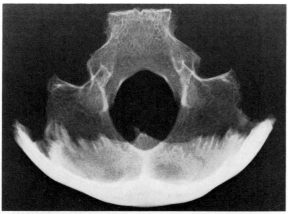 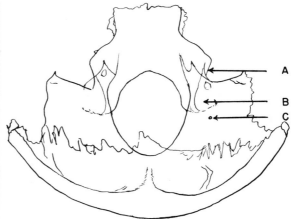

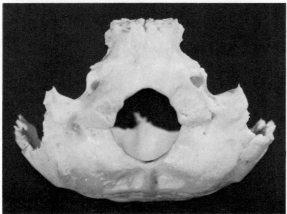

Fig 132.—Radiograph *(top)* and photograph *(bottom)* of inferior aspect of the occipital bone. Jugular notch; *(A)* occipital condyle; *(B)* posterior condyloid canal *(C)*.

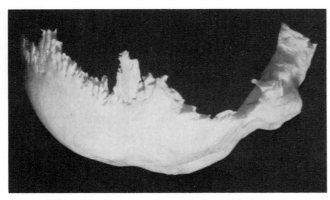

Fig 133.—Photograph of occipital bone in lateral view.

taken for a linear fracture of the parietal bone. The concave cerebral surface exhibits digital markings, pacchionian depressions, and grooves for the meningeal vessels and the sagittal and lateral sinuses.

The parietal bones articulate with each other in the midline along the sagittal suture. They also articulate with the frontal bone at the coronal suture, with the occipital bone at the lambdoidal suture, and with the greater sphenoidal wings and the temporal bones at the sphenoparietal, squamosal, and parietomastoid sutures. The parietal bones are best studied on the lateral roentgenogram.

Occipital Bone

The occipital bone forms the back and the posterior half of the base of the skull (Figs 130 and 131). It consists of four parts that surround the foramen magnum:

(1) the basiocciput, (2) and (3) the lateral portions, and (4) the squamous portion.

Following obliteration of the spheno-occipital synchondrosis, the basilar portion of the occipital bone fuses anteriorly with the body of the sphenoid. The roughened external surface presents the pharyngeal tubercle in the midline for insertion of the tendinous raphe and superior constrictor of the pharynx (Fig 132). The concave, smooth cerebral surface forms the posterior half of the clivus, the lateral border of which is grooved by the inferior petrosal sinus (Fig 132).

The lateral portions fuse with the basiocciput anteriorly and with the squamous portion posteriorly. The occipital condyles, which articulate with the superior facets of the atlas, are located on the inferior surface of the lateral portions (Fig 133). The hypoglossal canal (anterior condyloid canal) for the 12th cranial nerve is located at the base of the condyles. A small posterior condyloid canal for an emissary vein is frequently also present behind the condyles. The sides of the condylar portions form the jugular process that contains the jugular notch. This notch and a corresponding notch on the temporal bone form the jugular foramen that transmits the internal jugular vein, the 9th, 10th, and 11th cranial nerves, and the meningeal branches of the ascending pharyngeal and occipital arteries. The jugular process is grooved by the sigmoid sinus as it passes out of the foramen.

The large squamous portion, which forms the posterior part of the base and vault of the skull, articulates with the mastoid portion of the temporal bone at the

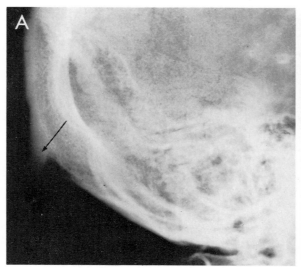

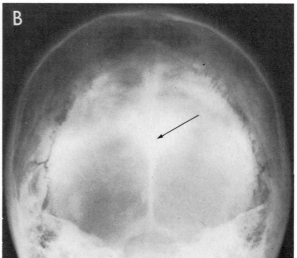

Fig 134.—External occipital protuberance *(arrow)*. **A,** lateral view. **B,** Towne view (different case).

occipitomastoid suture and with the parietal bone at the lambdoidal suture. Midway between its summit and the foramen magnum is the prominent external occipital protuberance (Fig 134). The internal occipital protuberance occupies a corresponding position on the cerebral surface. The internal surface of the squama is divided into four fossae, which are separated by bony ridges and grooves for the transverse, occipital, and sagittal sinuses. The confluence of the sinuses is known as the torcular Herophili. The upper two fossae receive the occipital lobes, while the lower two accommodate the cerebellar hemispheres.

The occipital bone is best studied in the Towne projection. The condyloid canals and jugular foramina cannot always be seen on a single projection. It may be necessary to take multiple films in the anteroposterior position with varying degrees of angulation in order to visualize all of these structures.

Sphenoid Bone

The wedge-shaped sphenoid bone lies between the horizontal portion of the frontal bone and the basiocciput at the base of the skull. It forms a large part of the middle fossa and also contributes to the lateral portion of the skull. It consists of a body, paired greater and lesser wings, and two pterygoid processes on either side (Figs 135 to 139).

The sphenoidal body, which contains the sphenoidal sinuses, forms the center of the middle cranial fossa. The sphenoidal sinuses are usually divided asymmetrically by a septum that presents as the sphenoidal crest

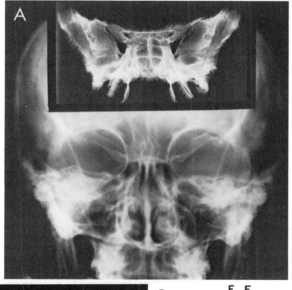

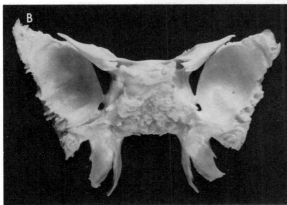

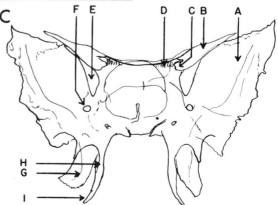

Fig 135.—A, radiograph of skull in Caldwell projection with insert of isolated sphenoid bone in same projection. **B,** photograph, and **C,** line drawing of sphenoid bone in Caldwell projection. Diagram shows the greater *(A)* and lesser *(B)* wings, anterior clinoid process *(C),* dorsum sellae at base of posterior clinoid process *(D),* sphenoidal fissure *(E),* foramen rotundum *(F),* lateral *(G)* and medial *(H)* pterygoid plates, and hamular process *(I).*

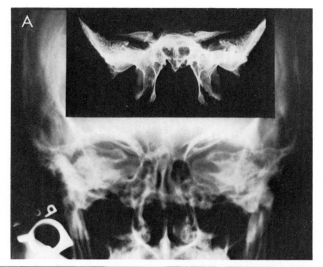

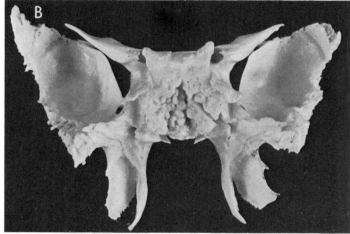

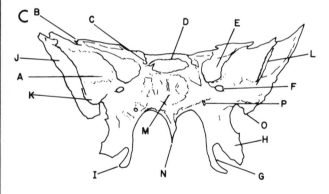

Fig 136.—A, straight posteroanterior projection of skull with insert of isolated sphenoid bone in same projection. **B,** photograph and **C,** line drawing of sphenoid bone in same projection showing spheno-maxillary surface *(K)*, squamozygomatic surface *(L)*, sphenoid sinus *(M)*, rostrum *(N)*, spine *(O)*, and vidian canal *(P)*.

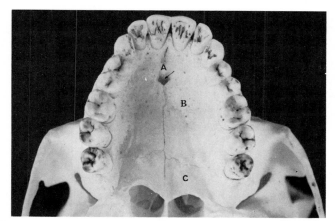

Fig 149.—Photograph of palatine bone and maxilla. Note incisive foramen *(A)*, maxilla *(B)*, and palatine bone *(C)*.

moid and the nasal cartilage. The nasal bones can be visualized in the lateral, Waters, and axial views (Fig 148).

Lacrimal Bones

The lacrimal bones are small, thin, flat bones on the medial wall of the orbits between the frontal process of the maxilla and the lamina papyracea of the ethmoid. They can be identified in the Caldwell view and in detailed films of the orbits.

Inferior Nasal Conchae

The inferior nasal conchae (inferior turbinates) are thin, scroll-like bones attached laterally to the conchal crests of the maxillae and palatine bones at the level of the lower third of the nasal cavity bilaterally. They articulate with the uncinate process of the ethmoid bone anterior to the opening of the maxillary sinus. The inferior turbinates are readily seen in the various posteroanterior projections and in the lateral view.

Palatine Bones

The flat palatine bones are located between the maxillae and the pterygoid processes of the sphenoid bone (Fig 149). Each consists of two plates arranged at right angles to each other: (1) the horizontal portion and (2) the vertical portion. The horizontal portions of both bones form the posterior part of the hard palate and articulate with the palatine process of the maxilla along the transverse palatine suture, thereby forming part of

the floor of the nose and the roof of the mouth. Their posterior free border is attached to the soft palate. The vertical portion covers the posterior part of the nasal surface of the maxilla, partially closing the opening of the maxillary sinus. Its inner surface lies in the lateral wall of the nasal cavity, while the outer surface is in the floor of the pterygopalatine fossa. The sphenopalatine foramen, which transmits vessels and nerves from this fossa to the nasal cavity, is found in its upper portion.

The Vomer

The vomer is a thin, flat plate of bone that forms the inferoposterior portion of the bony nasal septum. Its anterior border articulates with the cartilaginous nasal septum, its upper border with the perpendicular plate of the ethmoid, and its lower border with the nasal crest of the maxilla and the palatine bones. The vomer can be identified on submentovertical and lateral projections.

Zygomatic Bones

The zygomatic or malar bones form the prominence of the cheeks and part of the outer border and wall of the orbits. They articulate with the zygomatic processes of the frontal bone above, with the zygomatic processes of the temporal bones behind, with the maxillae anteriorly, and also with the zygomatic border of the greater sphenoidal wings.

The Maxillae

The paired maxillae containing the maxillary sinuses unite to form the upper jaw. They form the greater part

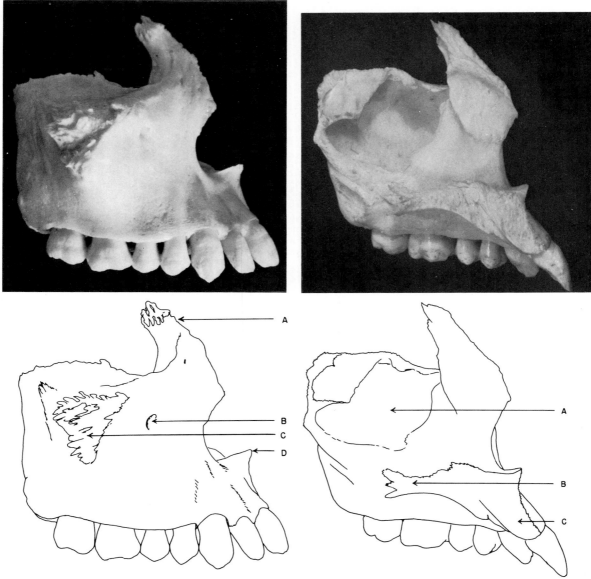

Fig 150.—Photograph of external surface of the maxilla *(left)* showing frontal process *(A)*, infraorbital foramen *(B)*, zygomatic process *(C)*, and anterior nasal spine *(D)*. Photograph of internal surface of the maxilla *(right)* showing maxillary antrum *(A)*, palatine process *(B)*, and alveolar process *(C)*.

of the skeleton of the upper face, part of the lateral walls and floor of the nasal cavity, the greater portion of the floor of the orbits, and part of the roof of the mouth. Each maxilla consists of a pyramidal hollow body and four processes: zygomatic, frontal, alveolar, and palatine (Fig 150).

The body of the maxilla has four main surfaces. The anterior facial surface contains the infraorbital foramen, just below the lower margin of the orbit, and the canine and incisive fossae, overlying the roots of the canine

and incisor teeth, respectively. The zygomatic process separates the anterior surface from the posterior surface, which is directed toward the infratemporal and pterygopalatine fossae. The orbital surface forms the floor of the orbit and is traversed by the infraorbital groove and foramen. The nasal surface forms part of the lateral wall of the nasal cavity.

The zygomatic process, which projects laterally between the anterior and posterior surfaces, supports the zygomatic bone. The frontal process projects up from

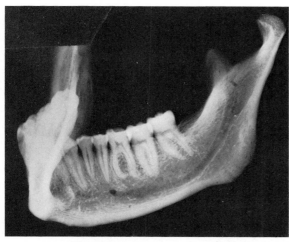 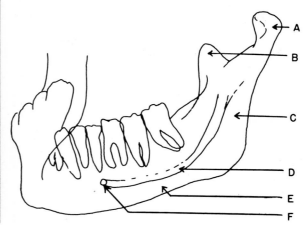

Fig 151.—Oblique radiograph of mandible showing condyle *(A)*, coronoid process *(B)*, ramus *(C)*, mandibular canal *(D)*, body of mandible *(E)*, and mental foramen *(F)*.

the upper anterior portion of the body, forming the inner margin of the orbit and part of the lateral wall of the nose. The alveolar process containing the sockets for the teeth of the upper jaw projects down from the inferior part of the body. The palatine process projects horizontally from the lower part of the medial surface to form the anterior two thirds of the hard palate; its smooth upper surface lies in the floor of the nasal cavity, while its lower surface forms the roof of the mouth. At the two ends of its medial border are the nasal crest and anterior nasal spine, which support the nasal septum.

The Mandible

The mandible forms the lower part of the face and the chin. It consists of two halves strongly fused in the midline at the symphysis. Each half has a ramus and a body, joined at an angle that varies with age and dentition. Thus, in the newborn skull, the ramus joins the body at an oblique angle, which only gradually becomes a right angle with age. The term "angle of the jaw," however, is applied to the prominence formed by the junction of the lower border of the body with the caudal margin of the ramus.

Each ramus ends above in two processes: the coronoid process in front and the condyloid process behind, separated by the sigmoid notch. The inner surface of the ramus presents the inferior dental (mandibular) foramen, from which the mylohyoid groove continues downward and forward to the body. The outer surface of the body presents the midline mandibular protuber-

ance, on either side of which is the mental foramen, the anterior opening of the mandibular canal that traverses the bone (Fig 151). Occasionally, there may be a bony spur (torus mandibularis) in the region of the canine and premolar teeth along the inner surface of the mandible at the anterior border of the mylohyoid ridge. This is best seen on an occlusal film as a small projection of bone on the lingual aspect of the mandible. The external oblique line is a smooth ridge coursing upward and backward from the body to become continuous with the front edge of the coronoid process.

ANATOMY OF THE SKULL IN THE CONVENTIONAL RADIOGRAPHIC PROJECTIONS

Lateral View

The lateral roentgenogram (Fig 152) provides a sweeping panorama of the cranial and facial bones. When viewed stereoscopically, it gives the viewer the impression of looking at a semitransparent globe with the various structures in true perspective. The contour, thickness, and texture of the various cranial bones, including the sella turcica, are clearly demonstrable. The facial bones can also be studied either by increased illumination or by underexposure. Large portions of the frontal and parietal bones and lesser portions of the sphenoidal, temporal, and occipital bones are demonstrated in this view. Localized normal thinning of the temporal squama, the inferior frontal, and inferior occipital regions is commonly seen.

The floor of the skull in this projection may be di-

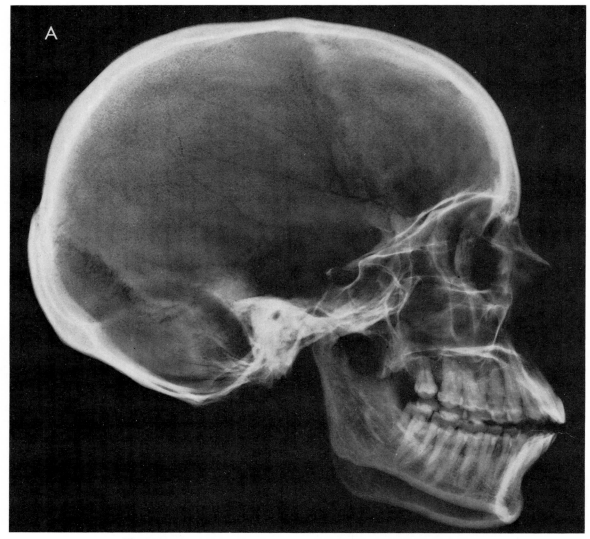

Fig 152.—Lateral projection (**A** and **B**) of adult skull. *(Continued)*

1 alveolar ridge of maxilla	13 coronal suture
2 anterior clinoid process	14 coronoid process of mandible
3 anterior border of pterygoid process	15 cribriform plate of ethmoid
4 anterior margin of frontal process of zygoma	16 dorsum sellae
5 anterior nasal spine	17 ethmoid air cells
6 anterior aspect of middle cranial fossa	18 floor of maxillary sinus
7 anterior wall of maxillary sinus	19 floor of sella turcica
8 anterior margin of foramen magnum	20 hard palate
9 body of zygoma	21 internal auditory canal
10 cerebral surface of orbital roof	22 lambdoidal suture
11 clivus	23 lateral portion of orbital floor
12 confluence of sinuses	24 lateral sinus

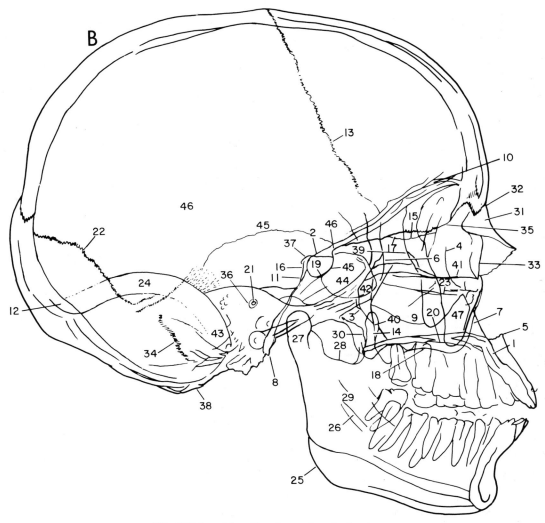

Fig 152 (cont.).—See legend on facing page.

25	mandibular angle	37	posterior clinoid process
26	mandibular canal	38	posterior margin of foramen magnum
27	mandibular condyle	39	posterior margin of frontal process of zygoma
28	mandibular notch	40	posterior wall of maxillary sinus
29	mandibular ramus	41	roof of maxillary sinus (medial portion of orbital floor)
30	medial pterygoid plate	42	pterygopalatine fossa
31	nasal bone	43	sigmoid sinus
32	nasofrontal suture	44	sphenoid sinus
33	nasomaxillary suture	45	squamosal suture
34	occipitomastoid suture	46	tuberculum sellae
35	orbital surface of orbital roof	47	zygomatic recess of maxillary sinus
36	external auditory canal		

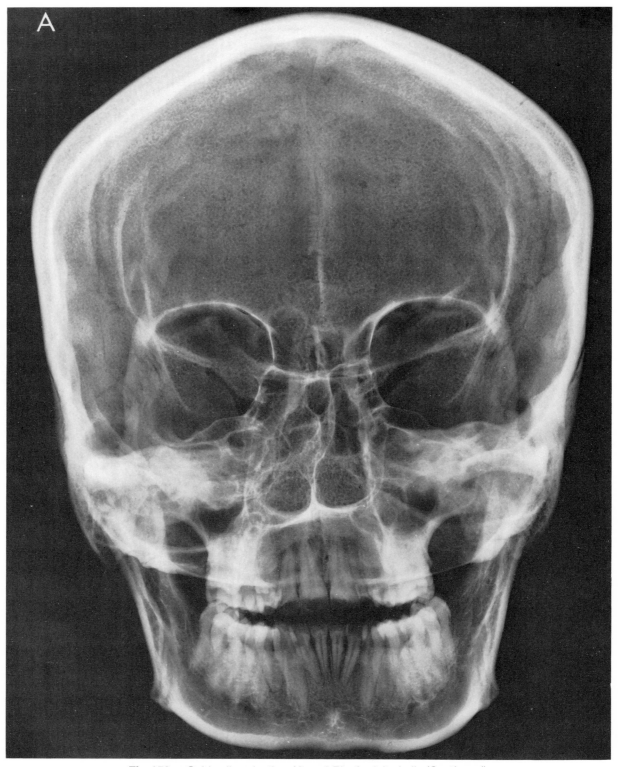

Fig 153.—Caldwell projection (**A** and **B**) of adult skull. *(Continued)*

1 alveolar ridge of maxilla
2 anterior portion of lamina papyracea
3 anterior portion of orbital floor
4 body of zygoma
5 crista galli

6 ethmoid air cells
7 ethmomaxillary plate
8 floor of sella turcica
9 foramen rotundum

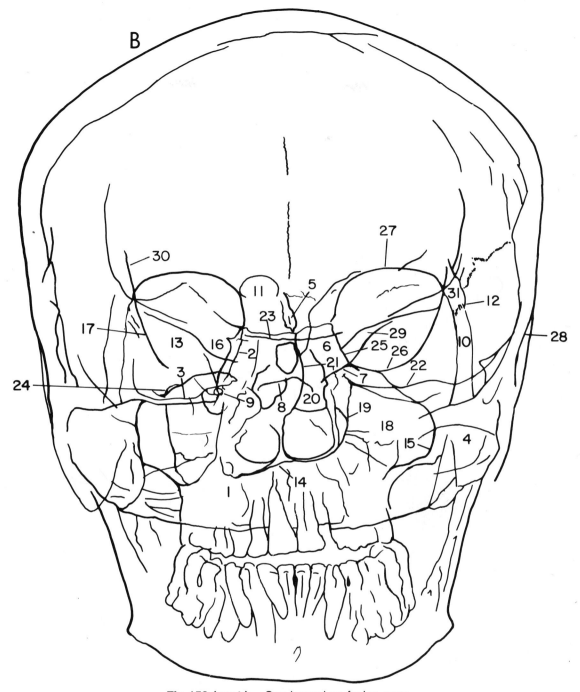

Fig 153 (cont.).—See legend on facing page.

vided into the anterior, middle, and posterior cranial fossae. The anterior fossa is bounded inferiorly by the orbital plate of the frontal bone, anteriorly by the vertical portion of the frontal bone, and posteriorly by the free margin of the sphenoidal wing. The deeper middle fossa contains the sella turcica, limited anteriorly by the tuberculum sellae and posteriorly by the dorsum sellae. The posterior clinoids may be seen at the superior angles of the dorsum sellae. The middle fossa is limited anteriorly by the sphenoidal wings and posteriorly by the petrous portions of the temporal bones and the dorsum sellae. The deep posterior fossa comprises the clivus and the occipital, temporal, and parietal bones. It is demarcated from the middle fossa by the dorsum sellae and petrous portions of the temporal bones. The petrous portion of the temporal bone is seen as a dense, white opacity anterior to the mastoid.

The lateral sinus can be visualized as a curved, wide radiolucent groove leading forward to the mastoid. The mastoid emissary vein is often seen in relationship to the sigmoid sinus. The external auditory meatus presents as a small radiolucent circle superimposed on the upper portion of the petrous bone. Frequently, the helix of the external ear casts a curvilinear shadow that is readily apparent. Air trapped within the folds of the external ear may produce a radiolucency that can be confused with the fourth ventricle during pneumoencephalography.

The following sutures are seen: (1) the coronal suture separating the frontal and parietal bones, often thin and nonserrated below the temporal line, simulating a fracture; (2) the lambdoidal suture between the parietal and occipital bones; (3) the zygomaticofrontal suture uniting the zygoma with the zygomatic process of the frontal bone; (4) the zygomaticotemporal suture between the zygomatic process of the temporal bone and the temporal process of the zygomatic bone; (5) the various sutures surrounding the greater sphenoidal wing, namely, the sphenozygomatic in front, the sphenofrontal and sphenoparietal above, and the sphenosquamosal behind; (6) the squamosal suture connecting the temporal squama with the lower border of the parietal bone (the squamosal suture continues behind into the parietomastoid suture between the mastoid process of the temporal bone and the posterior inferior margin of the parietal bone); and (7) the occipitomastoid suture between the occipital bone and the mastoid portion of the temporal bone. Not uncommonly seen is a narrow

cleft paralleling the clivus separating the basisphenoid from the petrous apex.

When the sutures of both sides of the skull are not perfectly superimposed upon each other, one suture may be projected anteriorly or posteriorly, superiorly or inferiorly to its mate of the opposite side. The suture closest to the film may be recognized by its relative sharpness and clarity.

Seen also in this projection are the zygomatic arch, the temporomandibular joint, the external auditory meatus, the various paranasal sinuses, the posterior nasopharynx, and the pterygopalatine fossa.

Caldwell Posteroanterior View

The Caldwell view (Fig 153) demonstrates the frontal bone and the orbits to excellent advantage. Because the petrous pyramids are projected onto the floor of the orbits, the sphenoidal fissures and the greater and lesser sphenoidal wings are clearly visualized. The lesser sphenoidal wing presents as a curvilinear bony ridge traversing the upper part of each orbit, extending superiorly and laterally beyond the lateral orbital wall. Crossing the outer third of the orbit is an oblique vertical white line, the linea innominata, produced by the projected cross section of the squamozygomatic surface of the sphenoid bone. The crista galli, which may be pneumatized to a varying degree, projects upward like an arrowhead from the superior end of the nasal septum. Seen also are the nose, the mandible, and the following sutures: nasofrontal, zygomaticofrontal, squamosal, and coronal, as well as some of the sutures of the orbit.

The orbits are rounded, symmetric cavities enclosed by four walls. The roof is formed by the orbital plate of the frontal bone and the lesser sphenoidal wing. The floor is formed by the maxilla, the palatine bone, and part of the zygoma. The medial wall is formed by the frontal, lacrimal, and ethmoidal bones and the body of the sphenoid. The lamina papyracea of the ethmoid bone, which comprises most of the medial orbital wall, is represented by two lines. The more medial line, representing the anteromedial margin of the orbit, is produced by the lacrimal bone and the anterior portion of the lamina papyracea. The line just lateral to it represents the posteromedial orbital margin, which is formed by the posterior portion of the lamina papyracea (Figs 154 and 155). The lateral wall is formed by the zygoma and the frontal bone anteriorly and by the greater

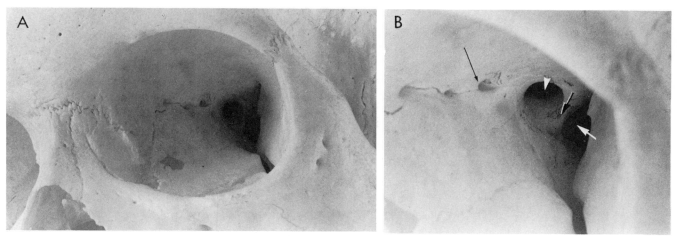

Fig 154.—Conventional **(A)** and close-up **(B)** photographs of left orbit of adult skull specimen; optic foramen *(arrowhead);* superior or-bital fissure *(thick white arrow);* optic strut *(thick black arrow);* ethmoidal foramen *(thin black arrow).*

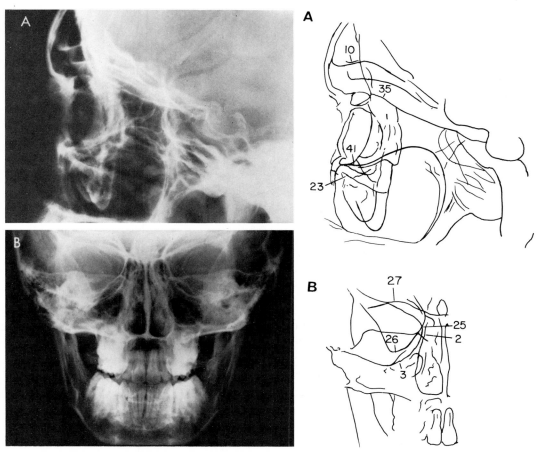

Fig 155.—Lateral **(A)** and Caldwell **(B)** projections showing details of orbital anatomy.

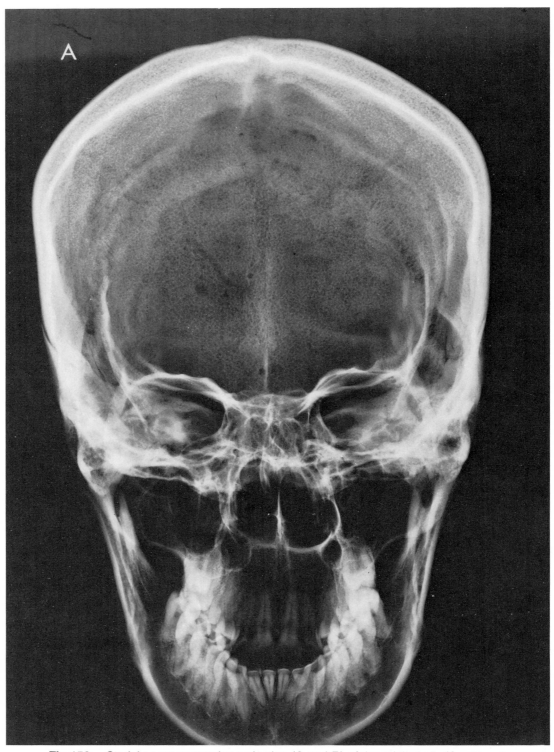

Fig 156.—Straight posteroanterior projection (**A** and **B**) of the adult skull. *(Continued)*

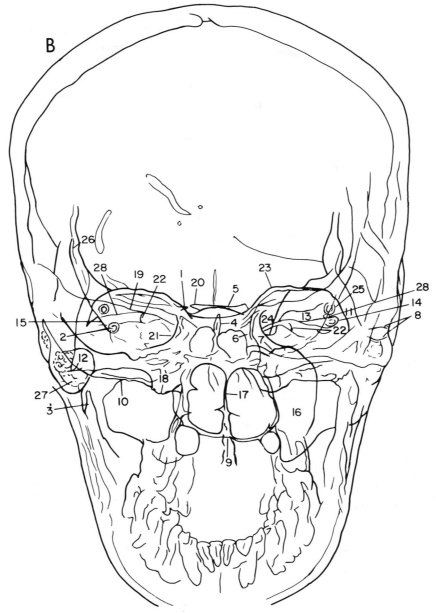

Fig 156 (cont.).—See legend on facing page.

1 anterior clinoid process	15 linea innominata
2 cochlea	16 maxillary sinus
3 coronoid process of mandible	17 nasal septum
4 crista galli	18 occipital condyle
5 dorsum sellae	19 petrous bone
6 ethmoid and sphenoid air cells	20 posterior clinoid process
7 ethmomaxillary plate	21 posterior portion of lamina papyracea
8 external auditory canal	22 posterior wall of internal auditory canal
9 floor of nasal fossa (hard palate)	23 roof of orbit
10 floor of posterior cranial fossa	24 superior orbital fissure
11 frontal process of zygoma	25 superior semicircular canal
12 head of mandibular condyle	26 temporal line of frontal bone
13 internal auditory canal	27 tip of mastoid process
14 lateral semicircular canal	28 vestibule

sphenoidal wing posteriorly. The following sutures are found along the orbital margins: zygomaticofrontal, laterally; frontomaxillary, medially; and zygomaticomaxillary, inferiorly. The anterior cranial fossa lies above the orbit and the maxillary sinus below it.

A crescentic radiolucent line resulting from air trapped in the upper eyelid is occasionally seen in the Caldwell or Waters projection. The trapped air may be located either in the conjunctival sac or between the skin folds of the open eyelid. This normal finding, which is accentuated in the presence of palpebral edema, should not be confused with air introduced into the orbital tissues as a result of trauma. The latter produces a more irregular shadow and is rarely confined to a crescent in the upper portion of the orbit (Fig 156).

Straight Posteroanterior View

The straight posteroanterior view is the best projection for studying the ear. In this projection (Fig 157), the petrous pyramids are projected onto the orbits. Within the inner and middle thirds of each petrous pyramid, the internal auditory canal can be seen as a horizontal, narrow radiolucent band. At the medial end of the canal is the internal auditory meatus. Laterally, the petrous ridges merge imperceptibly with the squamous and mastoid portions of the temporal bone. Also, the structures of the internal ear, especially the superior and lateral semicircular canals, the cochlea, and the vestibule, can be identified.

The frontal bone, the frontal and sphenoidal sinuses, and the anterior clinoid processes can also be seen. The coronal, sagittal, lambdoidal, and squamosal sutures are also visible in this projection.

Towne Anteroposterior View

The Towne view (Fig 158) demonstrates the occipital bone and the posterior part of the foramen magnum to best advantage. Frequently, the posterior arch of the atlas may be seen through the foramen magnum. In the newborn skull there is a normal cleft in this arch that usually disappears by the end of the second year. Occasionally, this cleft persists into adult life and should not be mistaken for a fracture. In addition, the triangular spinous process of C-2 and the dens can often be defined, superimposed on the sphenoidal sinus. The dorsum sellae is also commonly visible near the ventral margin of the foramen magnum. Likewise, the anterior

clinoid processes can be identified overlying the lateral margins of the foramen magnum.

The petrous pyramids extend outward from the anterior aspect of the foramen magnum. The internal auditory canal, the arcuate eminence, the tegmen tympani, and the superior semicircular canal are readily visualized, as well as the mastoid portion of the temporal bone and the posterior condyloid canals. Also recognized clearly are the lambdoidal, occipitomastoid, and parietomastoid sutures, the internal occipital protuberance and the cruciate ridge, as well as the grooves for the transverse dural sinuses.

Occasionally, the hair, particularly when braided or heavily oiled, casts a striking adventitious shadow that may be confusing (Fig 159,A). Other shadows cast by various superficial lesions and artifacts should not be confused with intracranial disease.

Base View

The roentgenogram of the base of the skull (Fig 160) demonstrates the maxillary teeth and the mandible anteriorly. On either side of the upper teeth are the maxillary sinuses. Superimposed on the middle of the upper teeth, crossing the symphysis of the mandible, is the nasal septum. Just behind the symphysis of the mandible is a dense line extending laterally from the nasal septum, which represents the posterior margin of the horizontal portion of the palatine bone. Occasionally, one can recognize the posterior palatine foramen anterior to the outer margin of this line. On either side of the nasal septum are the superimposed shadows of the nasal cavities, the turbinate bones, and the ethmoidal sinuses. Extending back from the posterior edge of the hard palate is the vomer. Superimposed on the vomer and posterior nares are the sphenoidal sinuses, on either side of which lie the medial and lateral pterygoid plates. The pterygoid fossa lies between the pterygoid plates. Occasionally, an oval-shaped, midline density representing the uvula is noted superimposed upon the clivus (Fig 161, top). Occasionally, a midline radiopacity may be seen at any age in the region of the hard palate, caused by a localized crest of the palatine bone along the median palatine suture. This bony elevation (torus palatinus) may increase in size until age 30 to 40, at which time growth ceases (Fig 161, bottom).

The base view is the projection par excellence for demonstrating the foramina of the middle fossa. Just behind and lateral to the pterygoid fossa is the foramen

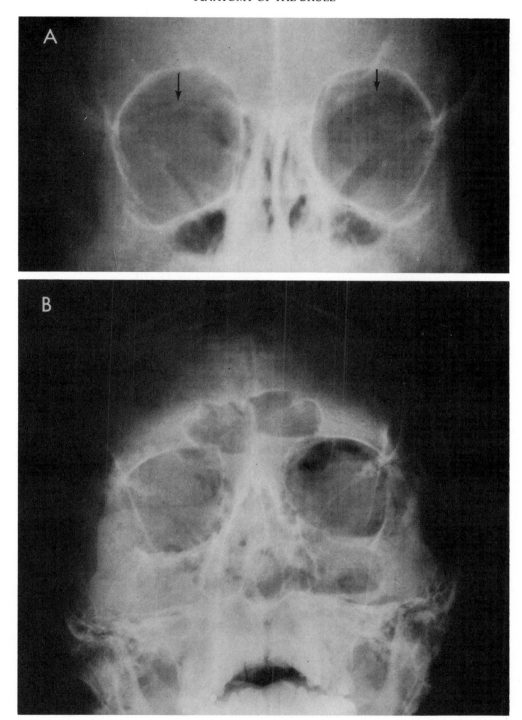

Fig 157.—**A,** *arrows* point to radiolucencies representing air trapped in the conjunctival sacs. **B,** bilateral orbital emphysema in a patient with severe facial trauma who suffered triple Le Fort fractures.

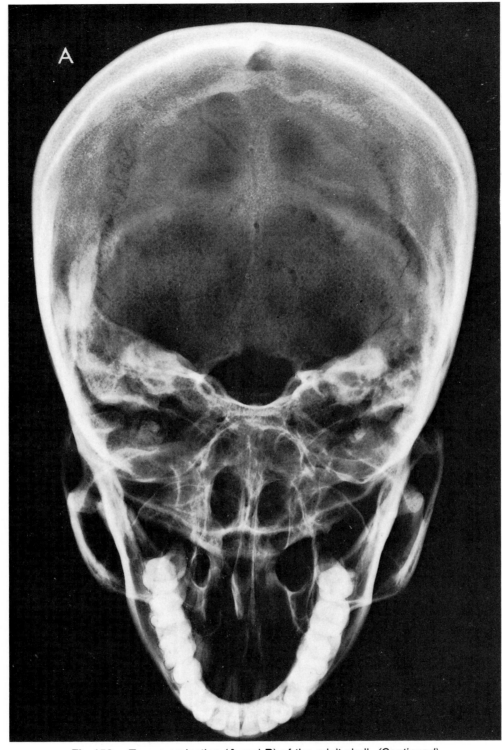

Fig 158.—Towne projection (**A** and **B**) of the adult skull. *(Continued)*

1	anterior clinoid process	7	foramen magnum
2	arcuate eminence	8	inferior orbital fissure
3	cochlea	9	infratemporal tubercle of greater sphenoidal wing
4	coronoid process of mandible	10	internal auditory canal
5	dorsum sellae	11	junction of roof and posterolateral wall of maxillary sinus
6	floor of middle cranial fossa	12	lateral semicircular canal

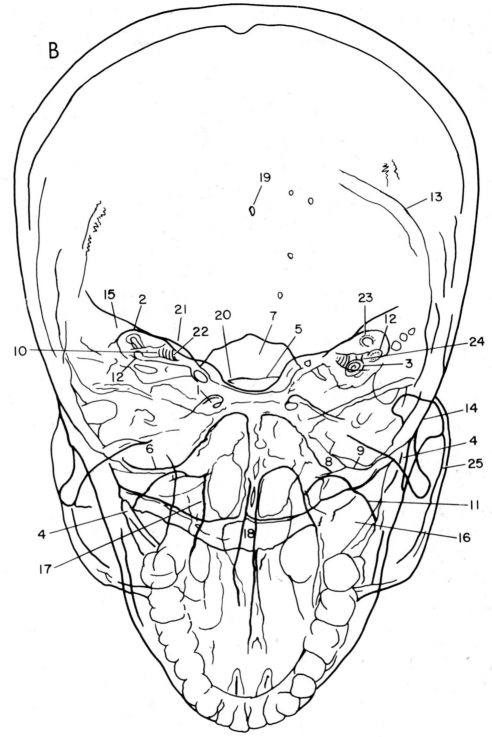

Fig 158 (cont.).—See legend on facing page.

13 lateral sinus	20 posterior clinoid process
14 mandibular condyle	21 posterior surface of petrous pyramid
15 mastoid antrum	22 posterior wall of internal auditory canal
16 maxillary sinus	23 superior semicircular canal
17 medial wall of maxillary sinus (lateral wall of nasal fossa)	24 vestibule
18 nasal septum	25 zygomatic arch
19 occipital foramen	

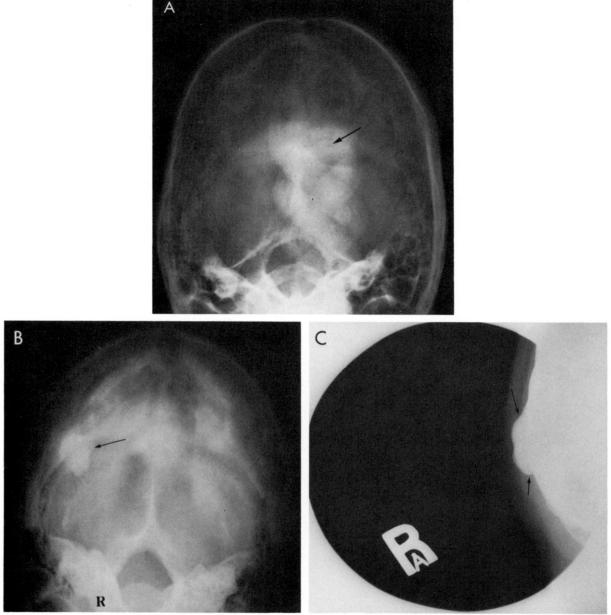

Fig 159.—**A,** adventitious density produced by hair braid *(arrow).* **B and C,** Towne **(B)** and tangential **(C)** projections clearly demonstrating an osteoma arising from the outer table of the right occipital bone *(arrows).* The superficial location can be recognized by tangential or stereoscopic films or by tomography.

ovale. Behind and lateral to the foramen ovale is the foramen spinosum. The foramen lacerum lies medial and slightly posterior to the foramen ovale at the anterior aspect of the apex of the petrous bone. The mastoid and petrous portions of each temporal bone, the internal auditory canal, the carotid canal, the jugular foramen, and the sigmoid sinus can all be visualized in this projection with varying degrees of clarity.

The temporal fossa lies behind the maxillary sinus, lateral to the posterior part of the body of the mandible. Superimposed on the temporal fossa is the curved, linear density of the lesser sphenoidal wing marking the boundary between the anterior and middle cranial fossae. Occasionally, the squamosphenoidal suture may be seen in the middle of the temporal fossa. Occasionally also, the sagittal suture is noted in the midline passing back from the region of the sphenoidal sinuses. Similarly, the irregular coronal suture is frequently noted superimposed on the structures of the base of the skull. These should not be mistaken for fracture lines. The zygomatic arches are demonstrable by increased illumination.

Just behind the clivus in the midline is the foramen magnum, which is usually partially obscured by the anterior arch of the atlas and the dens. The lateral masses of the atlas articulate with, and are superimposed upon, the occipital condyles. The transverse process of each lateral mass contains the foramen transversarium for the vertebral artery. To either side of the cervical spine, behind the petrous and mastoid portions of the temporal bones, are the posterior cranial fossae. The lambdoidal suture, the sigmoid and lateral sinuses, and the internal occipital protuberance can also be recognized in this region.

Waters View

The Waters posteroanterior projection (Fig 162) is the view par excellence for study of the orbital floor, the maxillary sinuses, and the facial bones. In the properly positioned radiograph, the petrous pyramid is projected below the floor of the maxillary sinus. The floor of the orbit is represented by two parallel lines transversely oriented. The superior line is the palpable anterior rim, while the inferior line corresponds to the floor of the orbit somewhat more posterior (1 cm) to the rim.

Optic Foramen View

In this view (Fig 163), the optic foramen is projected into the outer quadrant of the orbit. Inferior and lateral to the optic foramen is the superior orbital fissure. The roof of the optic foramen is formed by the superior root of the lesser sphenoidal wing, while the medial wall is formed by the sphenoidal sinus. Lateral to the optic foramen the lesser sphenoidal wing terminates in the anterior clinoid process. This projection is also useful to study the ethmoidal air cells.

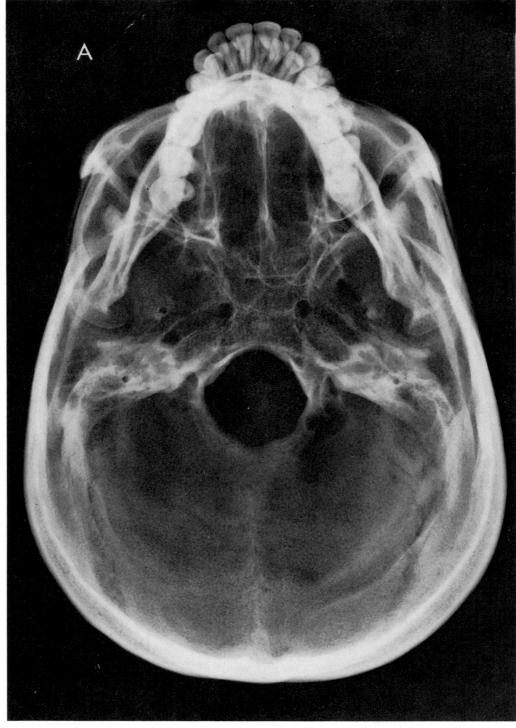

Fig 160.—Submentovertical projection (**A** and **B**) of the adult skull. *(Continued)*

1	anterior wall of middle cranial fossa	*7*	eustachian tube
2	body of zygoma	*8*	external auditory canal
3	carotid canal	*9*	foramen lacerum
4	clivus	*10*	foramen magnum
5	coronoid process of mandible	*11*	foramen ovale
6	ethmoid air cells and nasal fossa	*12*	foramen spinosum

118

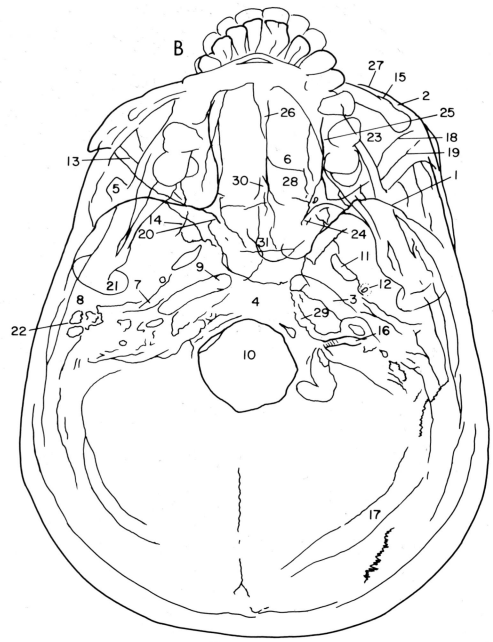

Fig 160 (cont.).—See legend on facing page.

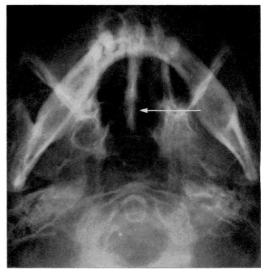

Fig 161.—Base view *(top)* showing contour of uvula projected onto air space of pharynx *(arrow)*. Base view *(bottom)* showing a torus palatinus *(arrow)*.

REFERENCES

Gregg H.: The linea innominata. *Radiology* 55:274–276, 1950.

Etter L. E.: *Atlas of Roentgen Anatomy of the Skull.* Springfield, Ill., Charles C Thomas, Publisher, 1955.

Etter L. E.: Detailed roentgen anatomy of orbits. *Radiology* 59:489–503, 1952.

Etter L. E.: New method for roentgen anatomical study. *Am. J. Roentgenol.* 53:394–402, 1949.

Goldhamer K.: Normale anatomie des Kopfes im Roentgenbild. Leipzig, Thieme, 1931, vols. 1 and 2.

Kieffer S. A.: Orbit, in Newton T. H., Potts D. G. (eds.): *The Skull.* Book 2: *Radiology of the Skull and Brain,* vol. 1. St. Louis, C. V. Mosby Co., 1971.

Kieffer S. A.: Superior orbital fissure, ibid.

Pendergrass E. P., Schaeffer J. P., Hodes P. J.: *The Head and Neck in Roentgen Diagnosis,* ed. 2. Springfield, Ill., Charles C Thomas, Publisher, 1956.

Potter G. D., Trokel S. L.: Optic canal, in Newton T. H., Potts D. G. (eds.): *The Skull.* Book 2: *Radiology of the Skull and Brain,* vol. 1. St. Louis, C. V. Mosby Co., 1971.

Psenner L.: Die anatomischen varianten des Hirnschädels. *Fortschr. Geb. Röntgenstrahlen* 75:197–214, 1951.

Wigh R.: Air cells in great wing of sphenoid bone. *Am. J. Roentgenol.* 65:916–923, 1951.

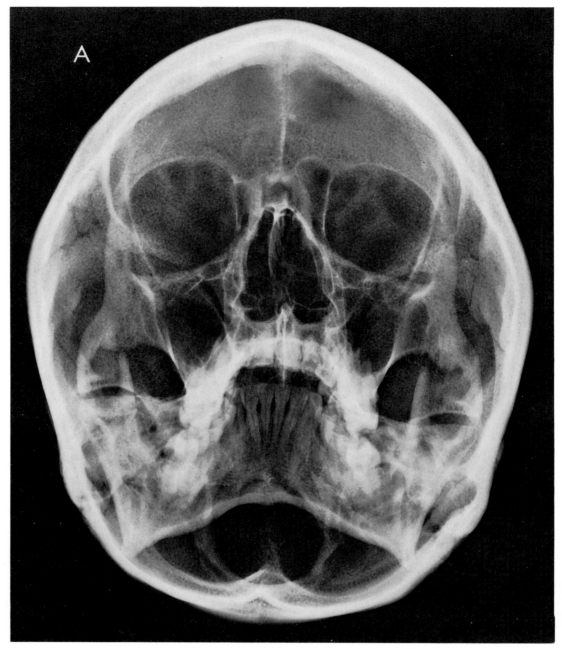

Fig 162.—Waters projection (**A** and **B**) of the adult skull. *(Continued)*

1	anterior ethmoid cells	
2	anterior rim of orbital floor	
3	anterior portion of lamina papyracea	
4	anterior portion of orbital roof	
5	body of zygoma	

6	coronoid process of mandible
7	ethmomaxillary plate
8	floor of orbit posterior to the anterior rim
9	foramen rotundum

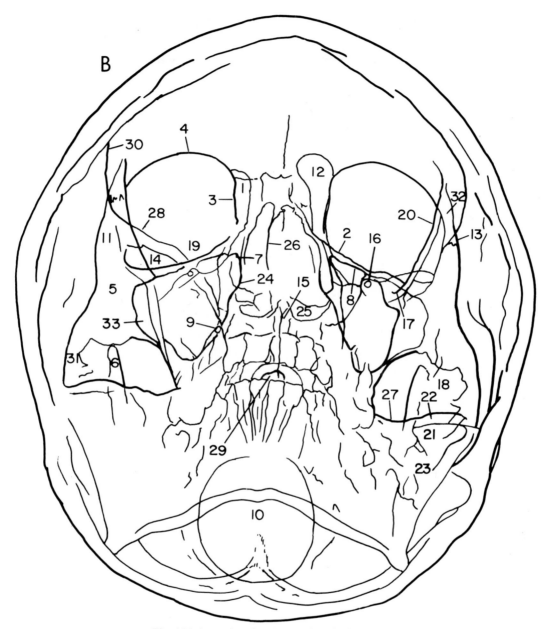

Fig 162 (cont.).—See legend on facing page.

10	foramen magnum	22	mandibular (glenoid) fossa
11	frontal process of zygoma	23	mandibular neck
12	frontal sinus	24	medial wall of maxillary sinus
13	frontozygomatic suture	25	nasal fossa
14	greater sphenoidal wing	26	nasal septum
15	hard palate	27	petrous ridge
16	infraorbital foramen	28	sphenoid ridge (most posterior portion of orbital roof)
17	infraorbital extension of linea innominata	29	sphenoid sinus
18	infraorbital fossa	30	temporal line of frontal bone
19	lesser sphenoidal wing	31	zygomatic arch
20	linea innominata	32	zygomatic process of frontal bone
21	mandibular canal	33	zygomatic recess of maxillary sinus

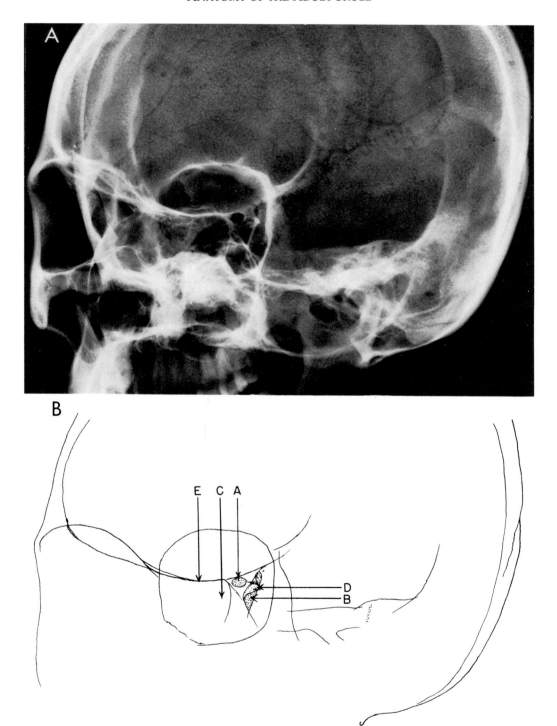

Fig 163.—Adult skull in Rhese projection for the optic foramen (**A** and **B**) showing optic foramen *(A)*, superior orbital fissure *(B)*, sphenoidal sinus *(C)*, anterior clinoid process *(D)*, and cribriform plate of ethmoid *(E)*.

8

Foramina, Fissures, and Canals

This chapter deals only with those cranial foramina that can be demonstrated on the roentgenogram. Careful scrutiny of these apertures may point the way to a correct diagnosis; for example, erosion of the foramina of the middle fossa may be the first clue to the presence of a nasopharyngeal tumor. In order to make an accurate comparison of the foramina on both sides, perfect centering of the skull and x-ray tube is essential. Minor degrees of rotation can produce artifactual differences between the two sides or obscure a real change.

Parietal Foramen

The parietal foramina are apertures frequently present in the upper posterior angle of the parietal bone somewhat lateral to the sagittal suture (Fig 164). They may be unilateral or bilateral, single or double, and equal or unequal in size (Fig 165). Either alone or in addition to the parietal foramen, there may be a single median sagittal foramen opening into the sagittal sulcus (Fig 166). The parietal foramen transmits an emissary vein (Santorini's) that connects the occipital veins with the superior sagittal sinus, and also a small anastomosis between the middle meningeal and occipital arteries. The vast majority (greater than 90%) of parietal foramina do not exceed 1 mm in diameter.

Uncommonly, the parietal foramina are markedly enlarged (Figs 167 and 168). The enlarged foramina are oval or rounded with smooth, beveled margins separated medially by a bony bridge. The foramina are capped by a fibrous membrane covered by normal scalp. A number of patients who were followed from birth had a midline gap between both parietal bones because of delayed ossification at that site. By the end of the second year of life, a midline bony bar usually developed, which split the defect into two parts. The osseous bridge was fully formed by age 3, after which there was minimal change in size or shape of the large bony defects. The defects can be readily differentiated

from burr holes and pathologic osteolytic lesions by their character and location. This anomaly has no clinical significance, although it has a definite hereditary tendency. It has been reported in a number of families, the best known of which is the Catlin family—hence the term "Catlin mark." Goldsmith traced 56 members of this family over a period of five generations and found enlarged foramina in 16 members.

Superior Orbital (Sphenoidal) Fissure

The superior orbital fissure is a curvilinear aperture leading from the middle fossa to the orbit. It is bounded by the lesser sphenoidal wing superiorly, the greater sphenoidal wing laterally, and the body of the sphenoid inferomedially. Through this aperture pass the third, fourth, and sixth cranial nerves, the ophthalmic division of the fifth cranial nerve, and sympathetic fibers from the carotid artery. The superior ophthalmic veins, the orbital branches of the middle meningeal artery, and the recurrent branch of the lacrimal artery also traverse the fissure (Figs 169 and 170). The fissure is inferolateral to the optic foramen, from which it is separated by a strut of bone projecting from the lesser sphenoidal wing. The foramen rotundum lies below the medial end of the fissure.

The configuration of the normal superior orbital fissure varies in size, shape, and symmetry. The normal fissure is characterized by a discrete, well-defined cortical margin. Kornblum and Kennedy studied the superior orbital fissure in 157 anatomical specimens and found an average length of 15 mm and width of 5 mm at the broadest point. Normal variations in shape included (1) the long, narrow fissure (12%), (2) the dumb-bell-shaped fissure (12%), (3) the cone-shaped fissure (11%), and (4) the most common configuration, narrow at the upper outer border and bulbous at the lower medial end (56%) (Fig 171). Approximately 9% of the fissures were asymmetric (Fig 172). Unilateral pneu-

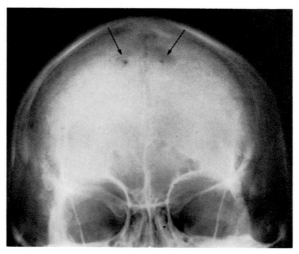

Fig 164.—Small symmetric parietal foramina on either side of sagittal suture *(arrows).*

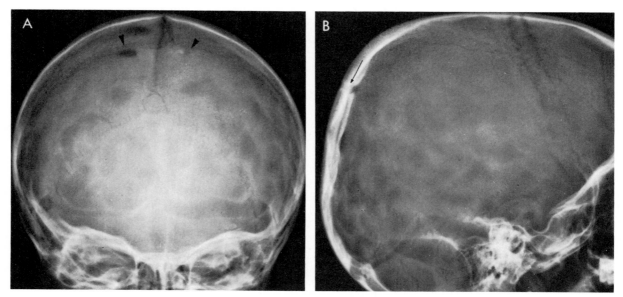

Fig 165.—Posteroanterior **(A)** and lateral **(B)** views in a child with asymmetric parietal foramina.

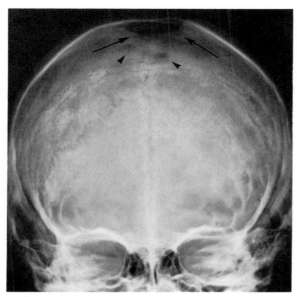

Fig 166.—Sagittal foramen *(arrows).* Note also small parietal foramina *(arrowheads).*

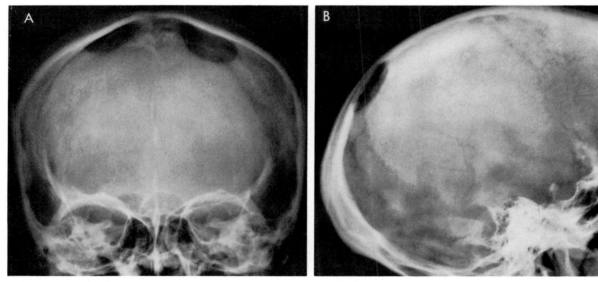

Fig 167.—Posteroanterior **(A)** and lateral **(B)** radiographs of skull of young woman showing large parietal foramina with characteristic convergence of inner and outer tables at thin margins of each opening.

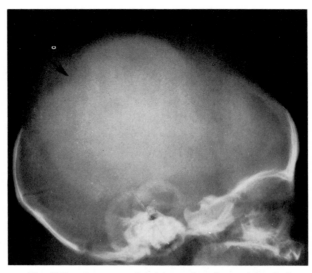

Fig 168.—Large parietal foramina *(arrow)* in skull of newborn daughter of patient in Figure 167.

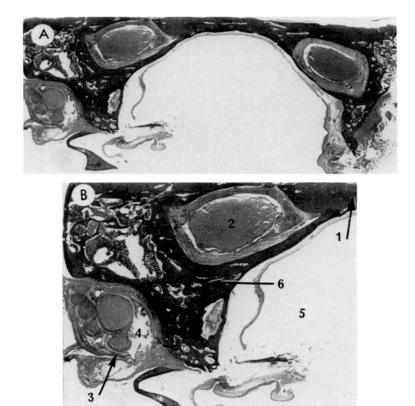

Fig 169.—Coronal section of adult skull specimen through the planum sphenoidale, optic foramina, and sphenoidal fissures. **A,** general view of both sides for orientation. **B,** enlargement for greater detail. Planum sphenoidale *(1);* optic nerve *(2);* sphenoidal fissure containing cranial nerves III, IV, and VI, and ophthalmic division of V *(3).* Anterior portion of cavernous sinus *(4)* lies medial to the cranial nerves. Sphenoidal sinus *(5);* optic strut *(6).* Paraffin-embedded section; hematoxylin eosin. (From Shapiro, R., and Robinson, F.: *Am. J. Roentgenol.* 101:814–827, 1967.)

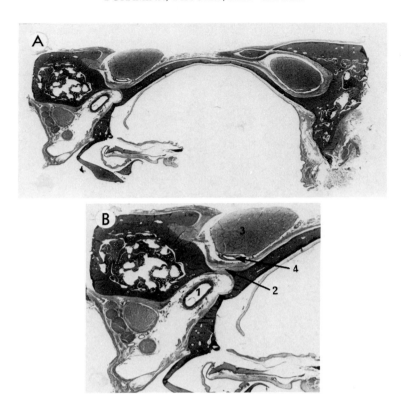

Fig 170.—Slightly more posterior coronal section through posterior rim of optic foramen showing relationship of internal carotid artery *(1)* to the sphenoidal fissure. **A,** general view of both sides. **B,** enlargement for detail. Note that most anterior portion of internal carotid artery projects into superior margin of sphenoidal fissure. This relationship accounts for bone erosion produced by intracavernous aneurysms of internal carotid artery and carotid-cavernous fistulas. In this plane, bony strut from lesser sphenoidal wing is incomplete *(2)*. Only periosteum separates optic nerve *(3)* and ophthalmic artery *(4)* from internal carotid artery. Paraffin-embedded section; hematoxylin eosin. (From Shapiro, R., and Robinson, F.: *Am. J. Roentgenol.* 101:814–827, 1967.)

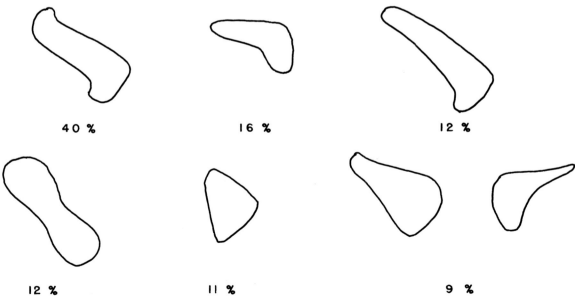

40 % 16 % 12 %

12 % 11 % 9 %

Fig 171.—Variations of normal sphenoidal fissures. (After Kornblum and Kennedy.) The first five types are right-sided fissures; the last two are a right and left pair.

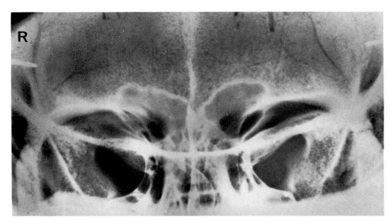

Fig 172.—Caldwell projection of adult dry skull showing asymmetry of sphenoidal fissures. Note well-defined cortical margins, hallmark of the normal fissure. (From Shapiro, R., and Robinson, F.: *Am. J. Roentgenol.* 101:814–827, 1967.)

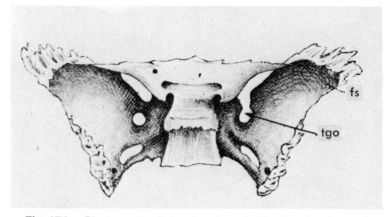

Fig 174.—Photograph of drawing from LeDouble showing unilateral communication of left sphenoidal fissure with foramen rotundum *(arrow)*. (From Shapiro, R., and Robinson, F.: *Am. J. Roentgenol.* 101:814–827, 1967.)

matization of the lesser sphenoidal wing by aberrant ethmoidal cells can result in significant fissural asymmetry (Fig 173).

Rarely, the superior orbital fissure may communicate with the foramen rotundum because of incomplete ossification of the chondral root of the greater sphenoidal wing and failure of its anterior portion to fuse with the postsphenoid (Fig 174). This anomaly represents the normal fetal state prior to the 12th week of gestation (foramen lacerum anterius). LeDouble described a specimen in which the sphenoidal fissure communicated with the optic foramen due to failure of development of the optic strut (Fig 175).

The superior orbital fissure is best demonstrated in

the Caldwell and the optic foramen projections. The head must be perfectly centered in the Caldwell projection since even slight rotation can produce artifactual differences in size and bony definition of the fissures. Overlying soft tissue swelling can also produce confusing differences in density. The pathologic fissure is characterized by loss of the sharp cortical margin, actual bone destruction, or erosion. The most common causes of pathologic fissural widening are carotid-cavernous fistula (Fig 176), aneurysm of the cavernous segment of the internal carotid artery (Fig 177), and lateral extension of a large pituitary adenoma. Other lesions include

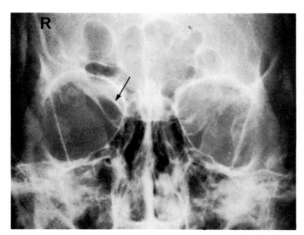

Fig 173.—Asymmetry of sphenoidal fissures and lesser sphenoidal wings due to ectopic ethmoidal cell formation *(arrow)* in right lesser sphenoidal wing. (From Shapiro, R., and Robinson, F.: *Am. J. Roentgenol.* 101:814–827, 1967.)

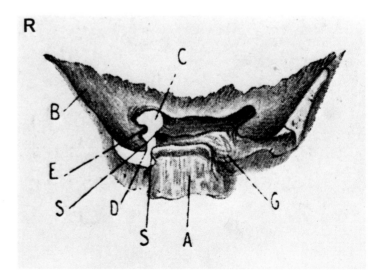

Fig 175.—Photograph of drawing from LeDouble showing communication of right sphenoidal fissure with optic foramen due to incomplete development of optic strut. (From Shapiro, R., and Robinson, F.: *Am. J. Roentgenol.* 101:814–827, 1967.)

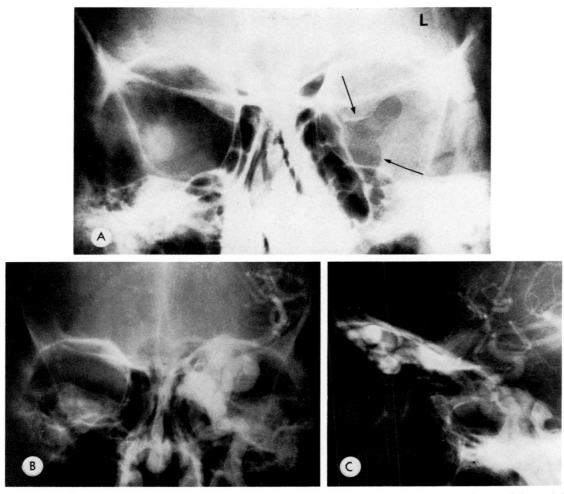

Fig 176.—Traumatic carotid-cavernous fistula of left orbit in 30-year-old man with discrete notching and erosion of superior and inferior medial margins of left sphenoidal fissure **(A).** Left carotid arteriogram demonstrating fistula with filling of the ophthalmic veins **(B** and **C).** (From Shapiro, R., and Robinson, F.: *Am. J. Roentgenol.* 101:814–827, 1967.)

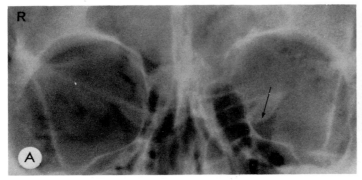
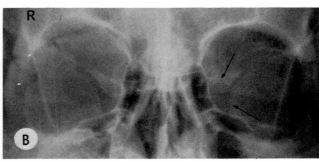

Fig 177.—Early subtle erosion of medial superior and inferior margins of left sphenoidal fissure *(arrow)* by intravenous aneurysm of internal carotid artery **(A).** Progression of bone changes six years later **(B).** (From Shapiro, R., and Robinson, F.: *Am. J. Roentgenol.* 101:814–827, 1967.)

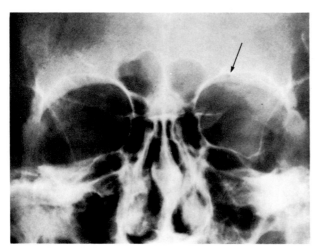

Fig 178.—Caldwell view showing supraorbital foramen bilaterally *(arrow).*

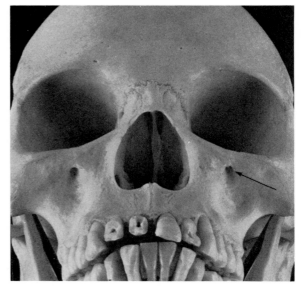

Fig 179.—Frontal photograph of adult skull showing infraorbital foramen *(arrow).*

angiofibroma of the nasopharynx, meningioma, primary or metastatic orbital tumors, and reticuloendotheliosis. A variety of diseases characterized by overgrowth of bone can produce narrowing of the fissure: fibrous dysplasia, Paget's disease, osteopetrosis, and meningioma.

Because of the many normal variations, the diagnosis of a pathologic superior orbital fissure should rarely be made in the absence of corroborative clinical evidence.

Supraorbital Foramen

At the junction of the inner and middle thirds of the orbital margin of the frontal bone is a notch, or foramen (Fig 178), which transmits the supraorbital vessels and nerve.

Infraorbital Foramen and Canal (Figs 179 and 180)

The infraorbital foramen is an aperture on the anterior aspect of the maxilla below the inferior orbital rim. The foramen transmits the infraorbital vessels and nerve. The foramen represents the anterior end of the thin-roofed infraorbital canal, which traverses the floor of the orbit to terminate posteriorly in the inferior orbital fissure. The inferior orbital fissure is a long cleft between the floor and lateral wall of the orbit that opens into the infratemporal fossa behind the maxilla. It transmits the maxillary nerve and its zygomatic branch, a few twigs from the sphenopalatine ganglion to the periosteum of the orbit, and a vein connecting the ophthalmic veins with the pterygoid venous plexus.

Optic Canal

The optic foramen is, in fact, a short canal with cranial and orbital ends, rather than a foramen. It courses laterally and slightly inferiorly in its passage from the middle fossa into the orbit. The optic canal is bounded medially by the body of the sphenoid, laterally by the superior orbital fissure, above by the superior root of

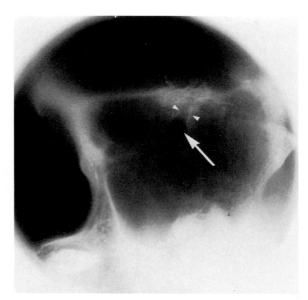

Fig 180.—Anteroposterior tomogram of isolated left maxilla showing distal end of infraorbital canal *(arrowheads)* and infraorbital foramen *(arrow).*

the lesser sphenoidal wing, and below by the inferior root of the lesser sphenoidal wing (optic strut). The optic strut separates the optic canal from the superior orbital fissure (Fig 181).

The optic canal is not perfectly circular throughout its course. Only the midportion is circular (average diameter, 5 mm); the cranial and orbital ends of the canal are oval. The long axis of the oval is oriented transversely at the cranial end (average size, 4.5 × 6.0 mm) and vertically at the orbital end (average size, 5 × 6 mm) (Fig 182). In the conventional optic foramen projection, the long axis of the canal should not exceed 6.5 mm. In this view, one is measuring for the most part the thicker, denser walls of the orbital end of the canal. Slight asymmetry of the canals is common, and a difference in size less than 1 mm is within normal limits. An optic canal is enlarged if it exceeds 6.5 mm in diameter or if it measures 2 mm more than the contralateral canal. An exception to this rule is the small optic canal resulting from enucleation early in life. The canal tends to be pear-shaped in young children, with a maximal normal diameter of 4 mm at birth, 5 mm at six months, and 5.5 mm by five years. According to Evans, the canal also grows in length during early childhood, from 2 mm in the neonate to 4 to 9 mm at five years.

In addition to routine optic foramen views, tomography at 1-mm intervals in the submentovertical projection is helpful (Fig 183). This is particularly useful in children to compare both sides. Sedatives may be desir-

LEFT

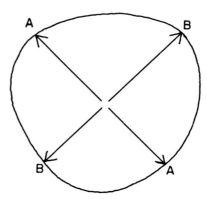

Fig 182.—Schematic diagram of diameters of optic foramen. (After Goalwin.)

able in younger uncooperative children to obtain films of good quality. Satisfactory tomography of the optic canal can also be carried out in the optic foramen projection, as suggested by Potter and Trokel.

The optic canal contains the ophthalmic artery as well as the optic nerve and its sheath surrounded by an extension of the subarachnoid space. The perioptic subarachnoid space is continuous with the intracranial subarachnoid space. The optic nerve lies above the ophthalmic artery.

There are two interesting normal variants: the key-

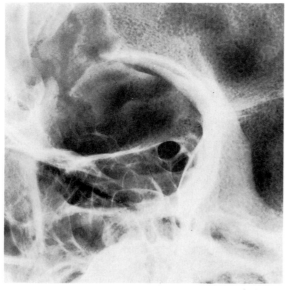

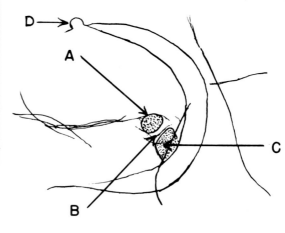

Fig 181.—Normal left optic foramen (dry skull). Note optic foramen *(A)*, optic strut *(B)*, medial end of superior orbital fissure *(C)*, and supraorbital notch *(D)*.

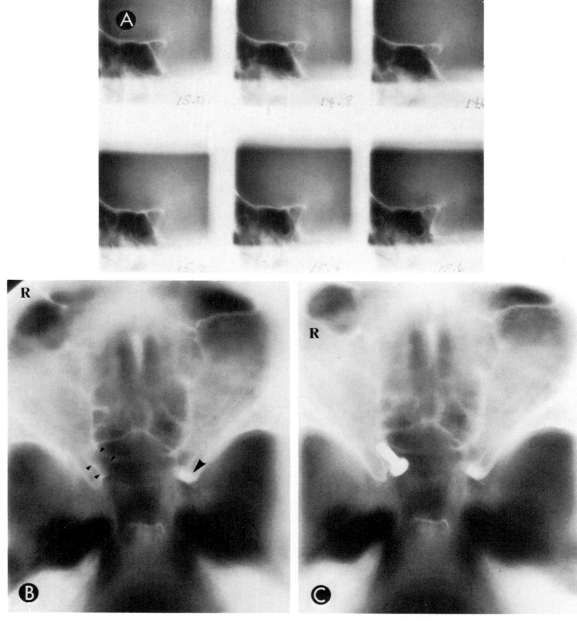

Fig 183.—A, tomograms in Rhese projection of a normal optic canal showing variable shape of canal as it passes from orbital end (14.6) to cranial end (15.6). **B,** tomograph of dried adult skull in sub-mentovertical projection showing left anterior clinoid process marked with a small metallic disc *(arrowhead).* The right optic canal is also well shown *(arrowheads).* **C,** the right optic canal is filled with a screw to identify its length.

hole canal (4%) and the figure-of-eight canal (1.2%). The keyhole anomaly, which may be unilateral or bilateral, is due to failure of development of the posterior segment of the optic strut (Fig 184). This creates a sulcus for the ophthalmic artery below the optic nerve. The figure-of-eight canal has a separate compartment for the ophthalmic artery below that for the optic nerve. These patients have duplication of the cranial opening of the canal, with the ophthalmic artery passing between the unfused anterior and posterior segments of the optic strut (Fig 185).

In the conventional optic foramen view, the canal is projected into the lower outer quadrant of the orbit. The normal canal has a smooth, sharply defined cortical

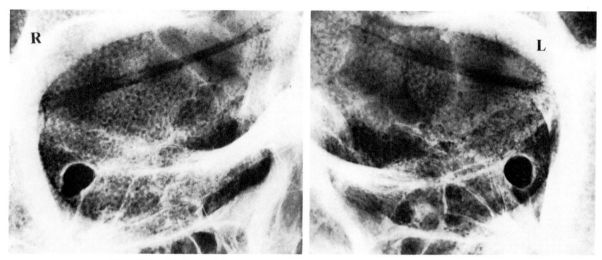

Fig 184.—Unilateral keyhole anomaly of optic foramen on right; left side is normal (dry skull). (From Kier, E. L.: *Invest. Radiol.* 1:346–362, 1966.)

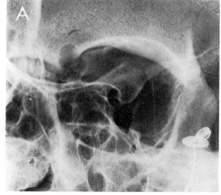

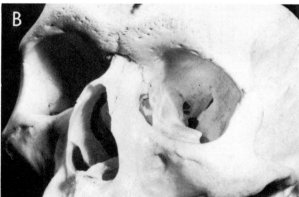

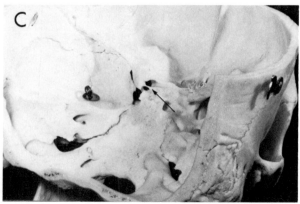

Fig 185.—Frontal radiograph **(A)** and photographs of orbital aspect **(B)** and endocranial aspect **(C)** of skull showing a figure-of-eight anomaly of optic foramen. Note that duplication is limited to cranial opening of optic canal *(arrow)*.

margin. The anterior clinoid process is often made up of cancellous bone surrounded by a cortical rim (Fig 186). Less commonly, the anterior clinoid process is pneumatized (Figs 187 and 188). In both instances, the cross section of the anterior clinoid process appears as a pseudoforamen lateral to the true optic canal. A good rule to follow in this situation is to assume that the most lateral "foramen" is either a pneumatized or cancellous anterior clinoid process. The "foramen" just medial to it represents the true optic canal. In those patients with pneumatization of the lesser sphenoidal wing, the optic canal is encircled by air cells.

Gliomas of the optic nerve usually enlarge the canal without eroding it (Figs 189 and 190). Erosion is more likely to be due to meningiomas arising in the nerve sheath, or aneurysms of the ophthalmic artery.

Caroticoclinoid Foramen (Canal)

Rostrally, the carotid groove terminates between the anterior clinoid process and the tuberculum sellae. When present, the middle clinoid process is represented on one or both sides by a small spicule of bone posterior and lateral to the tuberculum sellae. Ossification of the ligament between the anterior and middle clinoid processes results in the formation of the caroticoclinoid foramen. Osseous fusion of the middle and posterior clinoid processes produces two large foramina, which may be unilateral or bilateral. According to Keyes, some type of caroticoclinoid canal is found in approximately 35% of anatomical specimens, varying from a complete bony ring to an incomplete type with a gap between the anterior and middle clinoid processes.

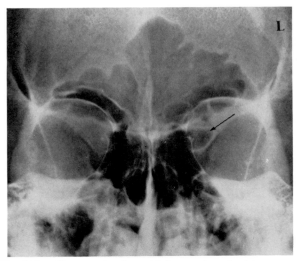

Fig 187.—Pneumatization of left anterior clinoid process.

In the conventional optic foramen view, the caroticoclinoid canal is projected upon the lateral wall of the orbit and cannot be recognized. In a slightly modified optic foramen view with the optic canal projected into the medial half of the orbit, the caroticoclinoid canal is visualized just lateral to the true optic canal. Similarly, in the lateral view, the caroticoclinoid foramen is superimposed upon the body of the sphenoid and cannot be readily identified. In an oblique lateral projection, however, the caroticoclinoid foramen can be seen lateral to the optic foramen (Figs 191 and 192).

Foramen for the Ophthalmomeningeal (Hyrtl's) Vein

Rarely, there is a small foramen in the greater sphenoidal wing, usually in the lateral half of the orbit (Figs

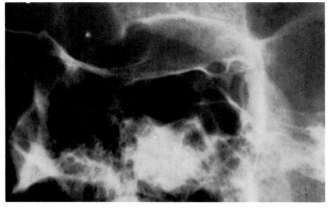

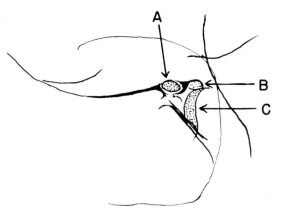

Fig 186.—Optic foramen view showing pseudoforamen (B) produced by cross section of anterior clinoid process. Optic foramen (A); superior orbital fissure (C).

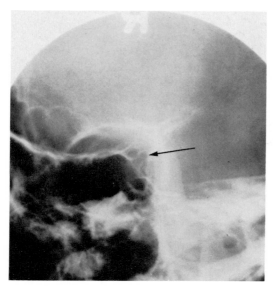

Fig 188.—Optic foramen view showing pneumatization of right optic strut *(arrow)*.

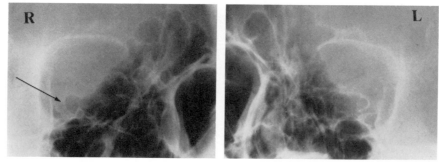

Fig 189.—Optic glioma of right orbit. Enlargement of right optic foramen *(arrow)* with preservation of normal cortical margins.

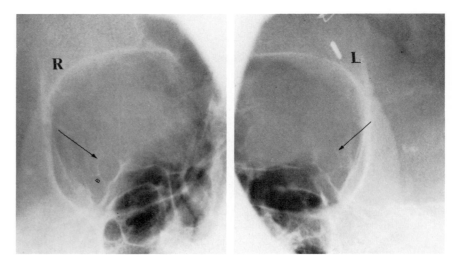

Fig 190.—Bilateral optic gliomas in a patient with neurofibromatosis. Note enlargement of both optic foramina *(arrows)*.

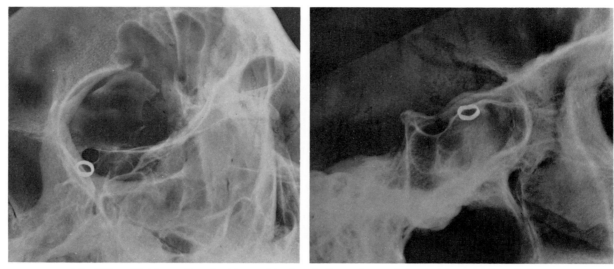

Fig 191.—Right caroticoclinoid canal in dry skull specimen. A lead strip was placed along
inner margin of opening, and films were made in optic foramen *(left)* and lateral *(right)* projections.

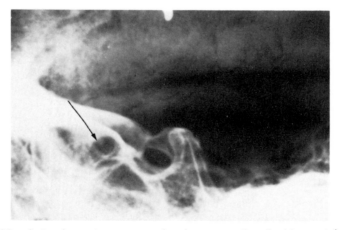

Fig 192.—Lateral roentgenogram showing a caroticoclinoid canal *(arrow).*

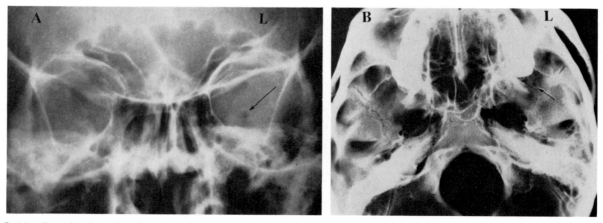

Fig 193.—**A,** Caldwell projection showing a foramen for ophthalmomeningeal vein of Hyrtl in left greater sphenoidal wing *(arrow).* **B,**
base view of dry skull with a foramen for ophthalmomeningeal *(arrow)*
vein of Hyrtl on left side.

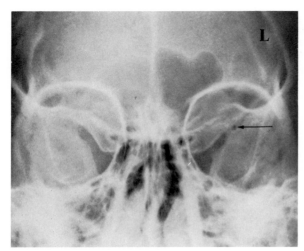

Fig 194.—Caldwell projection showing a tiny foramen in supero-medial aspect of left greater wing. Is this a foramen for the orbital branch of the middle meningeal artery or for the ophthalmomeningeal vein of Hyrtl?

193 and 194). The foramen may be found on one or both sides. The ophthalmomeningeal vein, which traverses the foramen, connects the orbital with the cerebral veins. The vein commonly drains into the sphenoparietal sinus, which anastomoses with the anterior portion of the cavernous sinus. The foramen should not be confused with the rare isolated ectopic ethmoidal cell in the greater sphenoidal wing. An isolated cell can be recognized by its well-defined mucoperiosteal border, characteristic of all normal pneumatized paranasal sinus cells (Fig 195).

More rarely still, there may be a separate small foramen in the greater sphenoidal wing for the orbital branch of the middle meningeal artery, which anastomoses with a lacrimal branch of the ophthalmic artery.

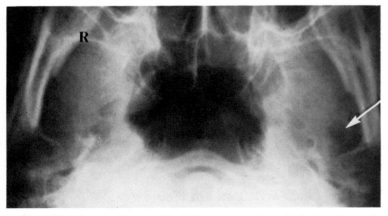

Fig 195.—Agger sinus cell in left greater sphenoidal wing (arrow). Note size of cell and its mucoperiosteal margin.

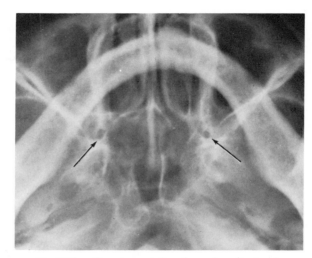

Fig 196.—Greater palatine foramina (arrows).

Greater Palatine Foramen

The greater palatine foramen is a small aperture in the posterolateral margin of the hard palate connecting the oral cavity with the pterygopalatine canal. It transmits the greater palatine artery and the greater palatine branch of the sphenopalatine nerve. It is best visualized in the underangulated submentovertical projection. In this view it can be recognized as a small (2 mm) foramen in the lateral aspect of the bony palate anterior to the medial pterygoid process (Fig 196).

Lesser Palatine Foramen

The lesser palatine foramen may exist singly or as multiple orifices posterior and slightly lateral to the greater palatine foramen (Fig 197). It transmits the lesser palatine nerve and small branches of the greater palatine artery.

Incisive Foramen

The incisive foramen is a midline opening in the maxilla just behind the central incisor teeth (Fig 198). In this opening the orifices of the lateral incisive canals (Stensen's foramina) may at times be seen, transmitting the nasopalatine nerve and a branch of the descending palatine artery. Occasionally, there are two additional orifices (Scarpa's foramina) in the midline for the nasopalatine nerves. All four of these openings lead into the nasal cavity. The incisive foramen is best visualized by means of special intraoral occlusal films.

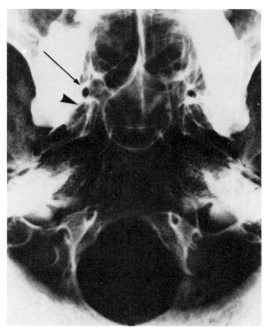

Fig 197.—Two lesser palatine foramina *(arrowhead)* in dry skull. Note also greater palatine foramen *(arrow)*.

Zygomaticofacial Foramen

The zygomaticofacial foramen is a tiny aperture on the malar surface of the zygoma slightly below the inferolateral margin of the orbit (Fig 199). It transmits the zygomaticofacial branch of the zygomatic nerve and a small branch of the lacrimal artery.

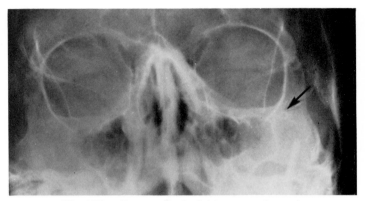

Fig 199.—Zygomaticofacial foramen *(arrow)*.

Ethmoidal Canals

The anterior and posterior ethmoidal canals are narrow tunnels which commence at the corresponding foramina between the superior and medial walls of the orbit (Figs 200 and 201). The canals run medially, between the ethmoidal labyrinth and the medial surface of the orbital plate of the frontal bone, to open into the cranial cavity. The large anterior canal transmits the anterior ethmoidal vessels and nerve; the latter is a continuation of the nasociliary nerve. The smaller posterior canal transmits the posterior ethmoidal vessels and nerve. The anterior canal opens on the lateral aspect of the midportion of the cribriform plate. The posterior canal opens at the junction of the cribriform plate with the anterior surface of the sphenoid bone.

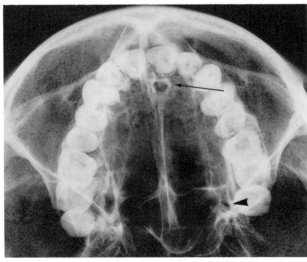

Fig 198.—Incisive foramen *(arrow)*. Note greater palatine foramen at level of last molar teeth *(arrowhead)*.

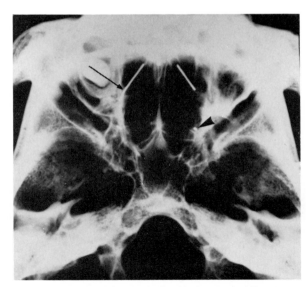

Fig 200—Base view of dry skull with long metallic pin traversing anterior ethmoidal canal *(arrow)* and small metallic marker in posterior ethmoidal canal *(arrowhead)*.

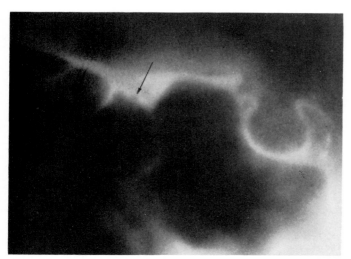

Fig 201.—Lateral tomogram showing posterior ethmoidal foramen *(arrow)*.

Foramina of the Skull Base

Prior to the 12th week of gestation, there are three prominent fenestrations at the base of the skull for various cranial nerves and blood vessels. These openings, which have their counterpart in the primitive mammalian skull, are as follows:

THE FORAMEN LACERUM ANTERIUS.—This hiatus between the orbitosphenoid (lesser wing) and alisphenoid (greater wing) persists as the superior orbital fissure for passage of cranial nerves III, IV, and VI, and the ophthalmic division of V.

THE FORAMEN LACERUM MEDIUS.—The opening between the basisphenoid and the periotic capsule is variously subdivided in different mammals. In man, it persists as the foramen lacerum medius, separated into a medial carotid canal and a lateral petrosphenoidal fissure for the greater superficial petrosal nerve.

THE FORAMEN LACERUM POSTERIUS.—The aperture between the basiocciput and the auditory bullae persists as the jugular foramen for transmission of cranial nerves IX, X, and XI.

These large fenestrations become subdivided by an ingrowth of bony spicules, leading to the formation of multiple discrete foramina in the floor of the skull. Various foraminal abnormalities result from failure of complete development of these bony spurs.

Foramen Rotundum

The foramen rotundum is a short canal in the anteromedial portion of the greater sphenoidal wing connecting the middle fossa with the pterygopalatine fossa. The canal, which runs obliquely forward and slightly downward, transmits the maxillary division of the trigeminal nerve and occasionally a few small veins that connect the cavernous sinus and the pterygoid venous plexus. The foramen rotundum lies directly below the medial end of the superior orbital fissure and is intimately related to the lateral wall of the sphenoidal sinus (Figs 202 to 204). Its size, according to Lindblom, varies roentgenologically from 3 × 3 mm to 4 × 5 mm. Since the

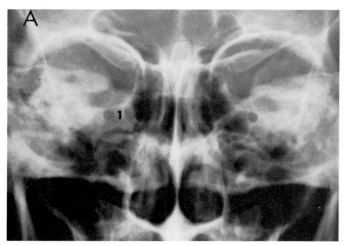
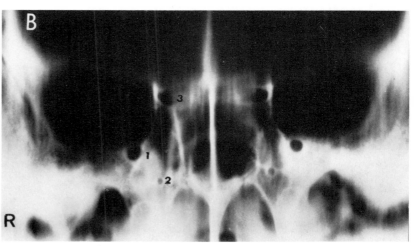

Fig 202.—Conventional roentgenogram in Caldwell projection **(A)** and tomogram in anteroposterior projection **(B)** showing foramen rotundum *(1)* in relation to floor of orbit. Note also the pterygoid canal *(2)* and optic foramen *(3)*. (From Shapiro, R., and Robinson, F.: *Am. J. Roentgenol.* 101:779–794, 1967.)

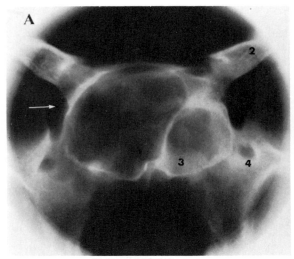

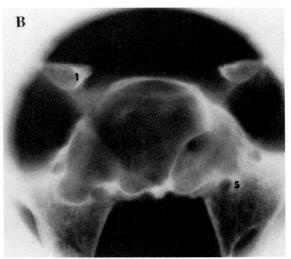

Fig 203.—Tomograms of isolated sphenoid bone in anteroposterior projection. **A,** a more anterior section. **B,** a more posterior section. Note anterior clinoid *(1)*, lesser sphenoidal wing *(2)*, sphenoid sinus *(3)*, foramen rotundum *(4)*, vidian canal *(5)*, and superior orbital fissure *(arrow)*.

course of the canal is angulated with respect to the plane of the skull base, the foramen rotundum is not demonstrated in the routine submentovertical projection. However, it may be visualized just below the medial aspect of the orbital floor in Caldwell and Waters projections and in anteroposterior tomograms.

Significant asymmetry of the foramen rotundum does occur, albeit uncommonly (Figs 205 and 206). This should be kept in mind when an enlarged foramen is encountered. The hallmark of the normal foramen is a sharply defined cortical margin. Taveras and Wood described a patient with symptoms compatible with a neurinoma of the maxillary nerve who had enlargement of the corresponding foramen rotundum. Surgical explo-

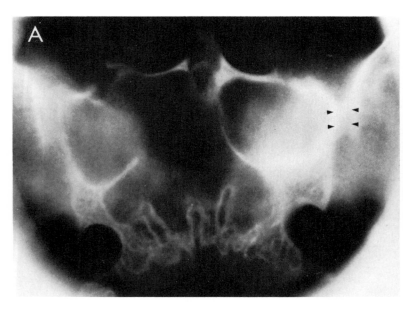

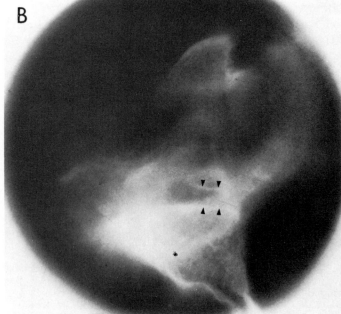

Fig 204.—**A,** tomogram of isolated sphenoid in the submentovertical projection showing course of foramen rotundum *(arrowheads)* as it passes from posterior to anterior. **B,** lateral tomogram of same specimen showing anteroposterior course of foramen rotundum *(arrowheads)*.

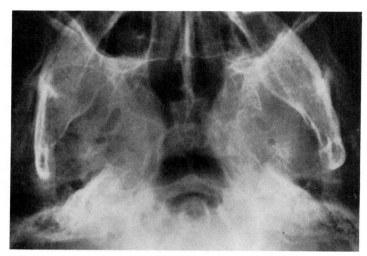

Fig 217.—Marked asymmetry of foramen ovale.

variations may be influenced both by differences in osteogenesis and by the venous channels passing through the foramen.

Foramen Spinosum

The foramen spinosum is a small orifice in the greater sphenoidal wing close to the sphenoidal spine and directly posterolateral to the foramen ovale. The round or oval foramen is usually 2 to 4 mm long, according to Lindblom. The foramen transmits the middle meningeal artery and the middle meningeal vein or veins that usually drain into the pterygoid plexus. The recurrent branch of the mandibular nerve also enters the skull through the foramen spinosum. A foramen larger than 5 mm in diameter should prompt one to exclude conditions associated with an enlarged middle meningeal artery (Fig 218).

The foramen spinosum in man is also subject to a number of variations related to incomplete osteogenesis or to aberrant development of the middle meningeal artery:

1. The foramen may be incompletely separated from, or remain confluent with, the foramen ovale (see Fig 215). This is due to incomplete osteogenesis rather than to anomalous vascular development.

2. In the presence of a primitive foramen lacerum medius, the foramen spinosum does not exist as a separate discrete orifice. It may be represented by a slight notch marking the site of entry of the middle meningeal artery into the skull. A partial foramen lacerum medius may communicate with either the foramen spinosum or the foramen ovale.

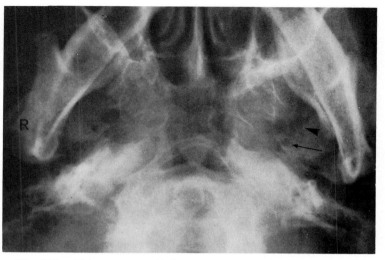

Fig 218.—Enlargement of left foramen spinosum *(arrow)* together with a dilated, tortuous meningeal vascular groove *(arrowhead)* in a patient with a large left pterional meningioma. (From Shapiro, R., and Robinson, F.: *Am. J. Roentgenol.* 101:779–794, 1967.)

3. The foramen spinosum may communicate with the canaliculus innominatus.

4. The foramen spinosum may have a more posterior location, abutting against the anterior margin of the petrous bone or opening into the petrosphenoidal fissure (Fig 219).

5. The foramen spinosum may be asymmetric (Fig 220). Included in this group is the small foramen spi-

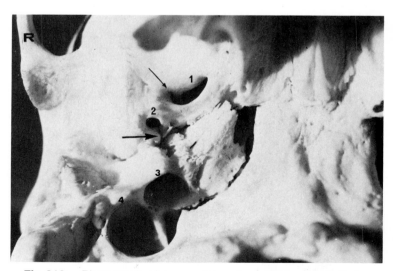

Fig 219.—Photograph of exocranial surface of base of skull showing foramen spinosum leading into petrosphenoidal fissure by a groove *(wide arrow)*. Note also the notch for accessory meningeal artery in foramen ovale *(thin arrow)*; foramen ovale *(1)*; foramen spinosum *(2)*; carotid canal *(3)*; and jugular foramen *(4)*. (From Shapiro, R., and Robinson, F.: *Am. J. Roentgenol.* 101:779–794, 1967.)

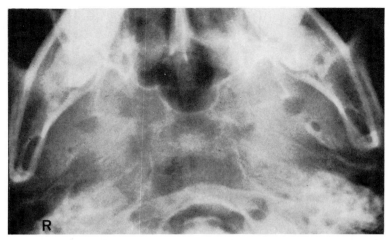

Fig 220.—Asymmetry of foramen spinosum (left larger than right) in a normal adult male. Foramen ovale is also asymmetric. (From Shapiro, R., and Robinson, F.: *Am. J. Roentgenol.* 101:779–794, 1967.)

nosum associated with a large accessory meningeal artery, which courses in a groove extending anterolaterally from the posterior margin of the foramen ovale.

6. Rarely, the foramen spinosum is absent in the presence of a normal foramen ovale (Fig 221). This is associated with anomalous origin of the middle meningeal artery, i.e., from the ophthalmic artery. Under

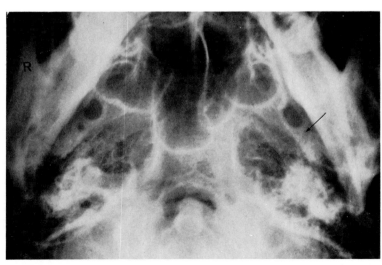

Fig 221.—Absence of left foramen spinosum *(arrow)* in a patient with marked pneumatization of paranasal sinuses and petrous bone. Multiple base views in varying degrees of extension failed to visualize a left foramen spinosum, thereby excluding spurious absence due to skull rotation or projection. This is usually associated with anomalous formation of the middle meningeal artery. (From Shapiro, R., and Robinson, F.: *Am. J. Roentgenol.* 101:779–794, 1967.)

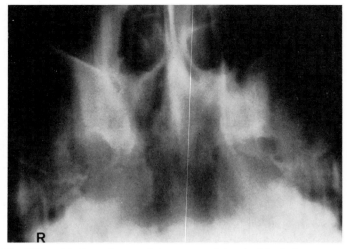

Fig 222.—Malignant neurolemmoma arising in Meckel's cave and invading right middle and posterior fossa. Tomogram clearly shows destruction of right middle fossa foramina. (From Shapiro, R., and Robinson, F.: *Am. J. Roentgenol.* 101:779–794, 1967.)

these circumstances, the middle meningeal artery enters the skull via the superior orbital fissure.

The middle fossa foramina may become enlarged, eroded, or destroyed by various pathologic processes, e.g., primary or secondary tumor, reticuloendotheliosis, and aneurysm (Figs 222 and 223). Contrariwise, the foramina can be narrowed by a variety of processes that produce sclerosis or new bone formation, e.g., fibrous dysplasia, Paget's disease, osteoblastic metastases, and osteopetrosis (Fig 224).

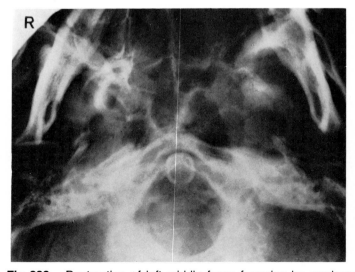

Fig 223.—Destruction of left middle fossa foramina by carcinoma of nasopharynx. (From Shapiro, R., and Robinson, F.: *Am. J. Roentgenol.* 101:779–794, 1967.)

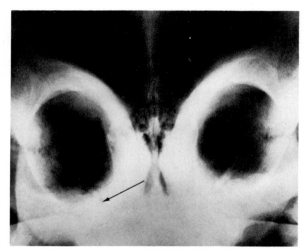

Fig 224.—Posteroanterior roentgenogram of postmortem specimen of skull of a 32-month-old girl with osteopetrosis. Note abnormally dense bone around base of skull, orbits, and face. Foramen rotundum is markedly constricted *(arrow)*. (Courtesy of Dr. M. H. Wittenborg.)

Pterygospinous and Pterygoalar Bars

The fascia separating the internal and external pterygoid muscles may calcify or ossify, giving rise to pterygospinous and pterygoalar bars. The pterygospinous bar is attached anteriorly to Civinini's spine (a small spur near the root of the posterior margin of the lateral pterygoid plate) and posteriorly to the sphenoidal spine, *medial to the foramen spinosum* (Figs 225 to 228). The space enclosed by the pterygospinous bar, i.e., the

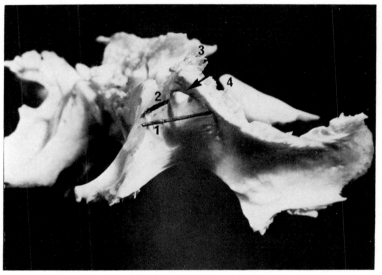

Fig 226.—Oblique-lateral photograph of isolated sphenoid bone seen from above, with metallic pin in position of pterygoalar bar *(1)* lateral to foramen ovale *(arrow)*. Note medial location of pin in position of pterygospinous bar *(2)*. Dorsum sellae *(3)*; anterior clinoid process *(4)*. (From Shapiro, R., and Robinson, F.: *Am. J. Roentgenol.* 101:779–794, 1967.)

pterygospinous foramen, is traversed by the pterygoid vessels and branches of the mandibular nerve supplying the internal pterygoid muscle. The pterygoalar bar attaches anteriorly to the root of the lateral pterygoid plate close to the attachment of the pterygospinous bar, and posteriorly to the undersurface of the greater wing,

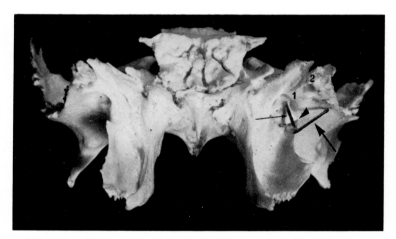

Fig 225.—Photograph of posteroinferior aspect of isolated human sphenoid bone with metallic pins placed in position of the pterygospinous *(thin arrow)* and pterygoalar *(thick arrow)* bars. Civinini's spine *(arrowhead)*; foramen ovale *(1)*; foramen spinosum *(2)*. Note the more medial position of pterygospinous bar. (From Shapiro, R., and Robinson, F.: *Am. J. Roentgenol.* 101:779–794, 1967.)

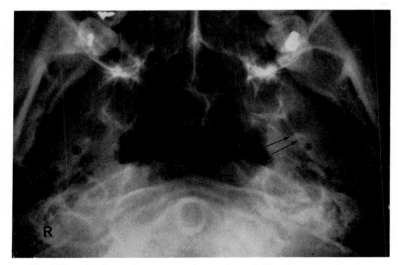

Fig 227.—Unilateral pterygospinous bar *(left)*. Note the characteristic insertion medial to foramen spinosum *(arrows)*. (From Shapiro, R., and Robinson, F.: *Am. J. Roentgenol.* 101:779–794, 1967.)

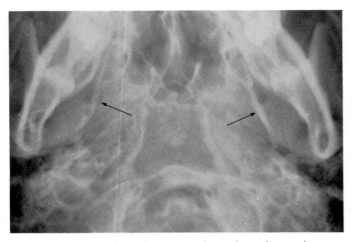

Fig 228.—Bilateral pterygospinous bars *(arrows).*

lateral to the foramen spinosum (Fig 229). The space enclosed by the pterygoalar bar, i.e., the pterygoalar foramen, provides passage for the major motor branches of the mandibular nerve supplying the muscles of mastication. A prominent lateral pterygoid plate can simulate a pterygoalar bar, but this can readily be recognized by tomography.

Since the pterygospinous bar has a more medial course, it does not compromise the foramen ovale. On the other hand, the pterygoalar bar can interfere with injection of the mandibular division of the trigeminal nerve. In Priman and Etter's material, complete ossification of the pterygospinous and pterygoalar ligaments

occurred in approximately 3% of skulls. Partial ossification of the pterygospinous ligament was noted in 8% and of the pterygoalar ligament in 14.4%. Calcification or ossification of either ligament can be unilateral or bilateral.

Pterygopalatine (Sphenomaxillary) Fossa

The pterygopalatine fossa (Figs 230 to 232) is a vertically oriented, narrow, triangular space bounded anteriorly by the posterior wall of the maxillary sinus, posteriorly by the root of the pterygoid plates, superiorly by the undersurface of the body of the sphenoid, and

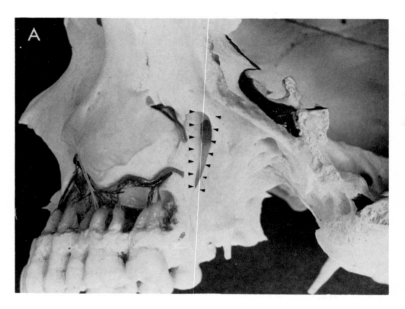

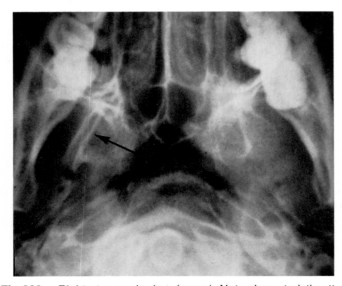

Fig 229.—Right pterygoalar bar *(arrow).* Note characteristic attachment lateral to foramen spinosum. (From Shapiro, R., and Robinson, F.: *Am. J. Roentgenol.* 101:779–794, 1967.)

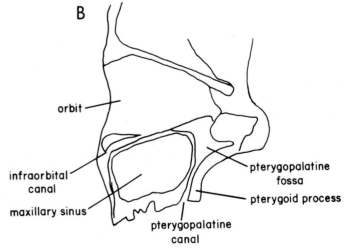

Fig 230.—**A,** lateral photograph of dry skull preparation with zygoma and mandibular removed to demonstrate pterygopalatine fossa *(arrowheads).* **B,** pterygopalatine fossa and adjacent structures.

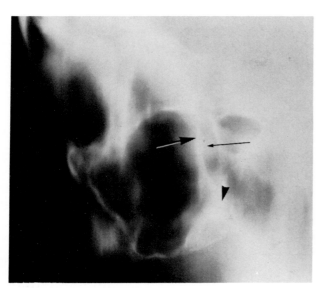

Fig 231.—Lateral tomogram showing pterygopalatine fossa *(thin arrow)*, posterior wall of maxillary sinus *(thick arrow)*, and anterior wall of medial pterygoid plate *(arrowhead)*.

medially by the vertical portion of the palatine bone. The fossa tapers inferiorly to become the pterygopalatine canal, which is traversed by the third portion of the internal maxillary artery, the maxillary nerve, and the sphenopalatine ganglion. The fossa communicates with the orbit via the inferior orbital fissure, with

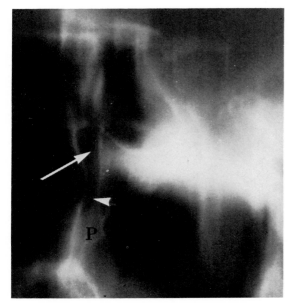

Fig 232.—Lateral tomogram through pterygopalatine fossa. Note that fossa *(arrow)* tapers at its lower end where it becomes the pterygopalatine canal *(arrowhead)*. Medial pterygoid plate is also clearly seen *(P)*.

the nasal cavity via the sphenopalatine foramen, and with the infratemporal fossa via the pterygomaxillary fissure.

Five foramina open into the pterygopalatine fossa: the sphenopalatine foramen on the medial wall of the fossa, the pterygopalatine canal inferiorly, and the foramen rotundum, the pterygoid (vidian) canal, and the pharyngeal canal on the posterior wall of the fossa. The most medial foramen opening onto the posterior wall is the pharyngeal canal. Lateral to it are the orifices of the pterygoid canal and the foramen rotundum.

Pterygoid (Vidian) Canal

The pterygoid canal is a short, narrow, horizontal tunnel in the common root of the pterygoid process and greater sphenoidal wing, connecting the pterygopalatine fossa anteriorly with the foramen lacerum posteriorly. The posterior opening of the canal lies below the foramen rotundum. The canal has a slight medial direction as it courses anteriorly (Fig 233). The pterygoid canal transmits the vidian nerve, which enters the sphenopalatine ganglion, and the vidian artery, which arises from the third part of the internal maxillary artery.

The pterygoid canal is best visualized by tomography in the anteroposterior projection (see Fig 203). It can also be seen at times in Waters and Caldwell views as a small (1 to 2 mm), rounded radiolucency with a sharply defined cortical outline.

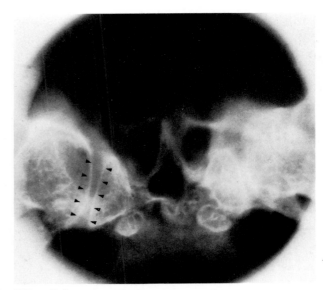

Fig 233.—Submentovertical tomogram of isolated sphenoid bone showing course of pterygoid canal *(arrowheads)*.

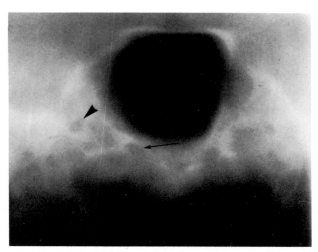

Fig 234.—Anteroposterior tomogram showing medial position of palatovaginal canal *(arrow)*. Note the more lateral location of vidian canal *(arrowhead)*.

Pharyngeal (Palatinovaginal) Canal

The pharyngeal canal is a short tunnel that traverses the vaginal process of the medial pterygoid plate, medial to the pterygoid canal (Fig 234). It transmits branches of the sphenopalatine artery and nerve to the roof of the nasal fossa.

Foramen Lacerum

The foramen lacerum is a short, wide aperture medial to the foramen ovale, bounded in front by the greater sphenoidal wing, behind by the apex of the petrous bone, and medially by the body of the sphenoid and basiocciput. The carotid canal opens into the foramen lacerum laterally, and the carotid groove begins on its anteromedial margin. The inferior aspect of the foramen lacerum is filled with cartilage. Traversing the foramen lacerum are a meningeal branch of the ascending palatine artery and the nerve of the pterygoid canal.

Carotid Canal

The exocranial end of the cartoid canal lies on the inferior surface of the temporal petrosa anterior to the jugular foramen (Fig 235). The canal runs upward for a short distance, then makes a 90-degree turn and passes medially and forward to terminate endocranially in the middle fossa at the petrous apex near the posterior margin of the foramen lacerum. The canal is traversed by the internal carotid artery, a few veins connecting the pharyngeal venous plexus with the cavernous sinus, and the internal carotid nerve, which is a continuation of the sympathetic superior cervical ganglion. According to Lindblom, the length of the canal is 3 to 4 cm; its width at the bend is 5 to 7 mm. The carotid canal can be visualized by conventional radiography in the submentovertical and Stenver projections. However, it is best demonstrated by tomography.

Jugular Foramen

The jugular foramen is a large aperture in the posterior half of the skull base behind the carotid canal. Its anterolateral wall is formed by the temporal petrosa, and its posteromedial wall by the occipital bone (Fig 236). A thin bony partition separates the jugular foramen from the carotid canal. The foramen varies considerably in size and shape, and there may be considerable asymmetry between the two sides (Figs 237 to 240). There are two principal reasons for the asymmetry: (1) variability in bone formation around the primitive fora-

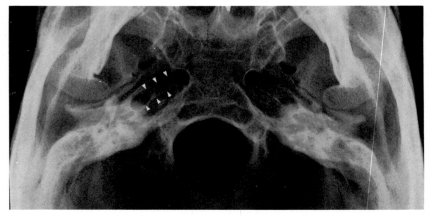

Fig 235.—Base view of dry skull showing exocranial course of carotid canal *(arrowheads)*.

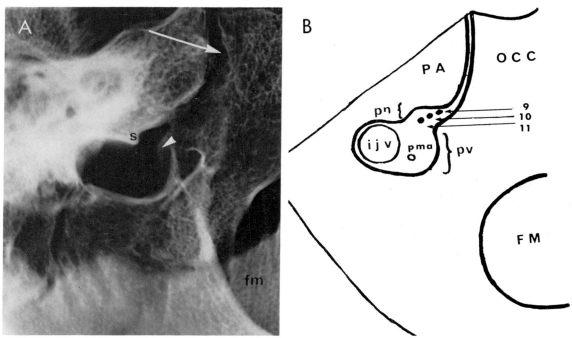

Fig 236.—A, submentovertical projection of articulated right temporal and occipital bones of dry skull showing jugular foramen. Note jugular process of occipital bone *(arrowhead)*, jugular spine of temporal petrosa *(S)*, foramen magnum *(fm)*, and petrooccipital fissure *(arrow)*. **B,** diagram of same specimen showing petrous apex *(PA)*; basiocciput *(OCC)*; foramen magnum *(FM)*; internal jugular vein *(ijv)*, posterior meningeal artery *(pma)*; pars vascularis *(pv)*; pars nervosa *(pn)*; and 9, 10, 11, cranial nerves. (From Shapiro, R.: *J. Neurosurg.* 36:340–343, 1972.)

men lacerum posterius, and (2) unequal development of the transverse dural sinuses. The second factor is usually more significant and is largely responsible for the major differences in the size of the jugular foramina in a given skull. Thus, when the transverse sinuses are equal in size, the jugular foramina are likely to be sym-

metric. When one transverse sinus is much larger than the other, the jugular foramen on the side of the large sinus is larger.

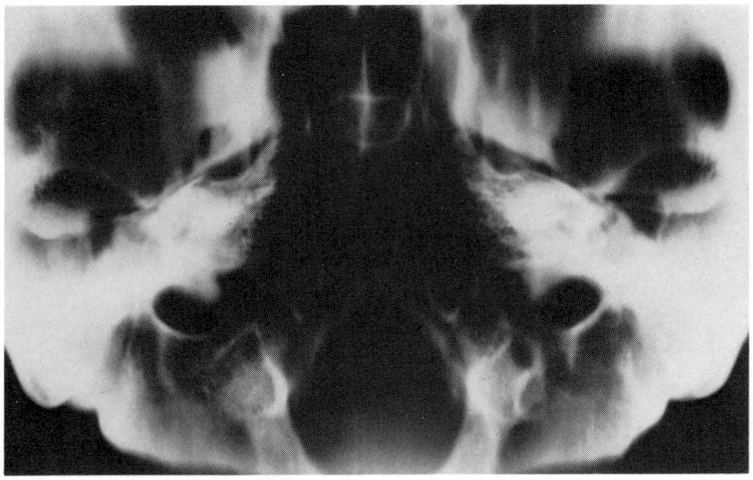

Radiologically, the jugular foramen is incompletely divided into two compartments by the constricted contour of the pars nervosa. Less commonly, there is a fibrous or bony septum connecting the jugular spine of the temporal petrosa with the jugular process of the occipital bone. The anteromedial compartment (pars nervosa) transmits the posterior end of the inferior petrosal sinus and the 9th, 10th, and 11th cranial nerves. The posterolateral compartment (pars vascularis) transmits the jugular vein and the meningeal branches of the occipital and pharyngeal arteries.

Both jugular foramina are best visualized simultaneously on a modified submentovertical projection (Eraso, 20 degrees; Kim and Capp, 37 degrees with the perpendicular). Each jugular foramen can also be seen in the Chaussé II projection, an oblique view which demonstrates only one foramen. This is a disadvantage because it is difficult to reproduce the projections perfectly. In the Chaussé II supine projection, the patient's head is rotated 10 degrees toward the side under study

Fig 237.—Submentovertical tomogram showing symmetric jugular foramina. (From Shapiro, R.: *J. Neurosurg.* 36:340–343, 1972.)

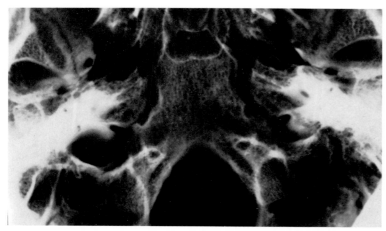

Fig 238.—Basal tomogram of dry skull showing gross asymmetry of jugular foramina. This normal variant is due to enlargement of right pars vascularis associated with large right lateral sinus. Note that pars nervosa is symmetric bilaterally. (From Shapiro, R.: *J. Neurosurg.* 36:340–343, 1972.)

and extended so that the central ray passes through the open mouth, perpendicular to a line joining the external auditory meatuses.

DiChiro et al. have described three principal pathologic configurations (Fig 241): The first is a generalized irregular enlargement of the entire foramen with ill-defined bone margins, seen in chemodectoma (Fig 242), metastatic tumor, and reticuloendotheliosis. The second is enlargement of the pars nervosa with preservation of

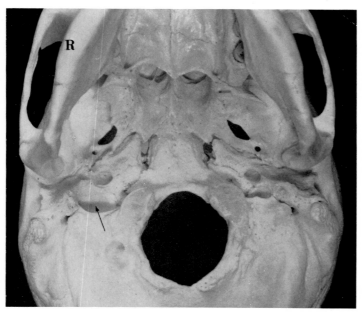

Fig 239.—Undersurface of a dry skull with "giant" jugular fossa on right side *(arrow).*

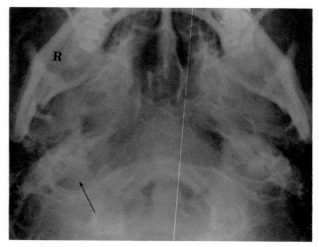

Fig 240.—Base view of skull of asymptomatic patient with a "giant" right jugular fossa *(arrow).*

the cortical rim of the foramen, due to neurinoma of the 9th, 10th, and 11th cranial nerves; large neurinomas may enlarge the entire jugular foramen, but the bony margins are well preserved. Finally, there is the sharply defined, smooth enlargement of the pars vascularis due to vascular malformations.

Internal Auditory Canal

The internal auditory canal is discussed in chapter 16, dealing with the ear.

Facial Canal

The facial canal is discussed in chapter 16.

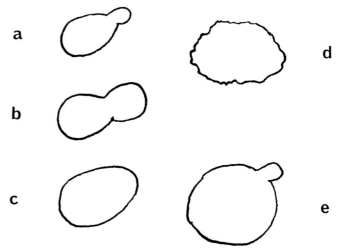

Fig 241.—Various jugular foraminal configurations: normal *(a);* neurinomas of cranial nerves IX, X, XI *(b,c);* chemodectoma and metastatic carcinoma *(d);* and vascular abnormality *(e).* (From Shapiro, R.: *J. Neurosurg.* 36:340–343, 1972.)

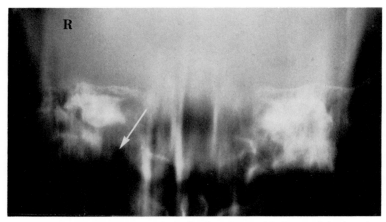

Fig 242.—Towne view of skull of patient with large right jugular chemodectoma. Note complete destruction of jugular foramen on involved side *(arrow)*.

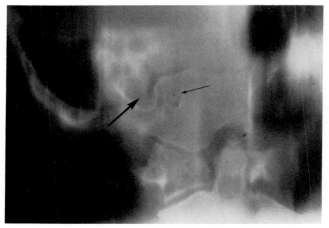

Fig 244.—Oblique tomogram showing relationship of hypoglossal canal *(thin arrow)* to jugular foramen *(thick arrow)*.

Hypoglossal Canal (Anterior Condyloid Foramen)

The hypoglossal canal is a short tunnel in the base of each occipital condyle. Its endocranial opening lies on the anterolateral aspect of the foramen magnum. The canal runs anteriorly and laterally to exit exocranially medial to the jugular foramen (Figs 243 and 244). The canal normally transmits the hypoglossal nerve, a meningeal branch of the ascending pharyngeal artery, and a small venous plexus. When a primitive hypoglossal artery is present, it also traverses the canal on its way to join the basilar artery. Occasionally, the internal as-

pect of the canal is partially or completely compartmented by a bony spicule, which separates the two bundles of the hypoglossal nerve. In the Towne projection, the hypoglossal canal is visualized superior to the foramen magnum at the base of each occipital condyle. However, the canal is best seen in the Stenver or reverse Stenver projection. According to Kirdani, the midportion of the normal canal tends to be round and varies from 4 to 11 mm in diameter (average, 6 mm). The canal may be asymmetric. The inner and outer

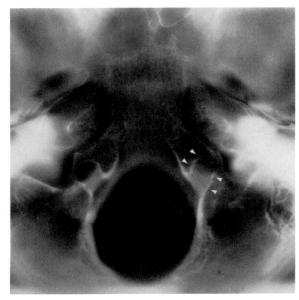

Fig 243.—Basal tomogram of dry skull showing course of hypoglossal canal *(arrowheads)*. (From Shapiro, R.: *Radiology* 133:395–396, 1979.)

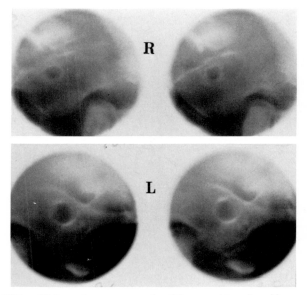

Fig 245.—Oblique tomograms of a 66-year-old male with persistent left primitive hypoglossal artery. Note normal size of right canal *(top)* and enlargement of left canal *(bottom)* with preservation of its cortical outline. (From Shapiro, R.: *Radiology* 133:395–396, 1979.)

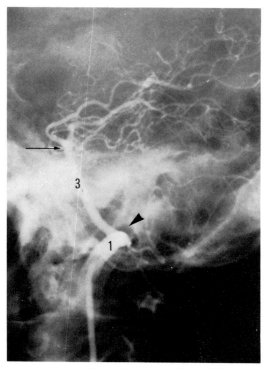

Fig 246.—Angiogram with catheter in left primitive hypoglossal artery *(1)*. Note artery passing thru enlarged hypoglossal canal *(arrowhead)*; basilar artery *(3)*; small aneurysm *(arrow)*. (From Springer, T. D., Fishbone, G., and Shapiro, R.: *J. Neurosurg.* 40:397–399, 1974.)

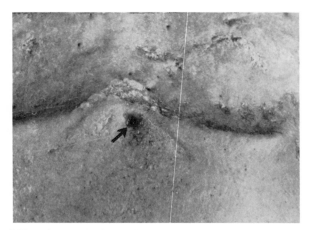

Fig 248.—Anatomical specimen with well-defined foramen emissarium occipitale *(arrow)*. (From O'Rahilly, R.: *Arch. Pathol.* 53:509–519, 1952.)

openings of the canal tend to be oval. The normal canal is characterized by a sharp, white cortical rim. The cortical margins are preserved in the presence of canal enlargement due to a persistent hypoglossal artery (Figs 245 and 246) or a neurinoma of the hypoglossal nerve. The cortical margins are lost in canal enlargement due to glomus jugulare tumors, chordoma, primary cholesteatoma, metastatic malignancy, reticuloendotheliosis, or osteomyelitis.

Posterior Condyloid Canal

Behind each occipital condyle is a depression (condyloid fossa) for the posterior margin of the superior facet

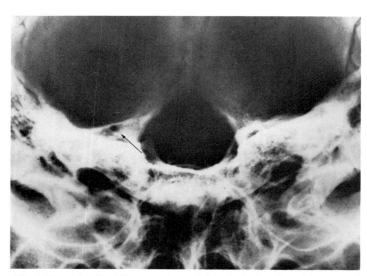

Fig 247.—Modified Towne view of dry skull showing right posterior condyloid canal *(arrow)*.

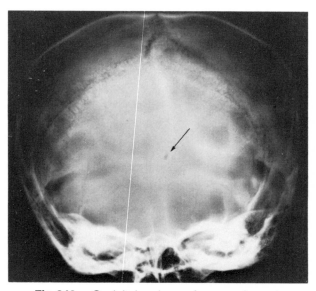

Fig 249.—Occipital emissary foramen *(arrow)*.

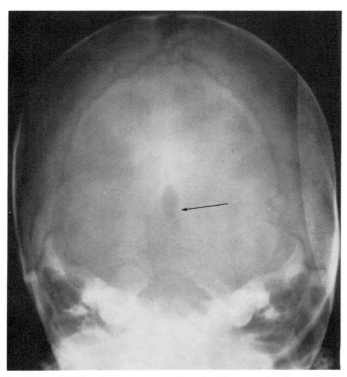

Fig 250.—Midline foramen associated with posterior fossa dermoid cyst. There were both intra- and extracranial components connected by a stalk that traversed the bony defect *(arrow)*.

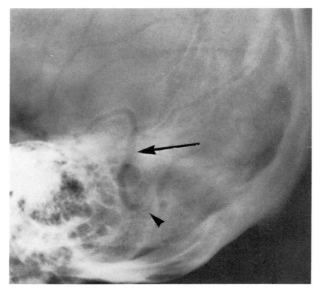

Fig 251.—Mastoid venous groove *(arrow)* and emissary foramen *(arrowhead)*.

of the atlas. Frequently, the floor of this fossa is perforated by the posterior condyloid canal, which transmits a vein connecting the suboccipital venous plexus with the lower end of the sigmoid sinus (Fig 247). This canal may be absent or present unilaterally or bilaterally. Roentgenographically, the canal is often visible in the submentovertical and modified Towne projections as a small, round radiolucency just lateral to the foramen magnum. When the groove for the sigmoid sinus is unusually deep, it appears as a well-defined, prominent radiolucency partially projected above the petrous pyramid lateral to the foramen magnum. This fossa for the sigmoid sinus should not be confused with the smaller posterior condyloid canal.

Foramen Emissarium Occipitale (Inioindineal Canal)

In the region of the internal occipital protuberance, there may be one or more small openings for emissary veins (Figs 248 and 249). These openings (i.e., inioindineal canals) must be differentiated from occipital meningoceles and from the rare midline posterior fossa dermoid cyst with external extension (Fig 250). In a study of 512 skulls, Sperino found a complete inioindineal canal in 44% and an orifice closed either externally or internally in 48%.

Foramen Mastoideum

The mastoid foramen is a canal in or near the occipitomastoid suture on a level with the external auditory meatus (Fig 251). In the lateral projection, it is S- or Y-shaped and varies considerably in size. It contains an emissary vein connecting the sigmoid sinus with the veins of the scalp, and also a small branch of the occipital artery.

REFERENCES

Allen W.: The varieties of the atlas in the human subject and the homologies of its transverse process. *J. Anat. Physiol.* 14:18–28, 1880.

Baylin G. J., Kerman H. D.: Roentgen examination of sphenoidal fissures. *South. Med. J.* 40:281–289, 1947.

Beutel A.: Pathologische veränderungen am canalis opticus. *Fortschr. Geb. Röntgenstrahlen* 48:576–584, 1933.

Bolk L.: Zur Frage der Assimilation des Atlas am Schädel beim Menschen. *Anat. Anz.* 28:497, 1906.

Boyd G. I.: Emissary foramina of cranium in man and anthropoids. *J. Anat.* 65:108–121, 1930.

Bystrow A. P.: Assimilation des Atlas und Manifestation des Proatlas. *Ztschr. Ges. Anat.* 95 (pt. 1):210–242, 1931.

Bystrow A. P.: Morphologische Untersuchungen über die occipital Region und die ersten Halswirbel der Säugetiere und des Menschen; die Assimilation des Atlas und deren Phylogenetische Bedeutung. *Ztschr. Anat.* 102:307–337, 1933.

Camp J. D., Allen E. P.: Microtia and congenital atresia of the external auditory canal. Demonstration of the external auditory canal by means of tomography. *Am. J. Roentgenol.* 43:201–203, 1940.

Camp J. D., Cilley E. I. L.: Significance of asymmetry of the pori acustici as an aid in diagnosis of eighth nerve tumors. *Am. J. Roentgenol.* 41:712–718, 1939.

Childe A. E.: Occipital vertebrae, in Golden R. (ed): *Diagnostic Roentgenology.* Baltimore, Williams & Wilkins Co, 1952, vol. 1, pp. 34BO–34BQ.

Chouke K. S., Hodes P. J.: Pterygo-alar bar and its recognition by roentgen methods in trigeminal neuralgia. *Am. J. Roentgenol.* 65:180–182, 1951.

Cushing H.: *Tumors of the Nervous Acusticus and the Syndrome of the Cerebello-Pontine Angle.* Philadelphia, W. B. Saunders Co., 1917.

DeBeer G. R.: The development of the vertebrate skull. Oxford, England, Clarendon Press, 1937.

DeFrue A., Wagenaar J. H.: Die Bedeutung der Porus Crotaphiticobuccinatorium und des Foramen pterygospinosum für Neurologie und Roentgenologie. *Fortschr. Geb. Röntgenstrahlen* 52:64–69, 1935.

DiChiro G., Fisher R. L., Nelson K. R.: The jugular foramen. *J. Neurosurg.* 21:447–460, 1964.

Dyke C. G.: Persistent craniopharyngeal canal, in Golden R. (ed.): *Diagnostic Roentgenology.* Baltimore, Williams & Wilkins Co., 1925, p. 30E.

Ebenius B.: Results of examination of the petrous bone in auditory nerve tumors. *Acta Radiol.* 15:284–290, 1934.

Engeset A., Torkildsen A.: On changes of the optic canal in cases of intracranial tumor. *Acta Radiol.* 29:57–64, 1948.

Eraso S. T.: Roentgen and clinical diagnosis of glomus jugulare tumors: Four cases and a new radiographic technique. *Radiology* 77:252–256, 1961.

Evans T. H.: Carotid canal anomaly: Other instances of absent internal carotid artery. *Med. Times* 84:1069–1072, 1956.

Farberow B. J.: Roentgenological diagnostics of the optic foramen. *Acta Radiol.* 18:594–606, 1937.

Fisher A. G.: Case of complete absence of both internal carotid arteries with a preliminary note on development of stapedial artery. *J. Anat. Physiol.* 48:37–46, 1914.

Gladstone R. J., Erichsen-Powell W.: Manifestation of occipital vertebrae and fusion of the atlas with the occipital bone. *J. Anat. Physiol.* 49:190–209, 1914–1915.

Gladstone R. J., Wakeley C. P. G.: Variations of occipital-atlantal joint in relation to metameric structure of cranio-vertebral region. *J. Anat.* 59:195–216, 1924–1925.

Glaesmer E.: Die Atlanto-occipital Synostose. *Anat. Anz.* 36:129–148, 1910.

Goalwin H. A.: Precise roentgenography and measurement of optic canal. *Am. J. Roentgenol.* 13:480–484, 1925.

Goalwin H. A.: The profile roentgenogram of the optic canal. *Am. J. Roentgenol.* 17:573–579, 1927.

Goalwin H. A.: One thousand optic canals. *J.A.M.A.* 89:1745–1748, 1927.

Goldsmith W. M.: The Catlin mark: The inheritance of an un- usual opening in the parietal region. *J. Hered.* 13:69–71, 1922.

Greig D. M.: Abnormally large foramina parietalia. *Edinburgh Med. J.* 34:629–648, 1927.

Greig D. M.: Congenital anomalies of the foramen spinosum. Edinburgh *Med. J.* 36:363–371, 1929.

Haas L. L.: The posterior condylar fossa, foramen and canal, and the jugular foramen. *Radiology* 69:546–552, 1957.

Hadley L. A.: Atlanto-occipital fusion, ossiculum terminale and occipital vertebra as related to basilar impression with neurological symptoms. *Am. J. Roentgenol.* 59:511–524, 1948.

Härtel F.: Röntgenographische Darstellung des Foramen ovale des Schädels. *Fortschr. Geb. Röntgenstrahlen* 27:493–495, 1919–1921.

Harwood-Nash D. C.: Axial tomography of the optic canals in children. *Radiology* 96:367–374, 1970.

Hawkins T. D.: Radiological investigation of glomus jugulare tumors. *Acta Radiol.* 5:201–210, 1966.

Heidsieck E.: Neue Beiträge zur Frage der Grenze zwischen Schädel und Wirbel-säule beim Menschen. *Anat. Anz.* 72:113–163, 1931.

Henderson W. R.: A note on the relationship of the human maxillary nerve to the cavernous sinus and to an emissary sinus passing through the foramen ovale. *J. Anat.* 100:905–908, 1966.

Hodes P. J., Pendergrass E. P., Dennis J. M.: Cerebellopontine angle tumors: Roentgenologic manifestations. *Radiology* 57:395–406, 1951.

Hodes P. J., Pendergrass E. P., Young B. R.: Eighth nerve tumors: Their roentgen manifestations. *Radiology* 53:633–665, 1949.

Holman C. B., Miller W. E.: Juvenile nasopharyngeal fibroma: Roentgenologic characteristics. *Am. J. Roentgenol.* 94:292–298, 1965.

Holman C. B., Olive I., Svien H. J.: Roentgenologic features of neurofibroma involving the gasserian ganglion. *Am. J. Roentgenol.* 86:148–153, 1961.

Jefferson G.: Radiography of the optic canals. *Proc. R. Soc. Lond.* 29:1169–1172, 1936.

Jefferson G.: On the saccular aneurysms of the internal carotid artery in the cavernous sinus. *Br. J. Surg.* 26:267–302, 1938.

Keyes J. E. L.: Observations on 4,000 optic foramina in human skulls of known origin. *Arch. Ophthalmal.* 13:538–568, 1935.

Khoo F. Y.: Giant jugular fossa with brief notes on the anatomical variations of the jugular fossa. *Am. J. Roentgenol.* 55:333–336, 1946.

Kirdani M. A.: The normal hypoglossal canal. *Am. J. Roentgenol.* 99:700–704, 1967.

Kollman J.: Varieten am os occipitale, besonders in der Umgebung des Foramen magnum. *Anat. Anz.* 27 (suppl.):231–236, 1905.

Kornblum K., Kennedy G. R.: The sphenoidal fissure: Anatomical, roentgenological and clinical study. *Am. J. Roentgenol.* 47:845–858, 1942.

List C. F.: Neurologic syndromes accompanying developmental anomalies of occipital bone: Atlas and axis. *Arch. Neurol. Psychiat.* 45:577–616, 1941.

McRae D. L., Barnum A. S.: Occipitalization of the atlas. *Am. J. Roentgenol.* 70:23–46, 1953.

O'Rahilly R., Twohig M. J.: Foramina parietalia permagna. *Am. J. Roentgenol.* 67:551–561, 1952.

Osborn A. G.: Radiology of the pterygoid plates and ptery-gopalatine fossa. *Am. J. Roentgenol.* 132:389–394, 1979.

Pancoast H. K.: Roentgen diagnostic significance of erosion of optic canals in study of intracranial tumors. *Ann. Surg.* 101:246–255, 1935.

Pancoast H. K.: Significance of petrous ridge deformation in roentgen-ray diagnosis and localization of brain tumors. *Am. J. Roentgenol.* 20:201–208, 1928.

Pendergrass E. P., Pepper O. H. P.: Observations on the pro-cess of ossification in the formation of persistent enlarged parietal foramina. *Am. J. Roentgenol.* 41:343–346, 1939.

Pepper O. H. P., Pendergrass P.: Hereditary occurrence of enlarged parietal foramina: Their diagnostic importance. *Am. J. Roentgenol.* 35:1–8, 1936.

Potter G. D.: The pterygopalatine fossa and canal. *Am. J. Roentgenol.* 107:520–525, 1969.

Priman J., Etter L. E.: Pterygospinous and pterygoalar bars. *Med. Radiogr. Photogr.* 35:2–6, 1959.

Radoïévitch S., Jovanovitch S.: La morphologie du canal Vi-dien et ses rapports avec les sinus paranasaux chez l'homme adulte et l'enfant. *Rev. Laryngol.* 76:481–492, 1955.

Radoïévitch S., Jovanovitch S., Lotritch N.: La morphologie du trou ovale et les rapports du nerf maxillaire inférieur avec le sinus sphenoidal. *Rev. Laryngol.* 77:11–19, 1956.

Renander A.: Anomalies roentgenologically observed of cran-iovertebral region. *Acta Radiol.* 10:502–513, 1929.

Rice R. P., Holman C. B.: Roentgenographic manifestations of tumors of the glomus jugulare (chemodectoma). *Am. J. Roentgenol.* 89:1201–1208, 1963.

Rischbieth R. H. C., Bull J. W. D.: The significance of en-largement of the superior orbital (sphenoidal) fissure. *Br. J. Radiol.* 31:125–135, 1958.

Schaaf J.: Die röntgenologische Darstellung des Foramen rotundum (canalis rotundus). *Fortschr. Roentgenstr.* 86:102–104, 1957.

Schmidt H., Driesen W.: Einseitige Erweiterung eines Fora-men ovale des Schädels. *Fortschr. Roentgenstr.* 86:508–511, 1957.

Schwartz C. W.: Tumors of the acoustic nerve from a roent-genological viewpoint. *Am. J. Roentgenol.* 47:703–710, 1942.

Shapiro R.: Compartmentation of the jugular foramen. *J. Neu-rosurg.* 36:340–343, 1972.

Shapiro R., Robinson F.: The foramina of the middle fossa: A phylogenetic, anatomic and pathologic study. *Am. J. Roent-genol.* 101:779–794, 1967.

Shapiro R., Robinson F.: Alterations of the sphenoidal fissure produced by local and systemic processes. *Am. J. Roent-genol.* 101:814–827, 1967.

Sondheimer F. K.: Basal foramina and canals, in Newton T. H., Potts D. G. (eds.): *The Skull.* Book 1: *Radiology of the Skull and Brain,* vol. 1. St. Louis, C. V. Mosby Co., 1971.

Sperino, quoted by LeDouble A.: *Traité des os du crane de l'homme.* Paris, Vigot Frères, 1903.

Strickler J. M.: New and simple techniques for demonstra-tion of the jugular foramen. *Am. J. Roentgenol.* 97:601–606, 1966.

Taylor F. R.: Hereditary enlargement of the parietal foramina. *Oxford Medicine* 5:1125–1126, 1940.

Towne E. B.: Erosion of the petrous bone by acoustic nerve tumor: Demonstration by roentgen ray. *Arch. Otolaryngol.* 4:515–519, 1926.

Travers J. T., Wormely L. E.: Enlarged parietal foramina. *Am. J. Roentgenol.* 40:571–579, 1938.

Valvassori G. E., Kirdani M. A.: The abnormal hypoglossal canal. *Am. J. Roentgenol.* 99:705–711, 1967.

Van Brücke H.: Über die Röntgendarstellung der Foramen Ovale. *Roentgenpraxis* 6:603, 1934.

Van der Hoeve J.: Roentgenography of optic foramen in tu-mors and diseases of optic nerve. *Am. J. Ophthalmol.* 8:101–112, 1925.

Wardwell G. A., Goree J. A., Jiminez J. P.: The hypoglossal artery and hypoglossal canal. *Am. J. Roentgenol.* 118:528–533, 1973.

White L. E.: An anatomical x-ray study of the optic canal in cases of optic nerve involvement. *Ann. Otol. Rhinol. Laryn-gol.* 33:121–140, 1924.

9

Vascular Supply to the Skull and Intracranial Structures

The skull and contents receive their blood from three principal sources:
I. Intracranial circulation
  A. Brain
    1. Arterial blood is carried to the brain by
      a. the internal carotid arteries
      b. the vertebral and basilar arteries
    2. The venous drainage consists of various cerebral and cerebellar veins and the dural sinuses. Since the latter are enclosed within dural reflections, they will be considered under meningeal vessels.
  B. Meninges
      The principal vessels of the meningeal system are the middle meningeal artery and its accompanying veins. In addition, branches of the ethmoidal, pharyngeal, and occipital arteries supply large portions of the meninges.
    1. Middle meningeal artery
    2. Meningeal veins
    3. Lacunae laterales
    4. Dural sinuses
II. Cranial (osseous) circulation
    The diploic veins are essentially nutrient vessels for the cancellous tissue of the calvaria.
III. Superficial (scalp) circulation
  A. The external carotid artery and superficial veins supply the superficial soft tissues, dura, and bone.
  B. The emissary veins link the blood supply of the scalp with the dural sinuses.
Although the inner and outer tables of the skull vault are grooved by arteries and veins, most of the vascular channels visualized are venous. There is a marked variability in the pattern of the radiolucent vascular channels seen in the normal skull. Whereas some skulls have only a few vascular markings, others are literally studded. The markings are not always bilateral or symmetric. At times, the prominence of the pattern, particularly in a vascular diploic skull, may be so striking as to suggest a vascular anomaly or neoplasm to the inexperienced. As a general rule, one should not be impressed by the number and size of the venous channels in the absence of a concomitant increase in number, size, or tortuosity of arterial channels. The presence of a concomitant increase is usually indicative of a meningioma or a vascular malformation. However, similar findings may be present in fibrous dysplasia and Paget's disease. Rarely, enlarged veins close to the midline are a clue to the presence of a falx meningioma that has occluded the superior sagittal sinus.

The principal arterial grooves in the inner table are produced by the anterior and posterior branches of the middle meningeal artery. Unlike veins, these structures are usually symmetric. As a rule, the arterial grooves tend to be straight, taper progressively, and branch dichotomously as they course peripherally toward the vertex of the skull. This is in contrast to venous grooves, which tend to be somewhat wider, relatively uniform in caliber, and more sinuous in their course. Often, the grooves for the middle meningeal arteries contain one or more accompanying meningeal veins. If the latter are large, the common vascular channel may be more venous than arterial in character. Diploic veins can be distinguished from superficial cerebral or meningeal veins because they are multidirectional and in direct contact with the bony trabeculae. Hence, they appear to lie within the bone without a sharp bone-vascular interface. On the other hand, the superficial cerebral and meningeal veins have a fixed direction, and are more or less surrounded by a bony shell that projects as a thin, white line around the vessel.

160

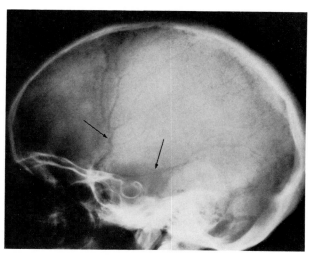

Fig 258.—Lateral roentgenogram showing grooves for anterior and posterior branches of middle meningeal artery *(arrows).*

more, fracture lines tend to be more radiolucent and more sharply defined than vascular channels.

The middle meningeal artery does not supply the medial portion of the anterior and middle fossae nor a great part of the posterior fossa. These areas are supplied by a number of smaller branches of the occipital, ascending pharyngeal, and ethmoidal arteries. However, the grooves for these minor meningeal vessels are normally too shallow and small to be recognized on the roentgenogram.

The meningeal arterial and venous channels may undergo striking enlargement and increased tortuosity in meningiomas and extensive cerebrovascular malformations.

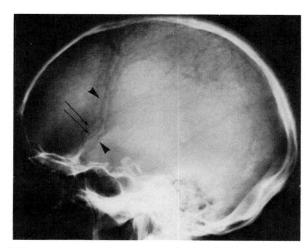

Fig 259.—Lateral roentgenogram demonstrating bilateral grooves for middle meningeal artery *(arrows)* and sphenoparietal sinus *(arrowheads).*

MENINGEAL VEINS

The meningeal veins that accompany the meningeal arteries are usually fairly small. Occasionally, however, the vein or veins accompanying the anterior branch of the middle meningeal artery may be larger than the artery. They may lie in a deep groove that passes up toward the vertex from their origin in the region of the lesser sphenoidal wing. These veins may be unilateral or bilateral, are commonly uniform in width, and may be bridged by bone for a varying distance, but unlike the artery do not branch dichotomously. As the veins approach the sagittal suture, they tend to become funnel-shaped before emptying into a lateral lacuna.

LACUNAE LATERALES (Fig 260)

The superior cortical veins empty directly into the superior sagittal sinus. On the other hand, the meningeal veins open into the lateral lacunae, which also receive blood from the diploic and emissary veins. The lacunae are essentially lateral projections of the lumen of the superior sagittal sinus between the two layers of dura. They are absent at birth, and the exact time of their development is not known. However, they increase in size with advancing years until the original series of cavities has been replaced by one or more lacunae on each side of the superior sagittal sinus. Sargent has described three such lacunae on either side of the midline: frontal, parietal, and occipital lacunae. The floor of the lacuna is almost entirely carpeted by pacchionian bodies, except for that portion traversed by the cerebral cortical veins on their way to the superior sagittal sinus.

The pacchionian bodies (arachnoidal granulations, or villi) are absent at birth and appear at approximately 18 months. They gradually increase in number, size, and extent with advancing years. They are most numerous in the region of the superior sagittal sinus. While a few villi project directly into the superior sagittal and other dural sinuses, the vast majority lie on the floor of the lateral lacunae. According to Key and Retzius, pacchionian bodies have also been found in relationship to the transverse sinus, cavernous sinus, superior petrosal sinus, and middle meningeal vein. Le Gros Clark has reported finding them in connection with the sphenoparietal and straight sinuses as well.

The pacchionian bodies are directly attached to the undersurface of the dura. Histologically, they appear as diverticulae of the subarachnoid space penetrating into

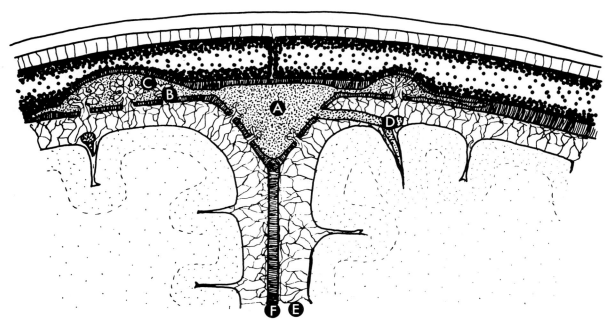

Fig 260.—Diagram showing relationship of cerebral and meningeal veins to lacunae laterales and superior sagittal sinus. Note superior sagittal sinus *(A)*; pacchionian granulation *(B)*; lacuna lateralis *(C)*; superior cerebral vein *(D)*; subarachnoid space *(E)*; and falx cerebri *(F)*.

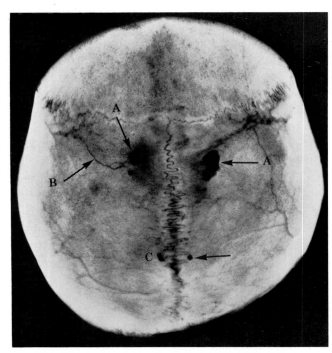

Fig 261.—Vertex of dry skull specimen demonstrating depressions produced by pacchionian bodies *(A)*. Meningeal vascular grooves *(B)* and parietal emissary foramina *(C)* are also shown.

the interstices of the dura, and are covered by a single layer of arachnoidal mesothelial cells. Occasionally, there is a small capillary in the cavity of the villus, and a capillary may also be seen leaving the villus on its way to the dura. In adults, small calcareous nodules may be found in the arachnoidal villi, but these are seldom recognized on the roentgenogram.

Roentgenologically, the pacchionian bodies and the lacunae in which they lie manifest themselves as irregularly rounded, sharply defined radiolucent depressions in the inner table of the skull (Figs 260 to 267). They are most frequently recognized just lateral to the superior sagittal sinus, although clusters are commonly seen in the occipital bone lateral to the midline. When they are located in relationship to other dural sinuses and are unusually numerous, they may be confused with areas of bone destruction resulting from conditions such as metastatic carcinoma and multiple myeloma. The differential diagnosis is simplified when a vascular channel leads directly to the radiolucency in question. At times, the pacchionian granulations may erode into and bulge the thinned outer table. Tangential views clearly show a smooth, funnel-shaped erosion widest at the inner table, which clearly indicates a benign process arising within the skull.

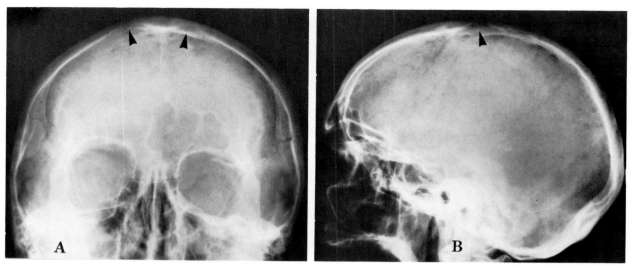

Fig 262.—Caldwell **(A)** and lateral **(B)** projections showing typical parasagittal pacchionian granulations with erosion of inner table *(arrowheads)*.

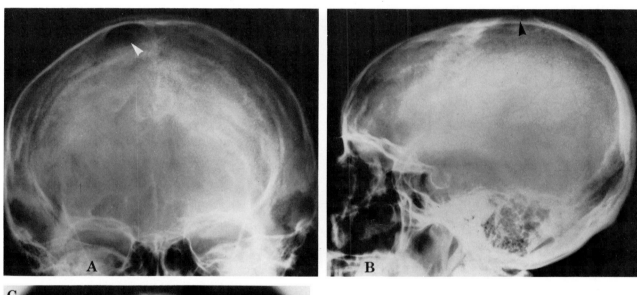

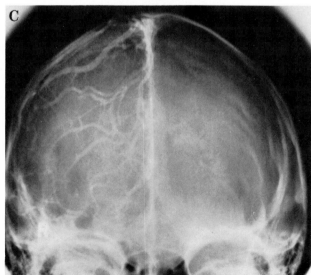

Fig 263.—Posteroanterior **(A)** and lateral **(B)** plain radiographs and anteroposterior angiogram in venous phase **(C)** in a 27-year-old male graduate student with palpable mass in right parasagittal area. Note marked erosion of inner table and diploë and the blistering outward of thinned outer table *(arrowheads)*. Note also the superficial cortical veins, lateral lacuna and superior sagittal sinus on the venogram, proving that bone defect is due to pacchionian granulation.

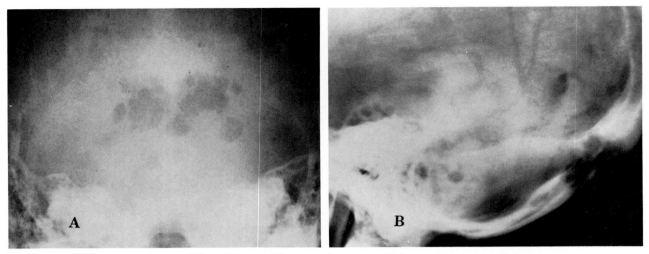

Fig 264.—Towne **(A)** and lateral **(B)** views showing multiple varying sized radiolucencies below transverse sinuses. Lateral view demonstrates erosion of all three tables of occipital bone.

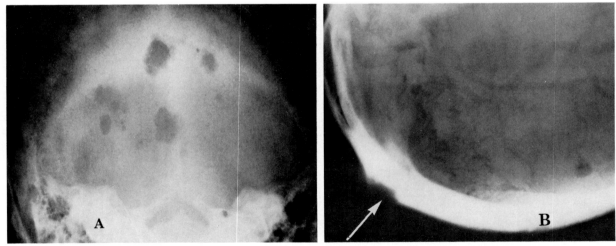

Fig 265.—Towne **(A)** and lateral **(B)** projections showing multiple pacchionian granulations in occipital bone with blistering *(arrow)* of outer table.

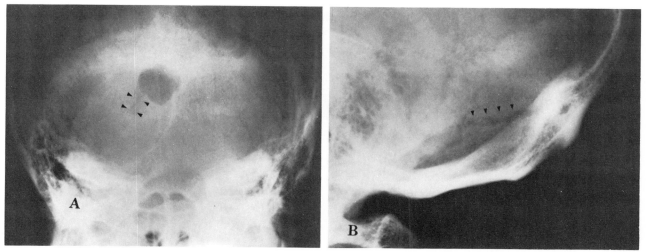

Fig 266.—Towne **(A)** and lateral **(B)** projections showing a single, large, somewhat lobulated midline occipital pacchionian granulation with an associated vascular channel *(arrowheads)*.

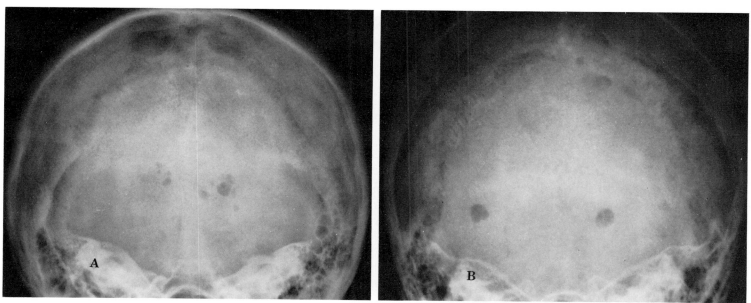

Fig 267.—Towne view in two different patients (**A** and **B**) demonstrating varying occipital radiolucencies produced by pacchionian granulations. Note distance from midline of right-sided radiolucency in **B**.

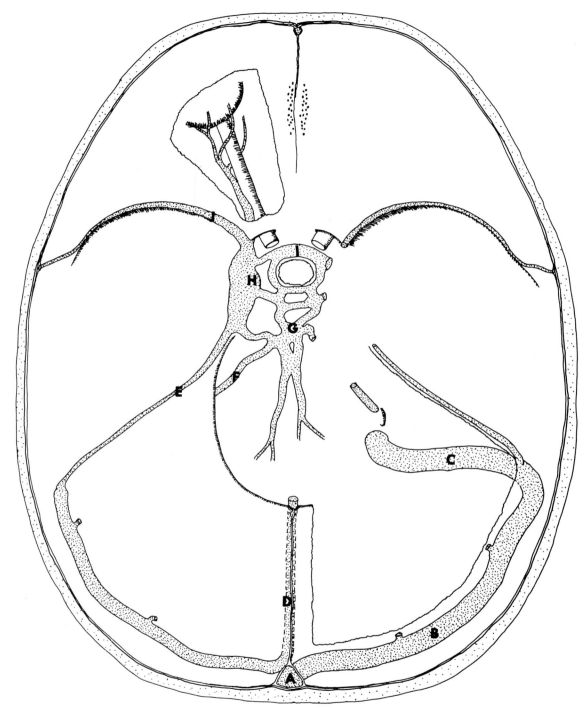

Fig 268.—Interior of skull showing the dural sinuses. Torcular Herophili *(A)*; lateral sinus *(B)*; sigmoid sinus *(C)*; straight sinus *(D)*; superior petrosal sinus *(E)*; inferior petrosal sinus *(F)*; basilar plexus *(G)*; cavernous sinus *(H)*; circular sinus *(I)*; and sphenoparietal sinus *(J)*, the lateral extension of which is commonly seen coursing up inner aspect of frontal bone anterior to middle meningeal artery groove.

DURAL SINUSES (Figs 268 and 269)

The dural sinuses are large, endothelial-lined, vascular channels that drain the veins of the brain, the orbits, and the emissary veins of the scalp. They lie between the two layers of the dura and, in turn, drain directly or indirectly into the internal jugular vein. Only the superior sagittal, sphenoparietal, transverse, and sigmoid sinuses have roentgenologically visible bone grooves that appear as broad, straight, or slightly curved rarefactions in the inner table. However, a brief description of all the dural sinuses is included for the sake of completeness and clarity.

Some of the cranial sinuses are paired, while others are unpaired. The unpaired sinuses are the superior and inferior sagittal, the straight, the basilar, and the anterior and posterior intercavernous. There are six paired sinuses: the transverse, occipital, sphenoparietal, cavernous, and superior and inferior petrosal.

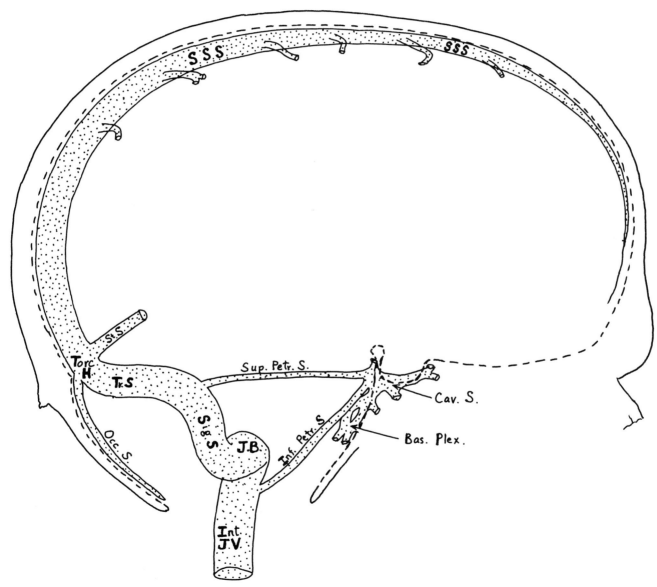

Fig 269.—Hemicranium in the lateral view showing dural sinuses: Superior sagittal sinus *(S.S.S.)*; torcular Herophili *(Torc. H.)*; transverse sinus (Tr. S.); sigmoid sinus (Sig. S.); jugular bulb *(J.B.)*; internal jugular vein *(Int. J. V.)*; straight sinus *(St.S.)*; occipital sinus *(Occ.S.)*; superior petrosal sinus *(Sup. Petr. S.)*; inferior petrosal sinus *(Inf. Petr. S.)*; cavernous sinus *(Cav. S.)*; and basilar plexus *(Bas. Plex.)*. Sphenoparietal sinus (not shown) usually extends from cavernous sinus to large lacuna lateralis near, but not directly into, superior sagittal sinus.

UNPAIRED SINUSES

SUPERIOR SAGITTAL (SUPERIOR LONGITUDINAL) SINUS.—The sinus begins in the anterior fossa near the foramen caecum, through which it communicates with the veins of the nasal cavity. The sinus extends posteriorly within the dorsally attached margin of the falx cerebri, grooving the frontal, parietal, and superior portions of the occipital bones. It terminates in the torcular Herophili, where it bends laterally to continue as one of the transverse sinuses. Although the superior sagittal sinus usually descends slightly to the right to terminate in the right transverse sinus, it may course to the left and end in the left transverse sinus. Occasionally, the superior sagittal sinus bifurcates and ends in both transverse sinuses (Figs 270 and 271).

The superior cerebral veins and the lacunae laterales are the main tributaries of the superior sagittal sinus. However, the superior sagittal sinus also communicates with the veins of the scalp through various emissary veins. The diploic veins may open into the superior sagittal sinus, although their principal drainage is into the lacunae laterales.

INFERIOR SAGITTAL (INFERIOR LONGITUDINAL) SINUS.—This sinus runs in the posterior half of the free margin of the falx cerebri to terminate in the straight sinus. Rarely, calcification in the walls of the inferior sagittal sinus may identify its position on the conventional roentgenogram.

STRAIGHT SINUS (SINUS RECTUS).—The straight sinus is formed by the union of the inferior sagittal sinus with the great cerebral Galen's vein. It lies in the median sagittal plane along the line of junction of the falx cerebri and the tentorium. It increases in caliber as it passes back to terminate in the transverse sinus opposite to that in which the superior sagittal sinus ends.

BASILAR PLEXUS.—The basilar plexus, which lies on the basiocciput, connects both inferior petrosal sinuses and anastomoses with the anterior spinal veins.

ANTERIOR INTERCAVERNOUS SINUS.—The anterior intercavernous sinus is a small channel connecting both cavernous sinuses in front of the hypophysis.

POSTERIOR INTERCAVERNOUS SINUS.—The posterior intercavernous sinus is a similar vessel connecting the cavernous sinuses behind the hypophysis. The anterior and posterior intercavernous sinuses and the cavernous sinuses are collectively termed the circular sinus.

PAIRED SINUSES

TRANSVERSE (LATERAL) SINUS.—The large transverse sinuses begin at the internal occipital protuberance, the right usually as the extension of the superior sagittal sinus, and the left as the continuation of the straight sinus. They curve laterally and forward to the base of the petrous bone, where they lie in the attached margin of the tentorium. They then leave the tentorium and

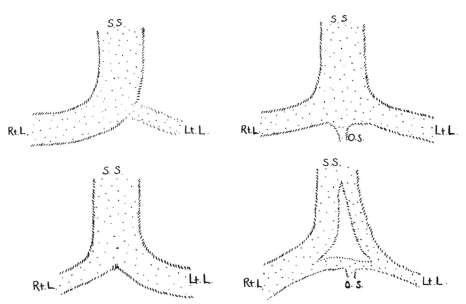

Fig 270.—Common normal variations of torcular Herophili. Note superior sagittal sinus (S. S.); right lateral (transverse) sinus (Rt. L.); left lateral sinus (Lt. L.); and the inconstant occipital sinus (O. S.).

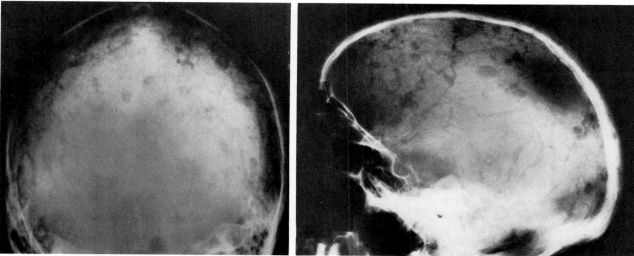

Fig 278.—Bilateral prominent diploic veins and lakes in skull of elderly woman who also has bilateral symmetric parietal thinning. There was no change in the appearance of the skull over a period of five years.

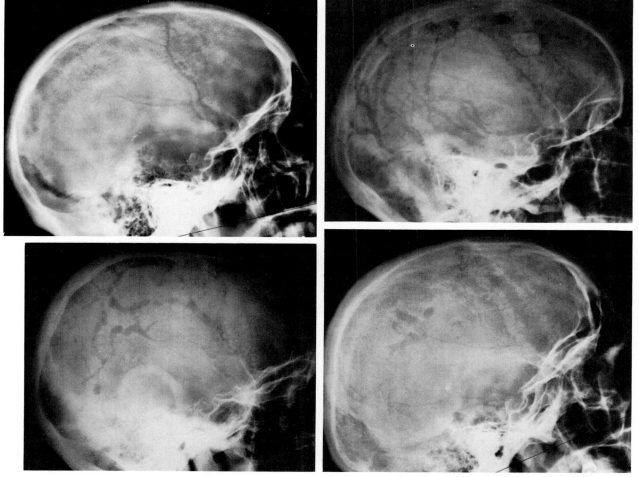

Fig 279.—Variations in appearance of diploic veins. Paucity *(top left);* a middle temporal arterial groove is also demonstrable. Rich diploic network *(top right).* Scattered diploic channels *(bottom left).* Localized, spiderlike parietal diploic veins *(bottom right).*

course of the diploic veins. A favorite site for this formation is the posterior parietal region, where the diploic veins frequently present a stellate, spidery configuration. The lakes usually do not exceed 2 cm in diameter. A common problem confronting the radiologist is the differentiation of a diploic venous lake from an osteolytic metastasis. The presence of a vascular channel draining into the lake, or a well-defined, albeit irregular, outline helps to distinguish the venous lake from the "moth-eaten," isolated metastatic focus. Tangential views may confirm the intradiploic location with intact inner and outer tables. However, even the experienced observer may have difficulty in differentiating multiple small lakes from multiple myeloma or metastatic tumor.

SUPERFICIAL CIRCULATION

The arterial blood supply to the soft parts of the skull is furnished by various branches of the external carotid artery. The superficial soft tissues of the head and face are drained by the frontal, supraorbital, angular, anterior and posterior facial, superficial temporal, internal maxillary, posterior auricular, and occipital veins. Since most of the large superficial vessels are external to the galea, they do not groove the outer table of the skull. There are, however, four exceptions worthy of note:

1. The deep groove for the occipital artery medial to the mastoid process is demonstrable roentgenologically.

2. More important is the middle temporal branch of the superficial temporal artery, which crosses the zygoma to pierce the temporal fascia and anastomose with the deep temporal branches of the internal maxillary artery. In its course it produces a vertical or semivertical groove on the external surface of the temporal squamosa unilaterally or bilaterally (Figs 280 to 282).

3. Anterior to the groove for the middle temporal artery, one may rarely find two other vascular grooves on the external surface of the temporal squamosa. These are for the anterior and posterior deep temporal arteries, which are branches of the second, or pterygoid, portion of the internal maxillary artery. Both deep temporal arteries arise in the region of the infratemporal fossa and course vertically upward beneath the temporalis muscle.

4. Occasionally, a branch of the middle meningeal artery grooves the inner surface of the temporal squamosa

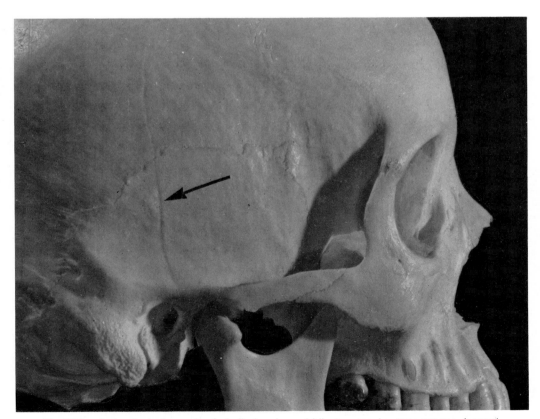

Fig 280.—Lateral photograph of skull showing middle temporal artery groove *(arrow).*

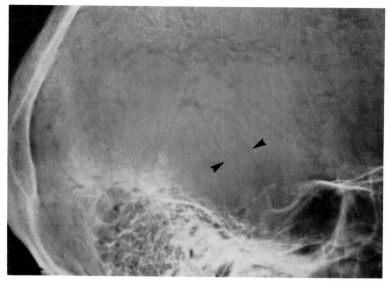

Fig 281.—Bilateral middle temporal artery grooves *(arrowheads)*.

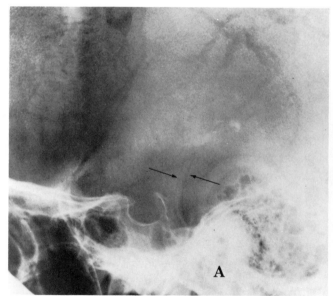

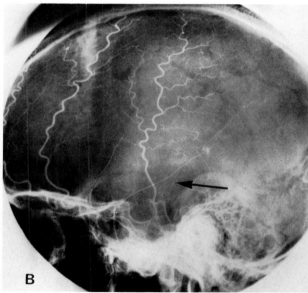

Fig 282.—Bilateral middle temporal artery grooves *(arrows)* shown on plain film **(A)**. Opacified right middle temporal artery can be seen lying in its vascular groove on selective right external carotid arteriogram **(B)**.

more posteriorly than usual. This vessel courses superiorly and caudad for approximately 4 to 5 cm in a shallow groove in the bone before entering the diploë, where it eventually loses its identity. The supraorbital artery may also groove the outer table of the vertical plate of the frontal bone on one or both sides (Fig 283).

When unilateral, any of these vascular grooves may readily be confused with a linear fracture of the skull (Fig 284). In general, the burden of proof is on the observer who calls one of these radiolucencies a fracture. In cases of trauma, the differential diagnosis may be extremely difficult or impossible. However, a new fracture line tends to be black and a vascular groove gray. Stereoscopy is often helpful in localizing the radiolucency to the inner or outer table.

The emissary veins link the dural sinuses with the veins of the scalp. Because they pass through the entire thickness of the skull, the radiolucent shadows cast on the roentgenogram are more pronounced and sharper than those of other vascular channels. The following are the most constant emissary vessels:

1. The mastoid emissary vein courses through the mastoid foramen to join the sigmoid sinus with the posterior auricular or occipital vein (Fig 285).

2. The parietal emissary vein passes through the parietal foramen and connects the superior sagittal sinus with the veins of the scalp. It passes through a small aperture in the superior, posterior, and medial portions of the parietal bone. Rarely, an inferior parietal emis-

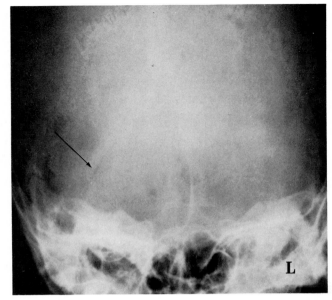

Fig 284.—Towne view of patient with fracture of right occipital bone *(arrow)*. Since there is no normal arterial groove in this area, the diagnosis of fracture should present no problem. In the frontal and temporal bones, however, it may at times be difficult to differentiate a fracture from an arterial groove.

sary vein is present, which passes through an inferior parietal foramen. It empties into the sigmoid sinus posterior to the mastoid process.

3. An occipital emissary vein is inconstantly present. It passes through the occipital protuberance, to join the confluence of sinuses with one of the occipital veins. In

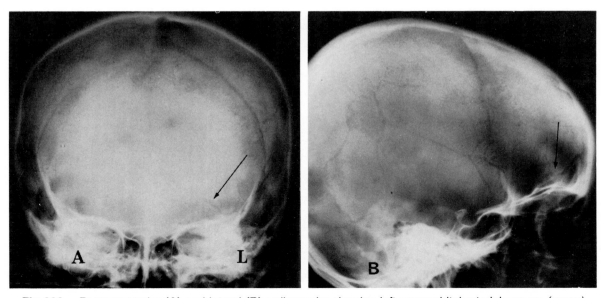

Fig 283.—Posteroanterior **(A)** and lateral **(B)** radiographs showing left supraorbital arterial groove *(arrow)*.

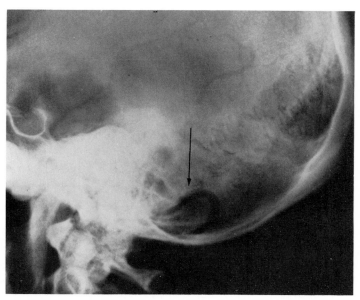

Fig 285.—Characteristic sinuous course of mastoid emissary vein *(arrow)*.

traversing the occipital bone, it communicates with the occipital diploic vein. Its foramen must be differentiated from the bony aperture that transmits the stalk connecting the rare posterior fossa dermoid cyst with its subcutaneous component. The constant midline position and larger size of the dermoid may permit a correct differential diagnosis.

4. When condyloid canals are present in the occipital bone, they are traversed by a condyloid emissary vein. The latter connects the corresponding transverse sinus with the deep veins of the neck.

5. Occasionally, a frontal emissary vein passes from the anterior end of the superior sagittal sinus through the foramen caecum to terminate in the veins of the nasal cavity or the angular vein.

6. Plexus of the hypoglossal canal: a network of veins traverses the hypoglossal canal to unite the homolateral transverse sinus with the vertebral veins and deep neck veins.

7. Emissary plexus of the foramen ovale: this plexus unites the cavernous sinus with the corresponding pterygoid plexus through the foramen ovale. Occasionally, the plexus of the foramen ovale is replaced or supplemented by an emissary vein passing through the foramen of Vesalius.

8. Two or more small veins course through the foramen lacerum to connect the cavernous sinus with the pterygoid plexus.

9. The internal carotid plexus accompanies the internal carotid artery through the carotid canal, connecting the cavernous sinus with the pharyngeal plexus or internal jugular vein.

Rarely, the communication between a dural sinus and the scalp veins may be unusually prominent, resulting in a large vascular pool known as a sinus pericranii. This is characterized by a more or less rounded defect, usually in the frontal or occipital bone close to the midline.

REFERENCES

Allen W. E. III, Kier E. L., Rothman L. E.: The maxillary artery: Normal radiographic anatomy. *Am. J. Roentgenol.* 118:517–527, 1973.

Breschet M. G.: *Recherches anatomiques, physiologiques et pathologiques sur le systeme veineux.* Paris, Villeret, 1829.

Coen B.: A communication as to the causation of large vascular grooves found on the inner aspect of the os parietale. *J. Anat. Physiol.* 48:293, 1914.

Ecker A.: *Normal Cerebral Arteriogram.* Springfield, Ill., Charles C Thomas, Publisher, 1951.

Ellsberg C., Schwartz C. W.: Increased cranial vascularity in its relation to intracranial disease. *Arch. Neurol. Psychiat.* 11:292–307, 1924.

Ersner M. S., Myers D.: An aid to interpretation of intracranial complications resulting from venous circulatory disturbance of the temporal bone: Offered by x-ray of the lateral sinus and jugular foramen. *Laryngoscope* 45:800–818, 1933.

Gathier J. C., Bruyn G. W.: The so-called condyloid foramen in the half axial view. *Am. J. Roentgenol.* 107:515–519, 1969.

Holmgren B. S.: Radiographic changes produced by intracranial arterio-venous aneurysms. *Acta Psychiatr. Neurol.*, suppl. 46:1946.

Jefferson G., Stewart D.: On the veins of the diploë. *Br. J. Surg.* 16:70–88, 1928–1929.

Knott F. F.: On the cerebral sinuses and their variations. *J. Anat. Physiol.* 16:27–42, 1882.

Kraus L., Werkner D. J.: Anatomische und rontgenologische Untersuchungen uber das Emissarium mastoideum. *Ztschr. Hals-Nasen und Ohrenheilkunde* 25:270–279, 1929–1930.

Krayenbuhl H., Richter H. R.: *Die Zerebrale Arteriographie.* Stuttgart, Georg Thiem, 1952.

Lapayowker M. S., Liebman E. P., Ronis M. L., et al.: Presentation of the internal carotid artery as a tumor of the middle ear. *Radiology* 98:293–297, 1971.

LeGros Clark W. E.: On the pacchionian bodies. *J. Anat.* 55:40–48, 1920–1921.

LeWald L. T.: Dilatation of diploic veins and other anatomical variations in the skull. *Am. J. Roentgenol.* 12:536–542, 1924.

Lima F. A.: *Cerebral Angiography.* London, Oxford University Press, 1950.

Lindblom K.: Roentgenographic study of vascular channels of the skull with special reference to intracranial tumors and arteriovenous aneurysms. *Acta Radiol.*, suppl. 30, 1936, pp. 1–146.

Nishikawa Y.: Über die röntgenographische Darstellung der Venenkanäle des Schädels. *Forschr. Geb. Röntgenstrahlen* 31:598–606, 1923–1924.

O'Connell J. E. A.: Some observations on the cerebral veins. *Brain* 57:484–503, 1934.

Rumbaugh C. L., Potts D. G.: Skull changes associated with intracranial arterio-venous malformations. *Am. J. Roentgenol.* 98:525–534, 1966.

Santagati F.: Roentgenographic anatomy of the vascular grooves and canals of the skull. *Radiol. Med.* 26:317–330, 1939.

Sargent P.: Some points in the anatomy of the intracranial sinuses. *J. Anat. Physiol.* 45:69–72, 1911.

Schüller, A.: Die röntgenographische Darstellung der diploëtischen Venenkanäle des Schädels. *Fortschr. Geb. Röntgenstrahlen* 12:232–235, 1908.

Schultze O.: Über sulci venosi meningei des Schädeldaches. *Z. Morphol. Anthropol.* 1:451–452, 1899.

Schunk H., Maruyama Y.: Two vascular grooves of the external table of the skull which simulate fractures. *Acta Radiol.* 54:186–194, 1960.

Schwartz C. W.: Vascular tumors and anomalies of the skull and brain from a roentgenographic viewpoint. *Am. J. Roentgenol.* 41:881–900, 1939.

Selander E.: The roentgen appearance of the anterior wall of the sulcus sigmoideus. *Acta Radiol.* 27:60–65, 1946.

Shearer W. S.: Cerebral angiography in intracranial vascular anomalies. *J. Fac. Radiologists* 3:242–253, 1952.

Streeter L.: The development of the venous sinuses of the dura mater in the human embryo. *Am. J. Anat.* 18:145–178, 1918.

Thompson I. M.: On certain grooves upon the deep aspect of the cranial vault. *Can. Med. Assoc. J.* 16:1194–1200, 1926.

Waltner J. G.: Anatomic variations of the lateral and sigmoid sinuses. *Arch. Otolaryngol.* 39:307–312, 1944.

Wanke R.: Zur Röntgenkunde der Gefässkandeder Diploë. *Fortschr. Geb. Röntgenstrahlen* 56:286–299, 1937.

Wickbom I.: Angiography of the carotid artery. *Acta Radiol.*, suppl. 72, 1948.

Woodhall B.: Variations of the cranial venous sinuses in the region of the torcular Herophili. *Arch. Surg.* 33:297–314, 1936.

Woodhall B., Seeds A. E.: Cranial venous sinuses: Correlation between skull markings and roentgenograms of the occipital bone. *Arch. Surg.* 33:867–875, 1936.

Woodhall B., Seeds A. E.: Cranial venous sinuses: Correlation between roentgenograms of the occipital bone and the Queckenstedt (Tobey-Ayer) Test. *Arch. Surg.* 37:865–870, 1938.

Yuhl E. T., Schmitz A. L.: The occipital emissary channel and increased intracranial pressure. *Acta Radiol.* 9:124–127, 1969.

10

Sutures

The cranial bones are joined by sutures (L. *sutura,* seam) in which the connecting tissue is a fibrous membrane, or by synchondroses (Gr. *syn,* together, + *chondros,* cartilage) in which the bones are united by a bar of hyaline cartilage. Both articulations are forms of synarthrosis characterized by absence of a joint cavity and a paucity of motion. At birth, the sutures and synchondroses are relatively wide seams. With advancing years, they tend to become obliterated, although this process is by no means uniform.

Normal development of the skull and its sutures depends upon several factors. The primary factor is the structure and growth of the early brain. The dura, in turn, reacts to this stimulus by billowing out from its attachments at the base of the skull in bandlike reflections, which correspond to the recesses of the growing brain. It is likely that the sites of ossification are influenced by the stretch-growth tensile forces in the dura. Ossification begins between the major dural reflections and spreads toward the reflections, leaving the sutures between the areas of ossific activity. Patients with severe congenital structural abnormalities of the brain, e.g., holoprosencephaly (single anterior ventricle), craniopagus, and dicephalus, clearly demonstrate that the sutures are related to the abnormal sites of dural reflection which, in turn, conform to the abnormal brain.

Premature closure of the fonticuli is common in microcephaly. Similarly, congenital cerebral hemiatrophy is associated with underdevelopment of the corresponding half of the skull. Scammon and Dunn have shown that growth of the brain may be graphically plotted as a parabolic curve, with the period of greatest growth occurring during the first two or three years. Since the rate of growth of the calvarium parallels that of the brain, there is only a slight increase in intracranial capacity and head size after age 3. This increase in head size is primarily due to thickening of the tables of the skull and development of the paranasal sinuses and facial bones.

Giblin and Alley demonstrated experimentally that skull growth occurs in two ways: (1) by accretion of bone along the external convex surface with simultaneous resorption from the inner concave surface, and (2) by growth in a lateral direction at the suture edges. Troitzky verified the occurrence of lateral growth of the cranial bones from the suture lines. This experimental observation is substantiated clinically by the absence of bone growth at the margins of a suture following synostosis.

GENERAL PATTERN OF SUTURE CLOSURE

Although closure of the sutures varies considerably in different parts of the skull, there are periodic bursts of activity involving all the sutures. Thus, there is a steady, progressive obliteration of all the sutures between ages 26 and 30, followed by a diminution of activity thereafter. Regardless of the state of fusion reached at that time, the sutures do not continue to close as rapidly after age 30 as they did before. However, minor periods of activity continue even into old age.

Todd and Lyons studied the sutures in a large number of skulls and noted the following patterns (Fig 286):

SAGITTAL SUTURE.—Closure begins at about age 22 in the obeliac portion, spreading to the rest of the suture by the end of the 23d year. There is a gradual increase in sutural fusion at age 26, a sharper rise at age 31, and complete union at age 35.

CORONAL SUTURE.—Closure commences at age 24, with gradual progression to age 26, and a steeper rise to age 29, followed by much slower activity until complete obliteration occurs at age 38.

LAMBDOIDAL SUTURE.—The lambdoidal suture closes

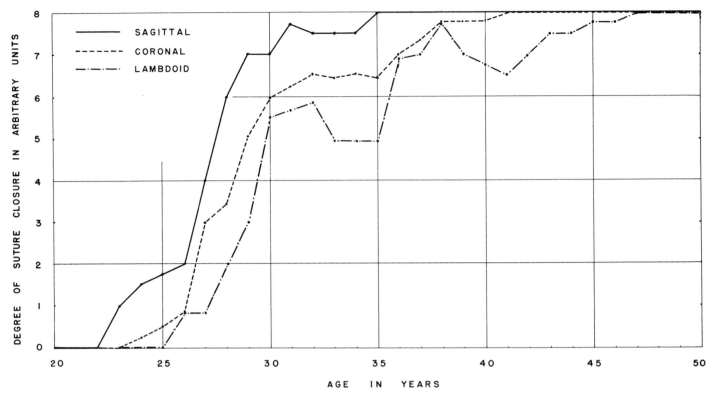

Fig 286.—Endocranial sutural closure patterns in white race stock.
(After Todd and Lyon.)

later than either the sagittal or coronal suture. This delay is appreciable throughout the course of obliteration. Closure begins at age 26, with a sharp rise at age 31, after which closure proceeds slowly to complete union at age 42. The asterionic portion does not completely fuse until age 47.

OCCIPITOMASTOID SUTURE.—This suture may be divided into three parts: the superior, middle, and inferior portions. The superior and middle portions begin to close at age 30, continuing until age 32, when obliteration becomes fairly stationary until age 45. From ages 45 to 64 there is a second burst of activity, followed by another period of relative quiescence, and terminated by a final spurt of activity at age 81. The inferior portion of the occipitomastoid suture begins to fuse at age 26, progressing briskly until age 30, when closure slows down until age 49. Then another slow plateau is reached until age 72, when complete union takes place.

SPHENOTEMPORAL SUTURE.—This suture may be divided into inferior and superior portions. The inferior part begins to unite at age 30 and progresses very slowly until

complete fusion at age 67. Obliteration of the superior part of the sphenotemporal suture commences at age 31. However, further significant union does not occur until age 63, when there is a sudden burst of activity. Beyond age 63 only minor progress is made.

SQUAMOSAL SUTURE.—Slight obliteration begins at age 37 but does not progress significantly until age 62, when there is a period of renewed activity. This is followed by a second period of quiescence until age 79, when further activity sets in, complete union occurring at age 81.

PARIETOMASTOID SUTURE.—Closure of this suture more or less parallels that of the squamosal suture.

SPHENOPARIETAL SUTURE.—Fusion begins at age 29, followed by almost immediate quiescence. There is a second burst of activity in the 50s, progressing steadily to complete union at age 65.

SPHENOFRONTAL SUTURE.—Closure commences at age 22, with a gradual rise in activity at age 26, followed by steeper progress at age 30. This, in turn, is followed by a period of oscillation until final closure at age 65.

INDIVIDUAL VARIATIONS IN CLOSURE

The individual sutures do not always follow the general patterns outlined above. Occasionally, one or more sutures may fuse prematurely (Fig 287). The suture most commonly implicated is the occipitomastoid, which may undergo unilateral or bilateral premature union in about 10% of children before the end of the sixth year. Partial or complete premature closure of the sagittal suture, which occurs in approximately 2.5% of children, tends to produce a scaphocephalic contour (Fig 288). Early partial or complete synostosis of the coronal suture is found less frequently (0.3% in Bolk's series of 1,820 infant skulls studied at the University of Amsterdam) (Figs 289 to 292). Rarer still is complete early fusion of the frontosphenoidal suture (0.2%), of the parietotemporal (squamosal) suture (0.15%), and of the sphenoparietal suture (0.05%). In the same anatomical collection, 1.3% of the skulls exhibited premature obliteration of two or more sutures (Fig 293). Bolk suggests that early physiologic obliteration of the sutures may be an atavistic trait, since the sutures in the ape close as soon as the skull is fully grown.

SCLEROSIS OF SUTURES

Occasionally, there is considerable sclerosis and condensation along various sutures, particularly the sagittal, lambdoidal, and coronal sutures (Figs 294 to 296). Although particularly striking at times, especially in patients with senile osteoporosis, the sclerosis has no known pathologic significance.

ENDOCRANIAL AND ECTOCRANIAL CLOSURE

The sutures begin to close on both the outer and inner aspects of the calvarium at about the same time. However, ectocranial fusion proceeds somewhat more slowly, shows more individual variation, and is generally not as complete as endocranial union. Furthermore, the sutures along the outer table are more or less serrated, while those on the inner table are comparatively straight. When the suture lines of the outer and inner tables do not exactly coincide, a double suture line is produced on the roentgenogram that may simulate a fissure fracture (Fig 297). A good rule of thumb is to refrain from making the diagnosis of a fissure fracture in a suture unless there is significant sutural diastasis (Fig 298). The normal coronal suture should not be mistaken for a fracture in the base view (Fig 299).

Rarely are the sutures of both sides of the skull perfectly superimposed on one another in the lateral projection. Consequently, both sutures may be visualized, one in front of the other. The suture closest to the film is narrower and more sharply defined than its fellow of the opposite side and should not be mistaken for a fracture line.

DELAYED CLOSURE

Occasionally, sutures that normally close early remain open in adult life. This occurs most frequently with the metopic suture, which divides the halves of the frontal bone. Normally, the metopic suture begins to unite toward the end of the first year of life, fusing completely by the end of the second year. However, in approximately 10% of skulls, this suture fails to become obliterated. The extent of persistence of the suture is very variable, e.g., it may be continuous from nasion to bregma (Fig 300), or it may persist only as a small segment anywhere along its course (Fig 301). The metopic suture may deviate slightly to one side and is generally associated with small frontal sinuses (Fig 302), which never extend across the suture line. This finding is helpful in differentiating a midline fracture of the frontal bone from an incompletely closed metopic suture. According to Torgersen, the tendency toward persistent metopism is inherited as a mendelian dominant trait. At times, a short vertical or transverse suture may be found just below the level of the frontal tuberosities, representing a remnant of the metopic fontanelle.

The spheno-occipital synchondrosis may also remain open throughout adult life, although it usually becomes obliterated before age 20 (Fig 303). This should be borne in mind so that an erroneous diagnosis of fracture may be avoided.

DIASTASIS OF SUTURES

It is important to pay attention to the width of the sutures, as sutural diastasis may be the first sign of increased intracranial pressure in children. Because bone growth along the sutural margins varies considerably in children, there are no well-defined criteria for minimal diastasis. Consequently, its early recognition may be most difficult, even for the experienced observer. In this regard also, it is important to have good lateral films, since oblique films may produce a spurious appearance of widened sutures (Fig 304). In borderline cases, serial studies may be helpful in resolving this

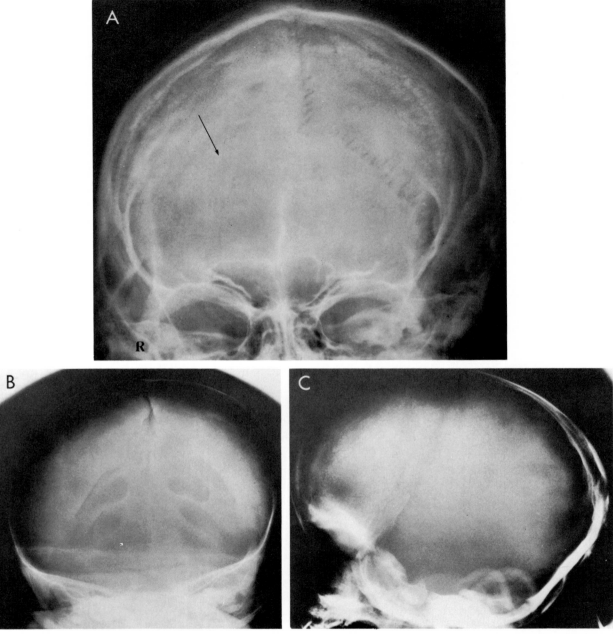

Fig 287.—**A,** posteroanterior projection in an adult demonstrating premature synostosis of the right lambdoidal suture *(arrow)* with slight plagiocephaly. **B,** Towne and **C,** lateral projections in a child with bilateral premature fusion of the lambdoidal sutures.

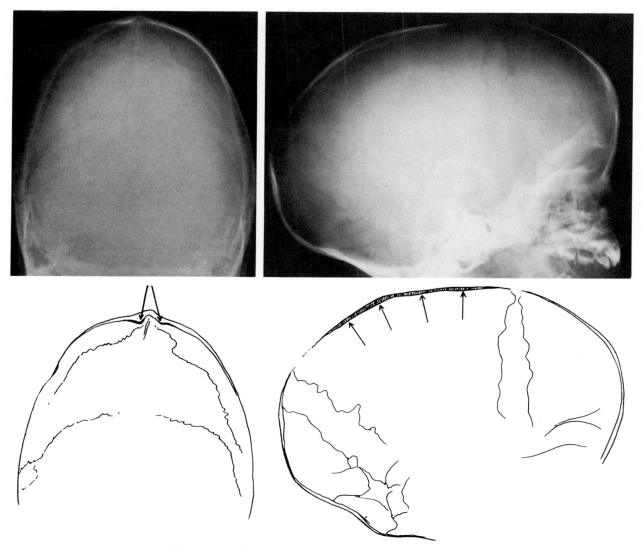

Fig 288.—Premature synostosis of sagittal suture with resultant scaphocephaly. Towne *(left)* and lateral *(right)* views. Elongated or dolichocephalic shape with a sagittal ridge or inverted "keel" is noted. However, characteristic abnormality is partial or complete absence of sagittal suture and inner table ridges *(arrows)* running front to back on either side of sulcus for sagittal sinus. This thickened ridge of bone can also be identified in lateral view but usually does not reach anterior and posterior fonticuli.

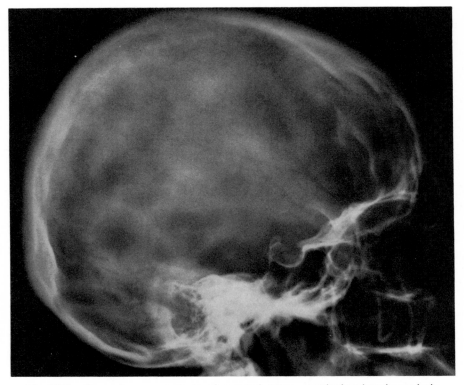

Fig 289.—Premature synostosis of coronal suture producing brachycephaly.

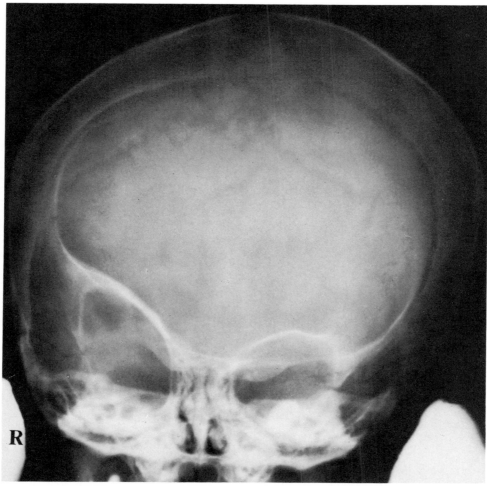

Fig 290.—Unilateral synostosis of right coronal suture with resultant plagiocephaly. Note harlequin appearance of orbit produced by elevated orbital roof and sphenoidal wings. Compare this with postoperative appearance (Fig 292).

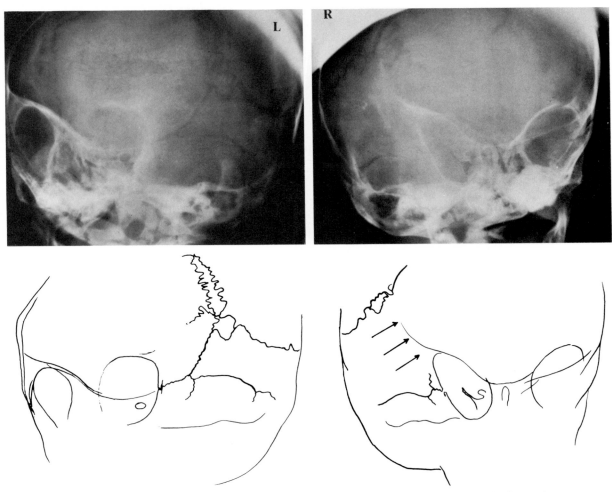

Fig 291.—Optic foramen views of same patient in Figure 290. Sutural absence in the region of pterion *(arrows)* indicates that adjacent sphenoidal suture is also fused.

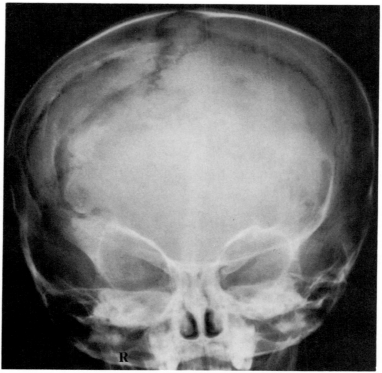

Fig 292.—Same patient as in Figure 290 18 months postoperatively. Frontal bone distortion has disappeared, but some degree of sphenoidal asymmetry persists.

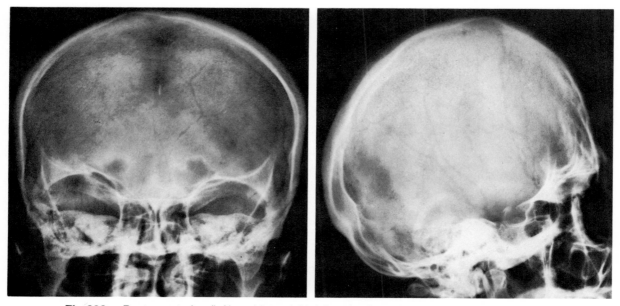

Fig 293.—Posteroanterior *(left)* and lateral *(right)* projections showing premature synostosis of coronal and sagittal sutures resulting in turricephaly. Patient also exhibits hypertelorism.

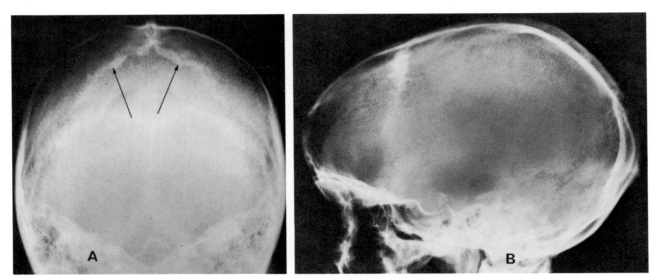

Fig 294.—Towne **(A)** and lateral **(B)** views showing coronal
sutural sclerosis in a normal 32-year-old woman.

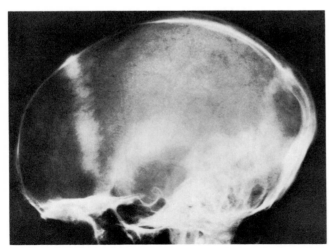

Fig 295.—Marked sclerosis of coronal sutures in a 33-year-old patient.

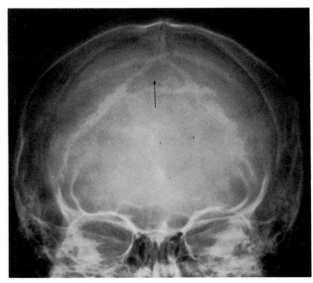

Fig 296.—Condensation (sclerosis) along suture lines. The patient,
a girl aged 14, also has an os incae *(arrow)* along lambdoidal suture.

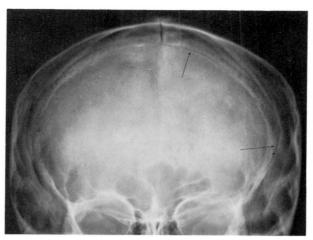

Fig 297.—Double suture line. Note straight endocranial portion *(arrows)*.

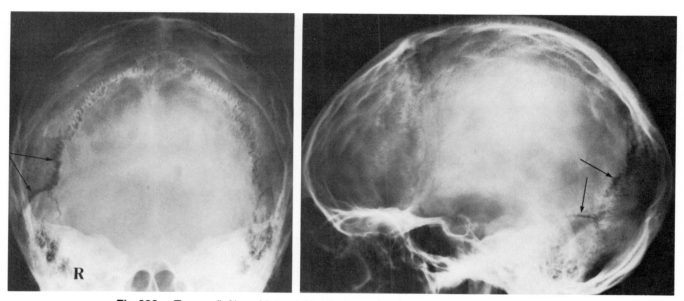

Fig 298.—Towne *(left)* and lateral *(right)* views showing diastasis of parietomastoid and inferior half of lambdoidal suture on right due to fracture *(arrows)*.

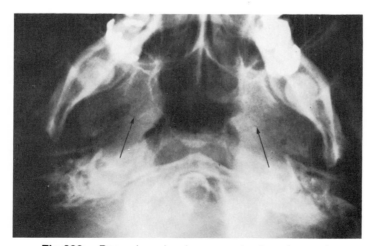

Fig 299.—Base view showing coronal suture *(arrows)*, which should not be confused with a fracture.

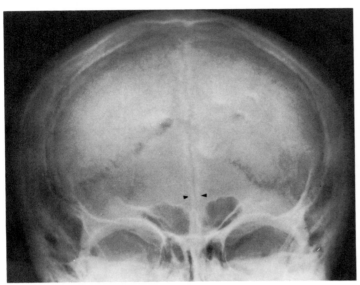

Fig 300.—Persistent metopic suture continuous from nasion to bregma. Note sutural sclerosis *(arrowheads)*.

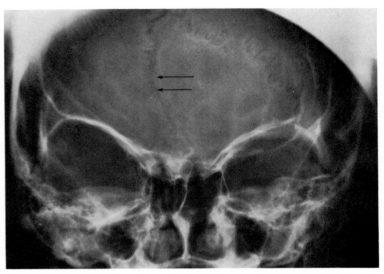

Fig 302.—Asymmetric metopic suture. At its inferior end it breaks up into several divergent sutures before reaching nasofrontal suture. Patient also exhibits hypertelorism.

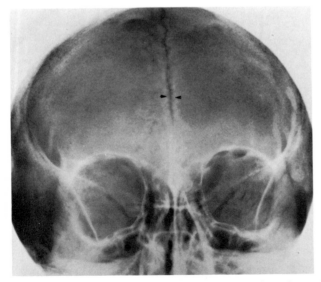

Fig 301.—Partial persistent metopic suture stopping short of nasion *(arrowheads)*.

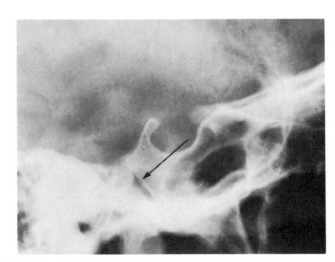

Fig 303.—Persistent spheno-occipital synchondrosis *(arrow)* in an adult.

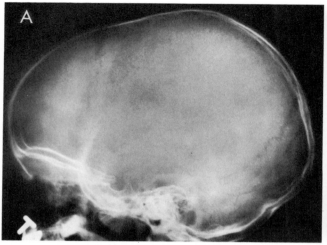

Fig 304.—Lateral roentgenograms in two normal children with long-term follow-up showing spurious widening of lambdoidal sutures **(A)** and of coronal sutures **(B)** due to slight obliquity in positioning of head.

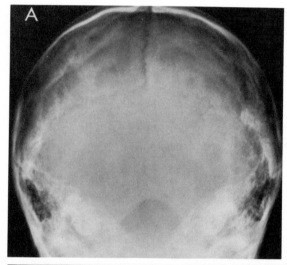

Fig 305.—Towne **(A)** and lateral **(B)** roentgenograms in a child with pontine glioma showing early sutural diastasis. Subtle changes are most evident in sagittal suture. Lateral ventriculogram **(C)** one month later shows obvious progressive diastasis of coronal sutures.

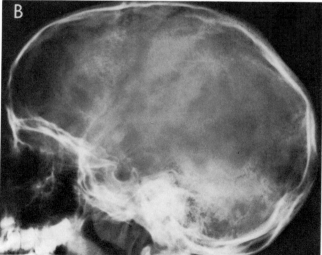

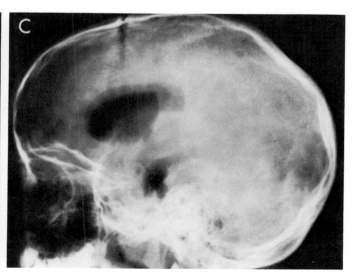

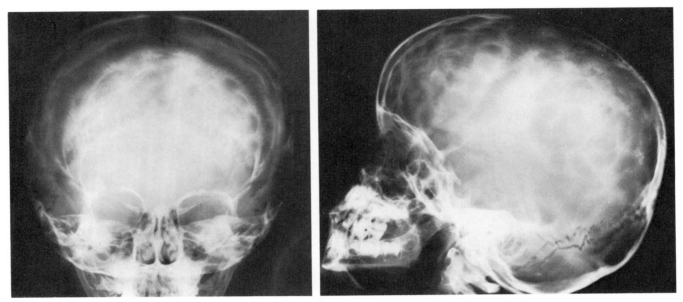

Fig 306.—Chronic increase in intracranial pressure with characteristic
sutural diastasis and increased convolutional markings.

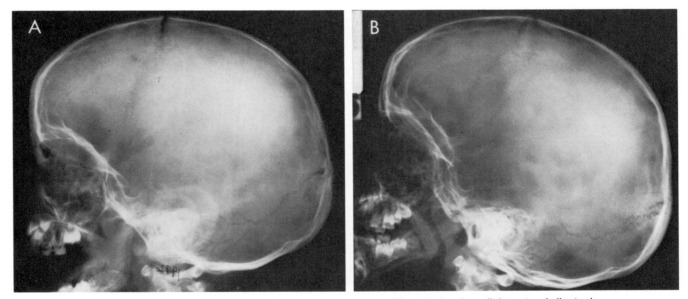

Fig 307.—Serial films in a child with cerebral gigantism (Sotos) showing slight sutural diastasis
over a three-year period. **(A),** 1969, at age 3 years 9 months; **(B),** 1972, at age 6 years.

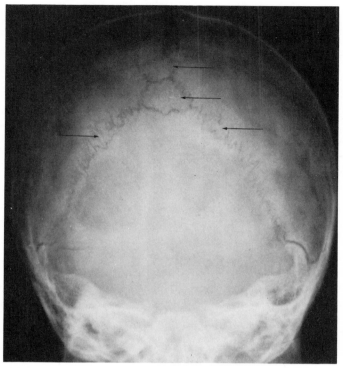

Fig 308.—Wormian bones along lambdoidal suture *(arrows).*

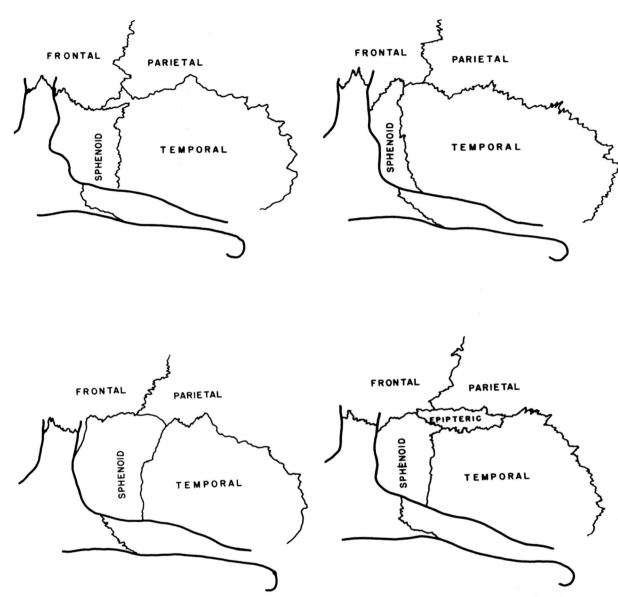

Fig 309.—Epipteric bones. (From Pendergrass, E. P., Schaeffer, J. P., and Hodes, P. J.: *The Head and Neck in Roentgen Diagnosis,* ed. 2. [Springfield, Ill., Charles C Thomas, Publisher, 1956].)

REFERENCES

Acken F.: Die Sutura frontalis im Röntgenbilde. *Fortschr. Geb. Röntgenstrahlen* 48:209–222, 1933.

Ashley-Montagu M. F.: The medio-frontal suture and the problem of metopism in the primates. *J. R. Anthropol. Inst. Great Britain and Ireland* 67:157–201, 1937.

Bass M. H., Caplan J.: Vitamin A deficiency in infancy. *J. Pediatr.* 47:690–695, 1955.

Bolk L.: On the premature obliteration of sutures in the human skull. *Am. J. Anat.* 17:495–523, 1915.

Bolk L.: On metopism. *Am. J. Anat.* 22:27–47, 1917.

Bryce T. H., Young M.: Observations on metopism. *J. Anat.* 51:153–166, 1916–1917.

Capitanio M. A., Kirkpatrick J. A.: Widening of the cranial sutures. *Radiology* 92:53–59, 1969.

Danelius G.: The occasional appearance of both inner and outer suture lines in roentgenograms of the skull simulating fissure fracture. *Am. J. Roentgenol.* 55:315–318, 1946.

DeLevie M., Nogrady M. D.: Rapid brain growth upon restoration of adequate nutrition causing false radiologic evidence of increased intracranial pressure. *J. Pediatr.* 76:523–528, 1970.

DuBoulay G.: The radiological evidence of raised intracranial pressure in children. *Br. J. Radiol.* 30:375–377, 1957.

Eisen D.: Cleidocranial dysostosis. *Radiology* 61:21–31, 1953.

Frederic J.: Untersuchungen über die normale obliteration der Schädelnähte. *Z. Morphol. Anthropol.* 9:373–456, 1906.

Giblin N., Alley A.: A method of measuring bone growth in the skull. *Anat. Rec.* 83:381–387, 1942.

Giblin N., Alley A.: Studies in skull growth: Coronal suture fixation. *Anat. Rec.* 88:143–153, 1944.

Hess L.: The metopic suture and the metopic syndrome. *Hum. Biol.* 17:107–136, 1945.

Hope J. W., Spitz E. B., Slade H. W.: Early recognition of premature cranial synostosis. *Radiology* 65:183–193, 1955.

Ingraham F. D., Alexander E. Jr., Matson D. D.: Clinical studies in craniosynostosis. *Surgery* 24:518–541, 1948.

Inman V. T., Saunders J. B. de C. M.: Ossification of the human frontal bone with specific reference to the presumed pre- and post-frontal elements. *J. Anat.* 71:383–394, 1937.

Irwin G. L.: Roentgen determination of the time of closure of the spheno-occipital synchondrosis. *Radiology* 75:450–452, 1960.

Knudson A. G., Rothman P. E.: Hypervitaminosis A. *Am. J. Dis. Chest* 85:316–334, 1953.

Laursen L.: Cranium bifidum occultum. *Nord. Med.* 14:1160–1161, 1942.

Limson M.: Metopism as found in Filipino skulls. *Am. J. Phys. Anthropol.* 7:317–324, 1924.

McLauren R. L., Matson D. D.: Importance of early surgical treatment of craniosynostosis: Review of 36 cases treated surgically during the first six months of life. *Pediatrics* 10:637–652, 1952.

Moss M. L.: The pathogenesis of premature cranial synostosis in man. *Acta Anat.* 37:351–370, 1959.

Moss M. L., Young R. W.: A functional approach to craniology. *Am. J. Phys. Anthropol.* 18:281–292, 1960.

Moss M. L.: Inhibition and stimulation of sutural fusion in the rat calvaria. *Anat. Rec.* 136:457–468, 1960.

Pendergrass E. P., Hodes P. J.: A mimicry of the turricephalic skull in children treated on a Bradford frame. *Radiology* 31:170–172, 1938.

Schultz A. H.: Metopic fontanelle, fissure and suture. *Am. J. Anat.* 44:475–499, 1929.

Sears H. R.: Some notes on craniostenosis. *Br. J. Radiol.* 10:445–487, 1937.

Shapiro R.: Anomalous parietal sutures and the bipartite parietal bone. *Am. J. Roentgenol.* 115:569–577, 1972.

Shapiro R., Robinson F.: The os incae. *Am. J. Roentgenol.* 127:469–471, 1976.

Simmons D. R., Peyton W. T.: Premature closure of cranial sutures. *J. Pediatr.* 31:528–547, 1947.

Sondheimer F. K., Grossman H., Winchester P.: Suture diastasis following rapid weight gain. *Arch. Neurol.* 23:314–318, 1970.

Soule A. B.: Mutational dysostosis. *J. Bone Joint Surg.* 28:81–102, 1946.

Terrafranco R. J., Zellis A.: Congenital hereditary cranium bifidum occultum frontalis. *Radiology* 61:60–66, 1953.

Todd T. W., Lyon D. W. Jr.: Endocranial suture closure. *Am. J. Phys. Anthropol.* 7:325–384, 1924.

Todd T. W., Lyon D. W. Jr.: Ectocranial closure in adult males of white stock. *Am. J. Phys. Anthropol.* 8:23–71, 1925.

Torgersen J.: Roentgenological study of the metopic suture. *Acta Radiol.* 33:1–11, 1950.

Torgersen J.: Hereditary factors in the sutural pattern of the skull. *Acta Radiol.* 36:374–382, 1951.

Troitzky W.: Zur Frage der Formbildung des Schädeldaches. *Z. Morphol. Anthropol.* 30:504, 1932.

Weinhold H.: Untersuchungen über des Wachstum des Schädels unter phys. und path. Verhältnisse. *Beitr. Path. Anat.* 70:311–342, 1922.

Welcker H.: *Untersuchungen über Wachstum und Bau des Menschlichen Schädels.* Leipzig, Wilhelm Engelmann, 1862.

11

Physiologic Calcification

Calcification in various intracranial structures is apparently normal. However, even so-called normal calcification may be associated with definite clinical syndromes, e.g., basal ganglia calcification and hypoparathyroidism. Some of the physiologic calcifications are of great value in the localization of intracranial mass lesions. It is important, therefore, to recognize and differentiate them from calcifications that are part of numerous pathologic processes. It is also important to recognize bony and soft tissue densities that may be confused with intracranial calcifications (Figs 317 to 319).

MENINGEAL CALCIFICATION

The most common site of intracranial calcification is the dura mater (L. *dura mater*, hard mother).

Falx Cerebri

The falx cerebri (L. *falx*, sickle) is a long, sickle-shaped reflection of dura separating both cerebral hemispheres in the midline. It is narrow anteriorly at its site of attachment to the crista galli and broadens as it passes posteriorly to attach to the upper central surface of the tentorium. The dorsal margin that attaches to the inner table splits into two layers to enclose the superior longitudinal sinus. The inferior longitudinal sinus courses along the free margin of the falx, where it terminates in the straight sinus.

It is well known that calcification of the falx is fairly common in adults. Not so well known, however, is that it also occurs in children. Indeed, I have seen calcification of the falx in a normal two-year-old girl. According to Balnitsky and co-workers, ossification is much more common than calcification in adults. Despite Robertson's claim that the normal uncalcified falx can be seen on a well-centered frontal film, I was unable to confirm this by radiographing a brain and its intact meninges in a water phantom (Fig 320). It is true that a thin, linear, midline density can often be visualized in the frontal projection. However, in my opinion, this density is not due to the normal uncalcified falx. It is probably related to the midline ridge of the inner table of the frontal bone to which the falx is attached.

Calcification or ossification may occur anywhere along the falx, although it is most common near the attached margin. In the frontal projection, the calcification may vary from a faintly visible, linear streak (Fig 321) to dense, broad plaques (Fig 322). These plaques are frequently triangular, with the base facing the midline (Fig 323). A favorite site for calcification is the region of the superior longitudinal sinus, where calcium may be deposited along either leaf or both leaves of the falx. When both leaves are calcified, they characteristically form a V shape, outlining the margins of the superior longitudinal sinus. In the lateral view, the calcification is seen with greater difficulty and tends to appear as a localized, frequently crescentic area of increased density in the frontal or anterior parietal region.

In the literature, one frequently finds the unqualified statement that the falx is a rigid structure that is not readily displaced. This is undoubtedly true of its attached margins. However, the free margin may be displaced by space-occupying lesions (Fig 324). Unfortunately, calcification usually occurs along the fixed attachments of the falx and hence is rarely helpful in indicating the presence of a space-occupying lesion. Occasionally, a displaced calcified falx may be the only roentgenologic clue of a mass lesion in patients without pineal or choroid plexus calcification.

Although most falcine calcifications have no diagnostic significance, calcification of the falx has been reported in pseudoxanthoma elasticum, a variety of hypercalcemic states, and the basal cell nevus syndrome. In the latter condition, the calcification tends to be extensive and quite exuberant (Fig 325).

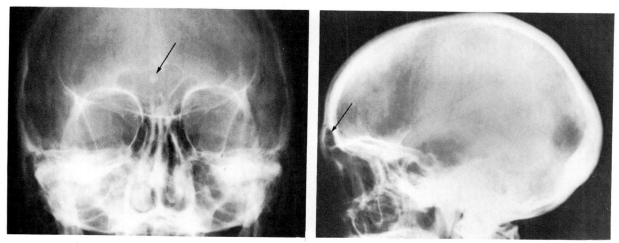

Fig 317.—Osteoma of frontal sinus *(arrow)* simulating calcified pineal gland on posteroanterior film.

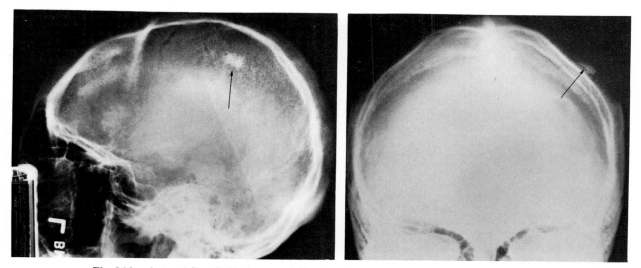

Fig 318.—Lateral film *(left)* shows calcific density in left parietal area. Underexposed frontal projection *(right)* clearly demonstrates intradiploic location of density *(arrow)*.

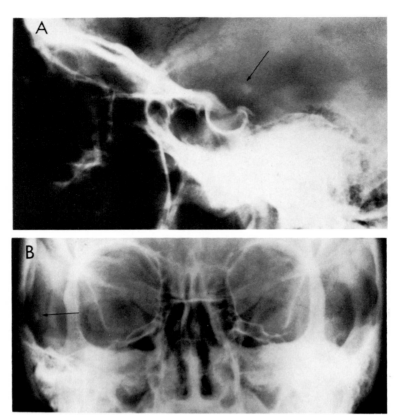

Fig 319.—Lateral film **(A)** demonstrates suprasellar calcification *(arrow)*. The Caldwell projection **(B)** indicates that the "suprasellar" density is actually a right temporal enostosis *(arrow)*.

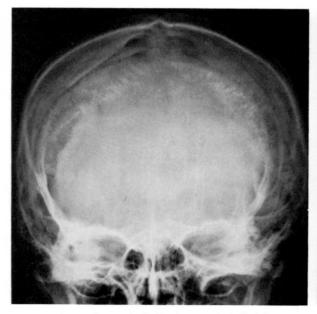
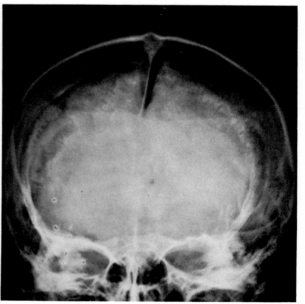

Fig 320.—Posteroanterior radiograph *(left)* of normal skull; falx cerebri is not visualized. Posteroanterior radiograph of same skull *(right)* outlining the falx after injection of air into subdural space. The falx, visible when air of lesser density surrounds it, is normally indistinguishable from surrounding structures.

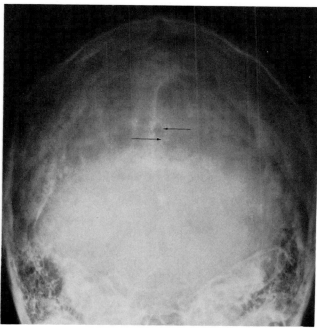

Fig 321.—Faint linear calcification of falx cerebri that is visible *(arrows)* even though skull is slightly rotated from a straight Towne view. There is sufficient dural calcium superimposed in a linear manner to cast a shadow recognizable on the roentgenogram.

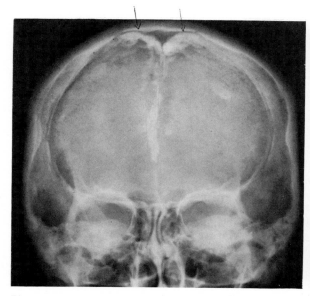

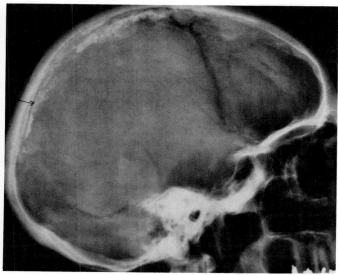

Fig 322.—The broad shaggy encrustations have a flat base on the dura and project into cranial cavity. Uncalcified dura can be seen as thin slit in midline and also over parasagittal region of vertex where it separates inner table from calcified plaques.

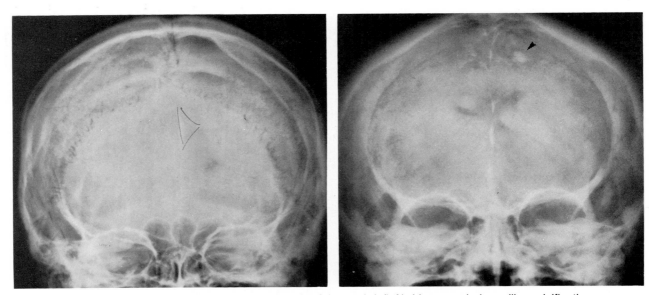

Fig 323.—Triangular calcified plaque along the falx cerebri *(left)*. Linear and plaquelike calcification of falx cerebri *(right)*. Note also flat plaquelike dural calcification *(arrowhead)*.

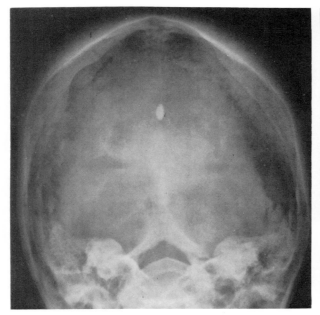

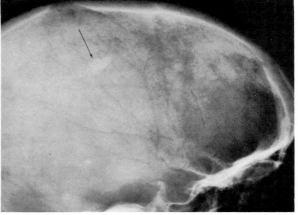

Fig 324.—The Towne view shows calcification along free margin of falx cerebri *(left)*. Lateral projection *(right); arrow* points to plaque that is prominent in the Towne view.

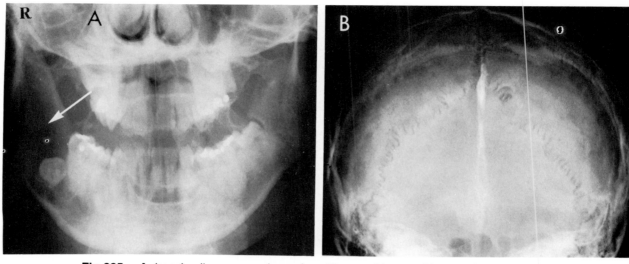

Fig 325.—A, basal cell nevus syndrome in a 23-year-old man with cyst of right mandible *(arrow).* **B,** the Towne view shows extensive calcification of the falx.

Tentorium Cerebelli

The tentorium (L. *tentorium,* tent) is a large, crescent-shaped reflection of dura that separates the cerebral hemispheres from the cerebellum (Figs 326 and 327). The apex of the tent lies anteriorly in the midline and contains the incisura tentorii cerebelli, the opening through which the brain stem passes. The tentorium slopes posteriorly and laterally to attach to the inner table of the parietal and occipital bones, where it encloses the transverse venous sinuses. Anterolaterally, the tentorium is attached to the superior surface of the petrous portion of the temporal bone, where it encloses the superior petrosal sinus. Beyond the apex of the petrous pyramid, the attached and free margins of the tentorium cross. The attached margins rise from an inferior position to insert into the posterior clinoid processes, while the free margins course above and insert into the anterior clinoid processes and tuberculum sellae (Fig 328).

Tentorial calcification is prone to occur at points of attachment. The most common sites are at the points of attachment of the tentorium to the clinoid processes. Thus, in the lateral roentgenogram, the steeply sloping calcifications represent the petroclinoid ligaments, while the more horizontal calcifications lie in the anterior free margin of the tentorium (Figs 329 and 330). Rarely, the falx cerebelli is calcified. Somewhat more commonly, calcification may occur at the apex of the tent and must then be differentiated from the pineal gland. This distinction can readily be made in the Towne projection, where the sloping obliquity of the tentorial calcification is evident (Figs 331 and 332). In the lateral view, stereoscopic films may be necessary to determine the exact site of the calcification. Occasionally, the tentorium is densely calcified (Fig 333). Tentorial calcification in children is considerably less common than in adults and is likely to be associated with various hypercalcemic states.

Other Dural Calcifications

Calcification of the dura mater may occur elsewhere in addition to the previously described sites. It is usually recognized in the lateral view as a thin plaque of increased density. Stereoscopic films are necessary to determine the location of the calcification (Fig 334).

Pacchionian Bodies

Calcification or actual ossification of the arachnoidal villi may occur in apparently normal persons, including older children. Cushing showed that this process begins as a proliferation of the arachnoidal mesothelium, followed by the deposition of calcium salts, particularly in the nuclei. The calcification is most often found just inside the inner table of the skull in the region of the superior longitudinal sinus. It tends to be more or less oval and may be associated with a typical pacchionian depression in the inner table.

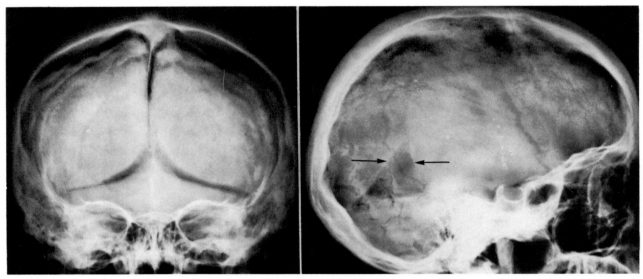

Fig 326.—Subdural air outlining tentorium and falx cerebri. Posteroanterior projection *(left)* again shows well-defined falx that is not visible in routine skull films. Lateral projection *(right)* shows two clearly defined margins. Anteriorly lies the free edge of tentorium *(double arrows)* at tentorial notch surrounding brain stem. Posteriorly lies the midline roof of posterior fossa where cerebral falx attaches to tentorium and envelops the straight sinus.

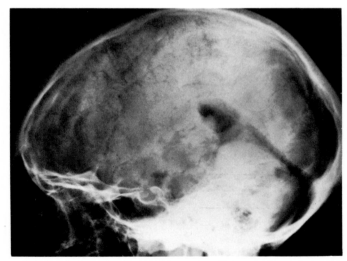

Fig 327.—Subdural air around cerebellum visualizing undersurface of tentorium.

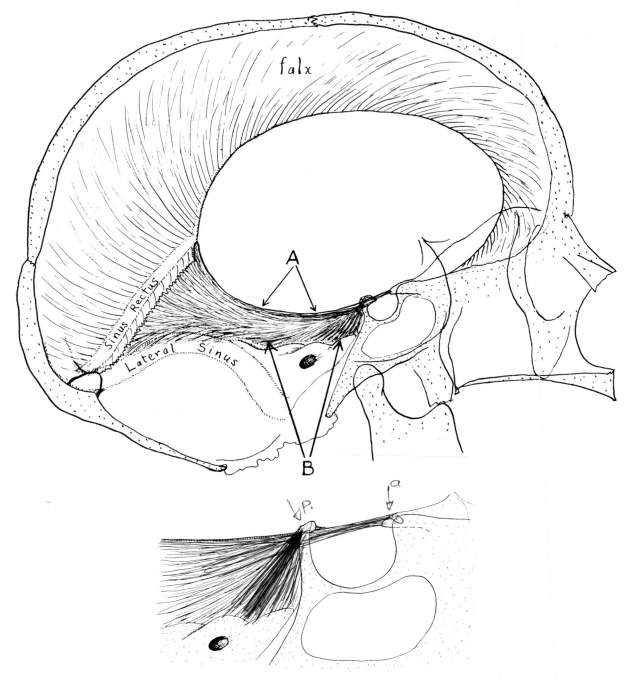

Fig 328.—Diagram *(top)* of cerebral falx and tentorial attachments to clinoid processes. Dura is viewed from right side after removal of right half of tentorium near sinus rectus. Note tentorial notch formed by free margin of tentorium *(arrow A)*; tentorial attachments along ir-regular surface of petrous ridge *(arrow B)*. Detail of the left tentorial attachments *(bottom)*. Fibers of free edge reach anterior clinoids by crossing superiorly and laterally to fibers of attached margin as the latter ascend to posterior clinoids.

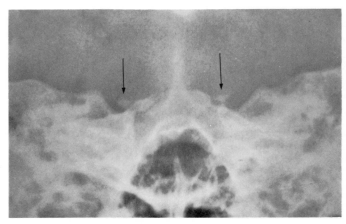 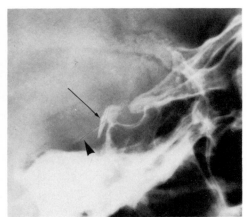

Fig 329.—Calcification of petroclinoid ligaments and anterior free margin of tentorium. Towne view *(left)* showing petroclinoid calcification *(arrows)* and dorsum sellae. Posterior clinoid attachment *(right; arrow).* Free margin of tentorial fibers going to anterior clinoids *(arrowhead).*

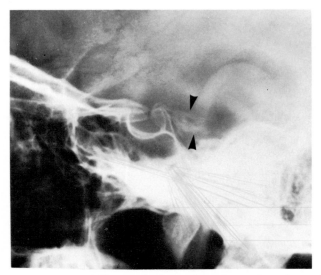

Fig 330.—Extensive calcification in free edge of tentorium *(arrowheads).*

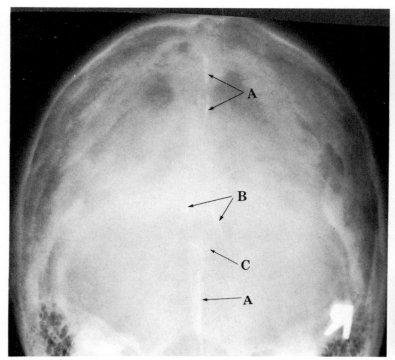

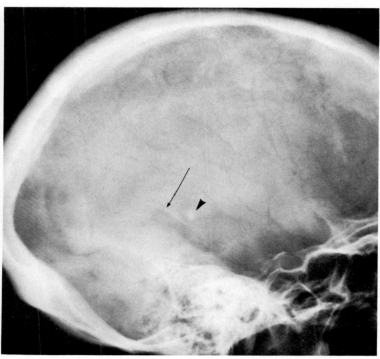

Fig 331.—Calcification in apex of tentorium; falx cerebri and pineal gland are also calcified. Towne view *(left)* showing falx calcification *(A)*, tentorial calcification *(B)*, and heavy pineal calcification *(C)*. Lateral view *(right)* showing calcification in posterior part of free margin of tentorium *(arrow)*; pineal gland *(arrowhead)*. (Courtesy of C. M. Nice, Jr.).

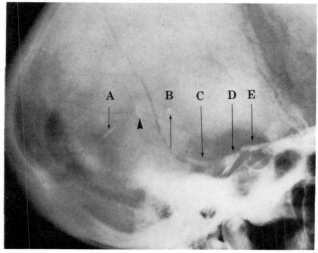

Fig 332.—Lateral view showing multiple tentorial and petroclinoid calcifications. Note junction of falx and tentorium at straight sinus *(A)*; pineal *(B)*; free margin of tentorium *(C)*; petroclinoid ligament *(D)*; interclinoid ligament *(E)*; and glomus of choroid plexus *(arrowhead)*.

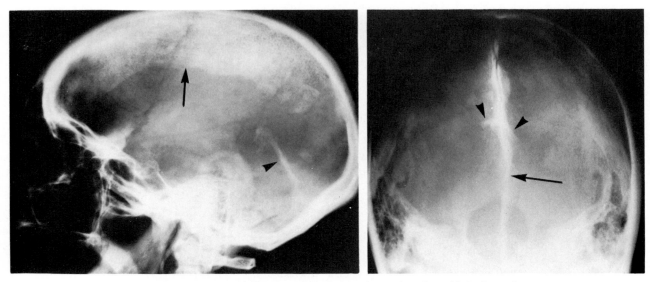

Fig 333.—Dense calcification of tentorium *(arrowhead)* and falx *(arrow).*

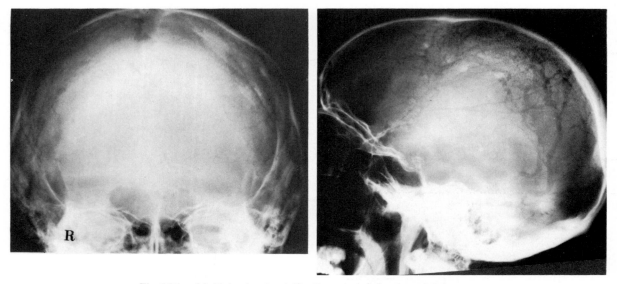

Fig 334.—Multiple dural calcifications in left frontoparietal area.

INTRACEREBRAL CALCIFICATION

Calcification of the Choroid Plexus

The choroid plexus (Gr. *chorion*, skin), so called by Galen because of its resemblance to the fetal membranes, consists of highly vascular folds of pia-arachnoid (tela choroidea, L. *tela*, web) that project into the ventricles. The plexus is covered by a layer of cuboidal ependymal cells that separates it from the ventricles and cerebrospinal fluid. There is plexus tissue in the body and temporal horn of the lateral ventricle and in the third and fourth ventricles. There is no plexus in the frontal or occipital horns of the lateral ventricle.

The plexuses are largest in the lateral ventricles, where they extend along the floor from the interventricular foramina to the atria. Here, each plexus makes a bend as it continues onto the floor of the temporal horn. The glomus (L. *glomus*, ball) is the expanded portion of the plexus commonly found just anterior to the atrium. Anteriorly, the plexuses of the lateral ventricles converge to pass through the interventricular foramina and then unite to form the choroid plexus of the third ventricle. This structure, which hangs from the roof of the third ventricle, extends from the interventricular foramina to the suprapineal recess. It is attached to the stria medullaris thalami on either side and to the commissure of habenulae posteriorly. The separate plexus of the fourth ventricle covers the lower half of the ventricular roof and extends into the lateral recesses.

Plexus calcification, long familiar to pathologists, was first described roentgenologically by Schüller. Although rare during the first two decades, it increases in frequency in the fourth decade and thereafter is roughly proportional to age. Its incidence has been variously estimated as 5 to 13% in normal adults and is approximately twice as common in males. I have seen it in normal children under age 5. However, it is uncommon prior to age 10 to 12. If the calcified glomus in a child is larger that 1.5 to 2.0 cm in diameter, a papilloma of the choroid plexus should be excluded.

The calcification is commonly bilateral, although it may be unilateral (Fig 335). It is usually confined to the glomus but may rarely occur in other portions of the plexus (Fig 336). Calcification in the choroid plexus of the third and fourth ventricles is rarely recognized roentgenologically (Fig 337). When present, the calcification tends to be linear. Zatz has reported unusual calcifications of the choroid plexus (in the third ventricle and in the temporal horn) in patients with neurofibromatosis. Extensive calcification of the lateral ventricles in these patients has also been reported.

Glomus calcification is characteristically round or kidney-shaped. It may range from a few faint specks or a cluster of punctate deposits to an irregular, dense, amorphous mass 1.5 cm in diameter (Fig 338). Although usually symmetric, it may vary from side to side (Fig 339). In the frontal projection, the calcified glomera, which lie 2.5 to 3.0 cm lateral to the midline, form the angles of an inverted isosceles triangle, with the pineal body as the apex (Fig 340). In the lateral view, the calcified glomus is located slightly above and behind the pineal body. The unilateral calcified glomus should ordinarily not be difficult to recognize because of its location and characteristic calcification. In rare instances, however, it may be difficult to differentiate the unilateral, faintly calcified glomus from the pineal body.

Slight displacement of the glomus should be interpreted with caution, particularly when the calcification is unilateral. Rotation of the skull can result in spurious displacement. In addition, the glomus may occasionally be pedunculated and mobile, shifting considerably with changes in position of the head (Fig 341). If these factors are excluded, a major distortion of the normal triangular relationship of the calcified glomera and pineal body can be regarded as evidence of an expanding or atrophic intracranial lesion. Likewise, marked displacement of a unilateral calcified glomus has similar significance. There is usually other evidence on the roentgenogram of an expanding lesion in addition to choroid plexus displacement. However, the latter may occasionally be the only roentgenologic evidence of an intracranial mass lesion on the plain skull films.

All the reported intracranial mass lesions producing choroid displacement have been located posteriorly in the parietal, occipital, posterior frontal, or temporal regions. In these sites, the mass presses directly upon and displaces the posterior portion of the lateral ventricle. Anterior tumors in the frontal or temporal lobes may produce little or no displacement of the choroid plexus.

Calcification of the Pineal Body

The pineal body (L. *pineus*, pine cone) is a small, cone-shaped structure that lies between the splenium of

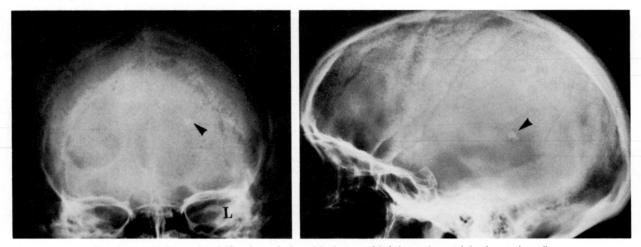

Fig 335.—Unilateral calcification of choroid plexus of left lateral ventricle *(arrowhead)*.
This should not be confused with displacement of pineal gland.

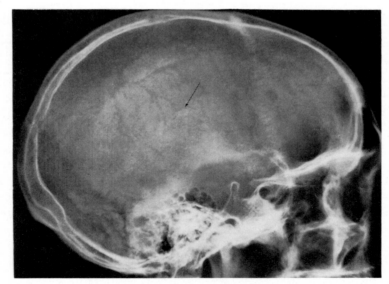

Fig 336.—Unusual location of calcification in choroid plexus of lateral ventricle *(arrow)*.

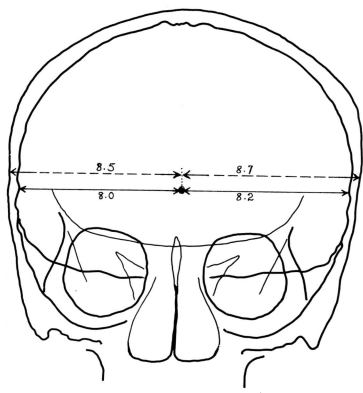

Fig 345.—Pineal measurements in frontal projection. Solid line measures distance from pineal to inner table; broken line measures distance from pineal to outer table of skull.

from the center of the calcified gland to corresponding, similar points on the inner or outer table of the calvarium (Fig 345). If the inner table is irregular and asymmetric, the outer table should be used as the reference point.

METHODS OF PINEAL LOCALIZATION

VASTINE-KINNEY METHOD.—In 1927 Vastine and Kinney measured 200 skull roentgenograms and first established a normal zone for pineal localization in the lateral view. These workers plotted the distance of the pineal body from the frontal bone against the sum of the distances from the pineal body to the frontal bone and to the occipital bone. This sum is approximately equal to the greatest anteroposterior diameter of the skull. These measurements, which indicate the pineal position in the anteroposterior axis, should be made from the center of the pineal calcification to the inner table of the frontal and occipital bones at their most distant points.

Vastine and Kinney also plotted the distance of the pineal body from the vault against the sum of the dis-

tances from the pineal body to the vault and to the basi-occiput. This sum is roughly equivalent to the vertical diameter of the skull. These measurements, which mark the pineal position in the craniocaudal axis, are made from the center of pineal calcification to the inner table of the vault and to the level of the base of the skull at their most distant points. The lines corresponding to all these diameters need not necessarily be continuous straight lines (Fig 346).

The normal pineal body is considered to lie between the diagonal lines on the Vastine-Kinney charts. A pineal body located outside the normal zone is regarded as displaced.

Dyke reviewed the Vastine-Kinney charts and noted that a number of normal pineal bodies fell in front of the normal zone. To remedy this difficulty, he advised moving the normal zone forward 4 mm (Fig 347). Stauffer has pointed out that 4 mm represents the average distance between the pineal body and the habenular commissure. Since radiologists were unaware of habenular calcification when the charts were constructed, it is reasonable to assume that these calcifications were included in the pineal measurements.

The weakness of the original Vastine-Kinney method and the Dyke modification is their failure to consider the great variability in shape of the normal skull. These graphs are purely linear, relating only to the anteropos-

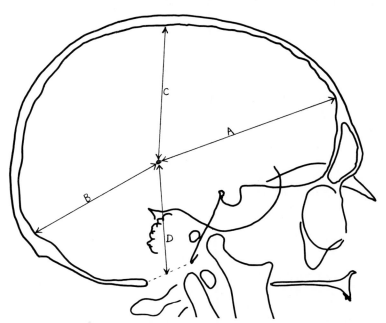

Fig 346.—Pineal measurements in lateral projection. Some tables and nomograms use the proportion A to B and C to D, while others use A to A + B and C to C + D.

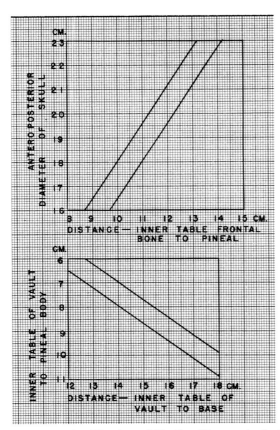

Fig 347.—Dyke's modification of Vastine-Kinney charts for pineal localization. This corresponds to the A to A + B and C to C + D measurements of Figure 346. Space between diagonal lines shows usual normal range of pineal position.

terior and vertical diameters. The original Vastine-Kinney charts are satisfactory for skulls with short anteroposterior diameters, while the Dyke modification is helpful when dealing with skulls with longer anteroposterior diameters. Dyke's modification is unsatisfactory for general use, however, because it increases the number of normal pineal bodies falsely displaced posteriorly.

To increase the accuracy of the Vastine-Kinney charts, one must take the shape of the skull into consideration.

PROPORTIONAL METHOD OF FRAY.—In an effort to improve the Vastine-Kinney charts, Fray suggested the proportional method. This method utilizes an elastic band of uniform stretch, with markers indicating the normal zones for the anteroposterior and vertical diameters. With zero at the inner table of the frontal bone and the end marker at the inner table of the occipital bone, the normal pineal body falls in the normal zone.

This method assumes that the distance of the pineal body from the frontal bone is 55 to 60% of the anteroposterior skull diameter. Similarly, it assumes that the pineal to vertex distance varies between 51 and 57% of the skull height.

Even though the proportional method eliminates the need for charts, it too fails to consider the variability in skull shape. Furthermore, the values of 55 to 60% and 51 to 57% are arbitrarily selected. In practice, I have not found that this method increases the accuracy of pineal localization.

CRANIOANGLE METHOD (Fig 348).—This method, also devised by Fray, avoids linear skull measurements. To identify displacement in the anteroposterior axis, it utilizes a transparent celluloid guide, with two ruled lines forming an angle of 8 degrees. The rule is placed with the vertex of the angle at the posterior margin of the foramen magnum. The main line passes through bregma (the junction of the coronal and sagittal sutures). The normal pineal body falls within the angle formed by the main baseline and its fellow. To determine up or down displacement, another angle of 11 degrees is placed with the vertex at the base of the anterior clinoid processes. The main line now passes through lambda (the junction of the lambdoidal and sagittal sutures). The normal pineal body falls within the angle.

I have had no personal experience with the cranioangle method. However, Fray himself stated that it was not as accurate as other methods in determining anteroposterior displacement, even though it might be useful in skulls of unusual shape.

DECRINIS AND RUSKEN'S METHOD.—DeCrinis and Rusken in Germany devised still another linear method for pineal localization. They determined three arbitrary distances from the pineal body to basal points in the cranium: (1) to the internal auditory meatus closest to the film (normal, 35 to 45 mm); (2) to the upper posterior border of the dorsum sellae (normal, 36 to 46 mm); and (3) to the tuberculum sellae (normal, 50 to 62 mm).

Several objections to this method can be raised. In the first place, it has all the disadvantages of any linear method. In addition, since the internal auditory meatus is located at a considerable distance from the midsagittal plane, the measurements may be inaccurate if a true lateral film is not obtained. Furthermore, the sella turcica varies considerably in shape and size and may not be a good anatomical landmark for this purpose.

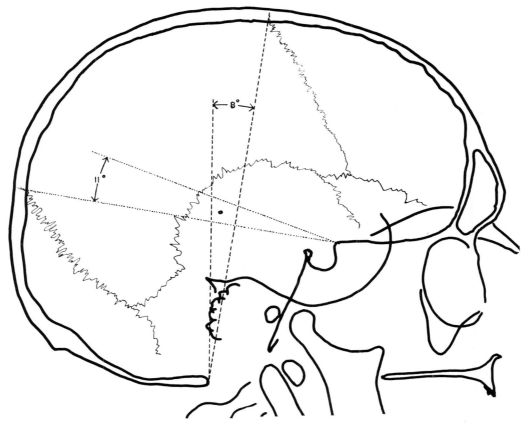

Fig 348.—Cranioangle method of localization. Baseline for antero-posterior displacement joins posterior margin of foramen magnum with bregma, and for vertical displacement joins tuberculum sellae with lambda.

LILJA'S METHOD.—Lilja in Stockholm made a detailed statistical study of pineal orientation in the skull, measuring the distances between the pineal body and numerous selected points in the calvaria, including the Vastine-Kinney points. He expressed his data as ranges of normal variation in the ratios of skull to pineal distance (from various points) to the anteroposterior and vertical diameters. This method has the distinct merit of indicating the statistical odds that a pineal body in any given location is normal or displaced. However, the exact positions of many of the focal points are difficult to determine on the roentgenogram.

ISLEY AND BAYLIN'S METHOD.—Isley and Baylin proposed a different approach to pineal localization. They drew a line from the nasofrontal articulation to a point midway between the anterior and posterior clinoid processes. A second line was drawn from the interclinoid point to the calcified pineal gland. The superior angle was measured with an angle-measuring device (normal, 138.5 to 157.5 degrees, with 95% confidence). The distance be-

tween the interclinoid point and the midpoint of the pineal calcification was also measured (normal, 3.9 to 5.3 cm, with 95% confidence) (Fig 349).

OON'S METHOD.—In 1964, Oon reviewed the various methods of pineal localization and found them to be either inaccurate or too cumbersome. He suggested drawing a line from the tuberculum sellae to basion. A perpendicular to this baseline is erected 1 cm caudal to the tuberculum sellae. A point is then measured on the perpendicular 5 cm from the baseline (Fig 350). The normal calcified pineal gland lies within 1 cm of this point (98% confidence).

While no method is perfect or entirely foolproof, I have found Oon's line to be simple and reliable and use it routinely.

Calcification of the Habenular Commissure

The epithalamus consists of the pineal body, the trigonum habenulae (L. *habena*, rein), and the posterior commissure. The pineal body arises as a diverticulum

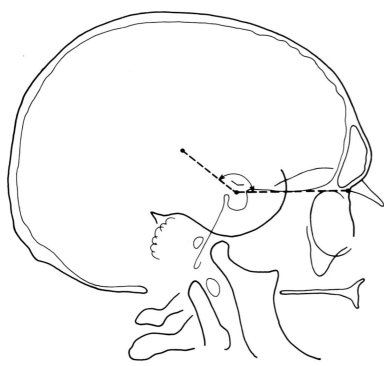

Fig 349.—Isley and Baylin's method of pineal localization.

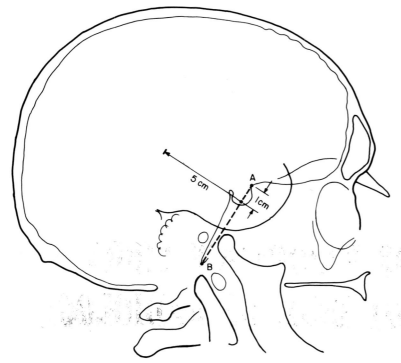

Fig 350.—Oon's method of pineal localization. A line is drawn from tuberculum sellae to basion. A perpendicular to this line is erected 1 cm distal to tuberculum. A point is measured on the perpendicular 5 cm from baseline. Normal pineal is within 1 cm of this point.

from the roof plate of the diencephalon. The superior portion of this diverticulum develops into the habenular commissure, while the inferior portion gives rise to the posterior commissure. The pineal stalk is thus connected to the posterior commissure, and also to the thalamus through the habenulae, which are direct extensions of the thalamic medullary striae. The habenular fibers from both sides decussate in front of the pineal stalk to form the habenular commissure (Figs 351 to 353).

Anatomists have been aware of habenular calcification for some time. However, this entity was unfamiliar to radiologists until the reports of Smith, and Stauffer, and Snow and Adams in 1953. The calcification is deposited in small neuroglial nodules between the decussating fibers of the habenular commissure and the overlying ependyma. Calcification has not been found in the posterior commissure. The calcification varies from a barely discernible fleck to a C-shaped mass of calcium covering the ventricular surface of the habenular commissure, anterior to the pineal gland. The open end of the C faces posteriorly. This characteristic appearance makes it possible to recognize the habenular commissure on the lateral skull roentgenogram. In the absence of pineal calcification, a calcified habenular commissure may be helpful in the diagnosis of intracranial mass lesions.

In Stauffer's series of 285 normal skull roentgenograms, approximately 31% showed habenular calcification, either alone or in conjunction with pineal calcification (Fig 354). In the autopsy series reported by Smith, of 123 brains examined, only 32% showed gross habenular calcification on roentgenograms, although 65% exhibited microscopic calcification.

Calcification of the Basal Ganglia

The basal ganglia are masses of gray matter embedded in the medullary white substance of the cerebral hemispheres. They consist of the caudate and lenticular (lentiform) nuclei, which together form the corpus striatum, and the amygdaloid nucleus (Fig 355).

The caudate nucleus (L. *cauda*, tail) is a pear-shaped structure with a bulbous head and a long, tapering tail. The head bulges into the frontal horn of the lateral ventricle, while the narrower portion forms the floor of the body of the ventricle. The tail continues downward onto the roof of the temporal horn, ending in the putamen as the amygdaloid nucleus.

The lenticular nucleus (L. *lens*, lentil), which lies lat-

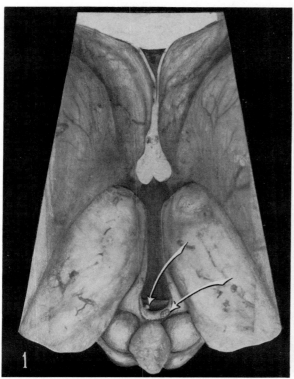
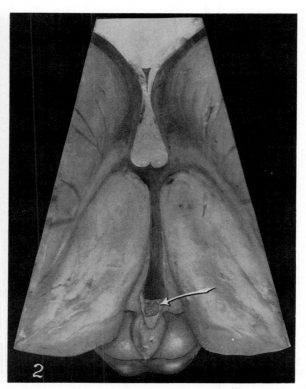

Fig 351.—**1,** dorsal aspect of forebrain with roof of third ventricle removed to show two small nodules on habenular commissure. **2,** similar view of another specimen with one large nodule on habenular commissure. (From Smith, C. G.: *Radiology* 60:647–650, 1953.)

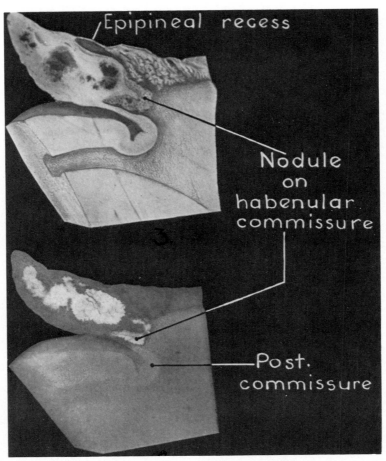

Fig 352.—Specimen and roentgenogram of midsagittal section of pineal gland and adjacent structures showing thickness and extent of large neuroglial nodule on habenular commissure. (From Smith, C. G.: *Radiology* 60:647–650, 1953.)

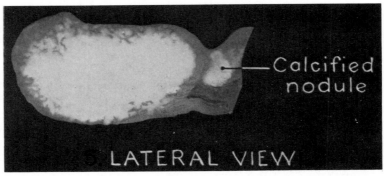

Fig 353.—Lateral roentgenogram of pineal gland and commissure of habenulae showing appearance of calcified neuroglial nodule covering only part of commissure. (From Smith, C. G.: *Radiology* 60:647–650, 1953.)

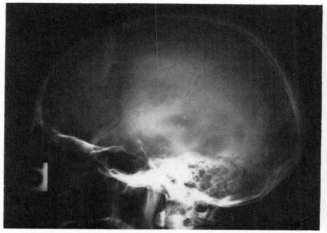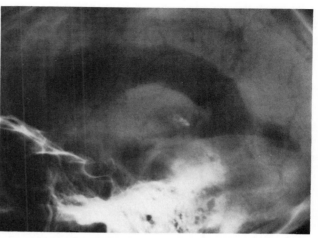

Fig 354.—Typical C-shaped calcification of habenular commissure *(left)*. Pneumoencephalogram showing calcified pineal gland and ha-benular commissure *(right)*. (From Stauffer, H. M., Snow, L. B., and Adams, A. B.: *Am. J. Roentgenol.* 70:83–89, 1953.)

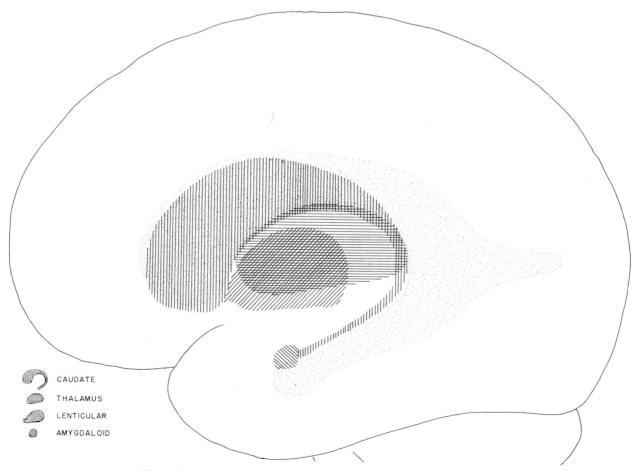

CAUDATE

THALAMUS

LENTICULAR

AMYGDALOID

Fig 355.—Basal ganglia in lateral view. Faintly stippled outline of lateral ventricle is shown for purposes of orientation.

eral to the caudate nucleus, does not extend as far forward or backward as does the caudate nucleus. It consists of two portions: (1) a larger lateral mass called the putamen (L. *putamen,* shell), and (2) two medial portions together termed the globus pallidus (L. *globus pallidus,* pale sphere). The internal capsule separates the lenticular nucleus laterally from the caudate nucleus and thalamus medially.

The amygdaloid nucleus (Gr. *amygdalē,* almond) is a rounded mass continuous with the tail of the caudate nucleus, located in the roof of the tip of the temporal horn of the lateral ventricle.

In 1935, Fritzsche observed calcification of the basal ganglia on the roentgenograms of three siblings. In the same year, Kasanin and Crank recorded the roentgenologic and pathologic findings in a single case. These authors did not mention the presence of parathyroid insufficiency, although the older literature contains isolated reports of the association of calcification of the basal ganglia with hypoparathyroidism.

In 1939, Eaton, Love, and Camp reported a group of 6 patients with bilateral symmetric calcification of the basal ganglia. Eight years later, Camp reviewed the Mayo Clinic experience of 12 cases of basal ganglia calcification associated with parathyroid insufficiency (Fig 356). Eleven of the twelve patients in this series had spontaneous hypoparathyroidism.

The calcification is not limited to patients with hypoparathyroidism but may also be found in patients with pseudohypoparathyroidism, in apparently normal persons, and in patients with a variety of pathologic conditions. It has been estimated that two thirds of the patients with bilateral symmetric basal ganglia calcification have hypoparathyroidism or pseudohypoparathyroidism. The remaining third of the patients comprise a heterogenous group, including patients with familial basal ganglia calcification, toxoplasmosis, encephalitis, tuberous sclerosis, and anoxia, and normal persons. The calcification is usually bilateral and symmetric, although Camp has observed two patients with minimal unilateral calcification.

The roentgenologic appearance of the calcification is quite characteristic. In the earliest stages, there are small, symmetric, discrete areas of increased density in the region of the basal ganglia. When the process is more pronounced, the irregular, discrete calcific deposits coalesce to form large, denser masses (Fig 357). Histologically, the densities noted on the roentgenogram represent calcification in and around the media of the smaller arteries. Ostertag believes that microscopic calcification in the globus palidus and the dentate nucleus is so common that it has no pathologic significance.

The bilateral symmetric character of basal ganglia calcification should differentiate it from calcified tumors. In case of doubt, air studies can be done for more accurate localization of the calcification. The anterior position of the calcification in the lateral roentgenogram distinguishes it from the glomus of the choroid plexus.

Calcification of the Dentate Nucleus

The dentate nucleus (L. *dens,* tooth) is a corrugated mass of gray matter embedded in each cerebellar hemisphere. The gray matter is folded on itself to enclose a

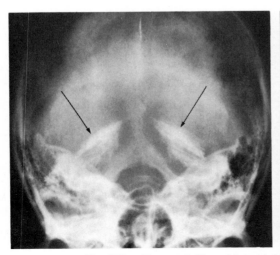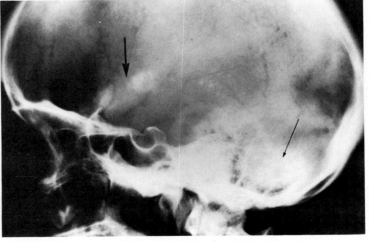

Fig 356.—Towne *(left)* and lateral *(right)* views in patient with hypoparathyroidism showing bilateral calcification of caudate nucleus *(thick arrow)* and dentate nucleus *(thin arrow).*

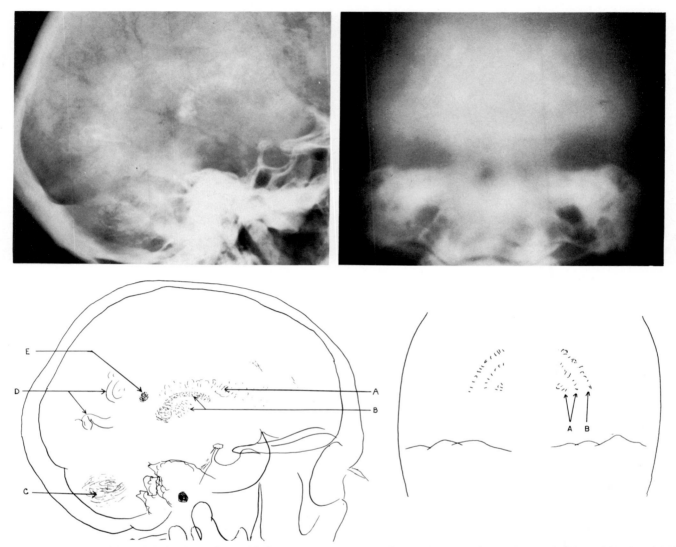

Fig 357.—Calcification of basal ganglia in patient with hypoparathyroidism. Lateral view *(left)* showing calcifications in caudate nucleus *(A)*, in lenticular nucleus *(B)*, in dentate nucleus and cerebellar folds *(C)*, within occipital cerebral gyri *(D)*, and in choroid plexus *(E)*. Anteroposterior laminograms *(right)* showing calcification in the lenticular nucleus; *A* is probably in globus pallidus and *B* in putamen.

central core of white matter. The fibers of the superior cerebellar peduncle pass out through the open medial end of the dentate nucleus.

The clinical significance of calcification in the dentate nucleus is not known. It was noted at autopsy by Mallory as early as 1896. In 1935, Fritzsche made the first roentgenologic observation of this condition in a report on symmetric calcification of the basal ganglia. Camp, and Rand, Olson, and Courville reported similar cases of cerebellar calcification associated with calcification of the basal ganglia. In 1952, King and Gould described two patients with isolated symmetric calcification of the dentate nucleus. Neither of these patients exhibited basal ganglia calcification or any obvious neurologic disorder.

The calcium deposits are of two types: (1) dense, serrated masses corresponding to the corrugated outline of the dentate nucleus, and (2) fine, linear calcifications in the surrounding white matter (Fig 358; see Fig 356 also).

Calcification of the Hippocampus

I have never seen calcification of the hippocampus in a normal patient. In 1949, Ramos E Silva reported bilateral hippocampal calcification associated with lipoid

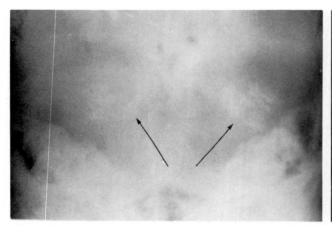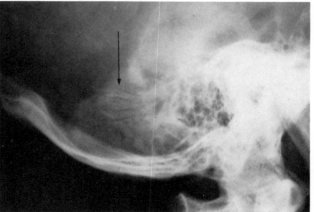

Fig 358.—Calcification of dentate nucleus. Anteroposterior lamino-gram *(left)* and lateral view *(right)*. Calcification is much heavier on left side. Asymptomatic patient was studied for a question of a frac-ture.

proteinosis. This observation has been confirmed by others. Hippocampal calcification, presumably due to anoxia, has also been reported in a three-year-old boy with seizures, mental retardation, and cafe-au-lait spots in the absence of lipoid proteinosis. Tomography helps to localize the calcification to the tip of the temporal lobes and more particularly to the region of the hippo-campal gyrus.

Calcification of the Pituitary Gland

Although calcification in pituitary (L. *pituita,* gelati-nous mucus) adenomas is familiar to pathologists, grossly recognizable calcification in the normal pituitary

gland is rare. I have observed this finding in only two patients, who had a normal sella turcica and no clinical or usual signs of pituitary dysfunction (Fig 359). What is commonly regarded as pituitary calcification is usu-ally an irregular hyperostosis of the inner table of the skull that is superimposed upon the sella turcica in the lateral view. Stereoscopic films and tomography readily demonstrate the lateral position of these bony plaques.

Calcification of the Internal Carotid Artery

Calcification in the internal carotid artery and its branches may occur as part of the aging process. In Dyke's series, it was noted in 1.3% of all skull roent-

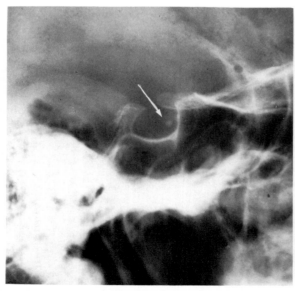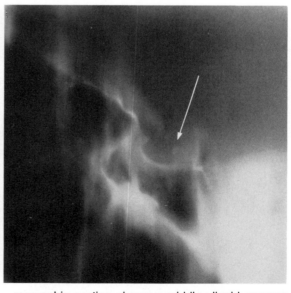

Fig 359.—Pituitary calculus in two patients. Calculus in film on the left was confirmed by stereoscopy and tomography. On the right, to-mographic section shows a middle clinoid process as well as a pitu-itary stone.

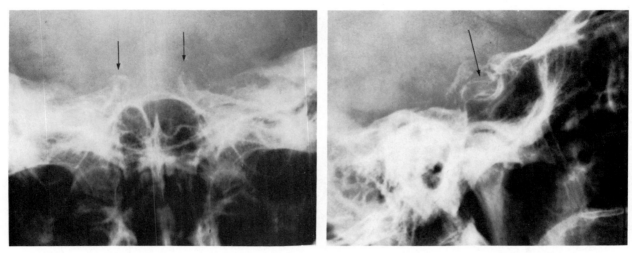

Fig 360.—Calcification of internal carotid arteries. Anteroposterior projection *(left);* lateral projection *(right).*

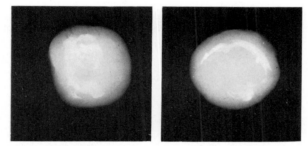

Fig 361.—Calcification of choroid and lens in an eye removed because of a metallic foreign body. Anteroposterior projection *(left);* lateral projection *(right).*

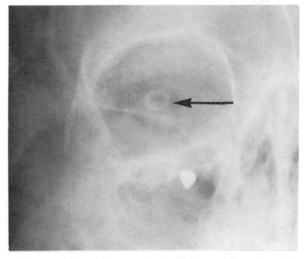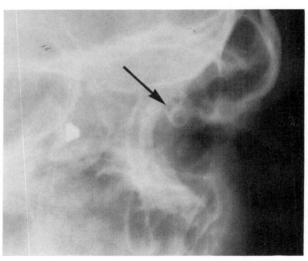

Fig 362.—Calcification in lens in a patient with traumatic cataract. Anteroposterior *(left)* and lateral *(right)* views showing shell-like calci-fication and a large extraocular metallic foreign body. (From Vogler, E.: *Fortschr. Geb. Roentgenstrahlen* 74:87–91, 1951.)

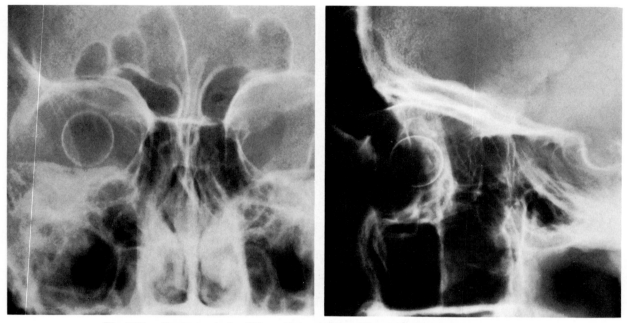

Fig 363.—Posteroanterior **(A)** and lateral **(B)** radiographs of a patient with right ocular prosthesis. Lateral view gives good indication of posterior extent of orbit.

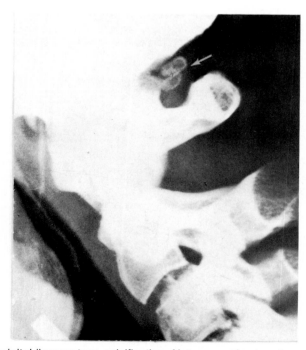

Fig 364.—Atlanto-occipital ligamentous calcification. Note several separate ossified bodies *(arrow).* (From Hadley, L. A.: *The Spine.* [Springfield, Ill., Charles C Thomas, Publisher, 1956].)

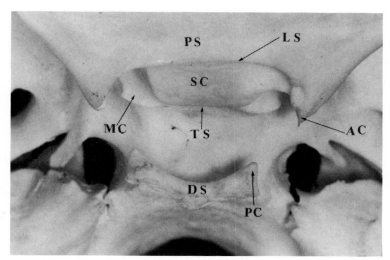

Fig 366.—Interior of base of dry skull delineating landmarks of sella turcica: anterior clinoid process *(AC);* dorsum sellae *(DS);* limbus sphenoidalis *(LS);* middle clinoid process *(MC);* posterior clinoid process *(PC);* planum sphenoidale *(PS);* sulcus chiasmatis *(SC);* and tuberculum sellae *(TS).*

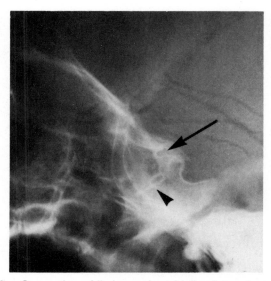

Fig 368.—Separation of limbus sphenoidalis at age 6 months, i.e., cleft for chiasmatic sulcus *(arrow).* Note that synchondrosis between presphenoid and postsphenoid centers is still patent *(arrowhead).*

sellar sphenoid depends upon the extent of posterior growth of the planum. The region of the presphenoid not overlapped by the planum becomes the chiasmatic sulcus. The length of the planum sphenoidale governs the width of the chiasmatic sulcus. A long planum is associated with a narrow chiasmatic sulcus and vice versa (Fig 371). During the stage of posterior growth of the planum, the chiasmatic sulcus is relatively long, well corticated, and clearly defined. The limbus sphenoidalis and tuberculum sellae are also well defined.

This appearance has unfortunately been called J-shaped or omega-shaped, because of the slope of the chiasmatic sulcus (Fig 372). The configuration of the sella resulting from erosion of the tuberculum or chiasmatic sulcus by an optic glioma has also been termed J-shaped or omega-shaped. These terms should be discarded because they are confusing and misleading. A long, sloping chiasmatic sulcus is pathologic only when erosion and abnormal bone modeling are present. The latter changes are usually associated with obvious abnormalities of the tuberculum sellae (Fig 373).

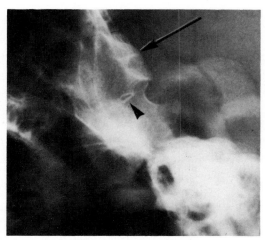

Fig 367.—Lateral view of neonatal skull showing normal high position of roof of optic canal *(arrow).* Note also synchondrosis between presphenoid and postsphenoid centers *(arrowhead).*

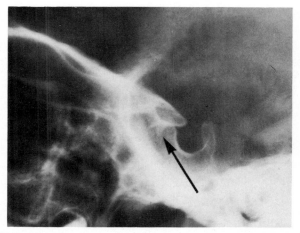

Fig 369.—Remnant of synchondrosis between limbus sphenoidalis and presphenoid *(arrow)* in a 6-year-old boy. Limbus is usually completely fused by this age.

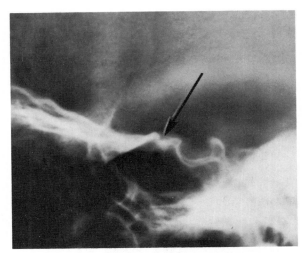

Fig 370.—Failure of fusion of limbus sphenoidalis in a 19-year-old man *(arrow)*. This should not be mistaken for a fracture.

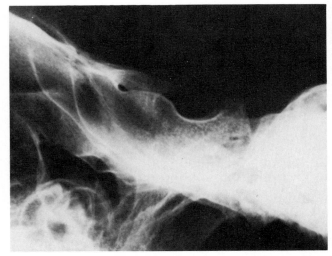

Fig 372.—Normal J-shaped sella in newborn (dried specimen).

Similarly, the normal high position of the roof of the optic canal in early infancy should not be mistaken for the planum sphenoidale, particularly in a film made with the head tilted (Fig 374). Angulation of the patient's head or of the x-ray tube results in spurious upward displacement of the optic canal, which can simulate the changes seen in optic glioma.

JUVENILE AND ADULT SELLA

Pneumatization of the sphenoid bone begins at age 2 to 4 years. Pneumatization progresses medially and posteriorly into the body of the sphenoid with considerable variability. It frequently extends beyond the body proper into the lingular and pterygoid processes and

into the greater and lesser wings. Pneumatization in adults usually stops at the spheno-occipital synchondrosis, although rarely it may extend into the basiocciput (Fig 375). The degree of pneumatization influences the position and appearance of the chiasmatic sulcus. With progressive extension of the pneumatization toward the tuberculum sellae, the chiasmatic sulcus tends to be less prominent and more vertically oriented. In general, when the chiasmatic sulcus is deeply concave, the limbus sphenoidalis tends to be prominent; when the sulcus is shallow, the limbus is less conspicuous.

The septa which partition the sphenoid sinuses are thought to represent bony remnants at the junction of various fetal ossification centers. Thus, the sagittal septum may well represent the fusion plane between both

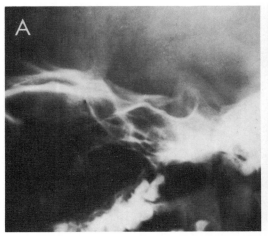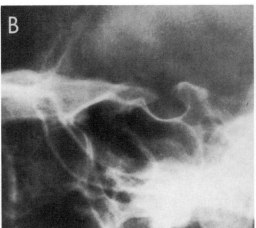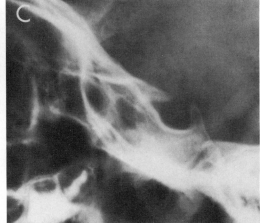

Fig 371.—Normal variations in planum sphenoidale. **A,** short horizontal planum in a child. **B,** short planum in an adult. **C,** vertical planum.

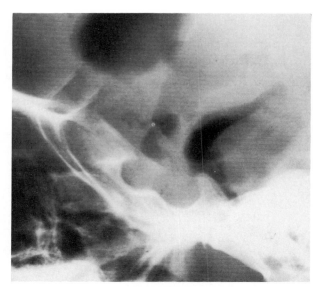

Fig 373.—Lateral film from pneumoencephalogram showing a pathologic J-shaped sella in a youngster with neurofibromatosis and bilateral optic gliomas. Note erosion and undercutting of planum as well as abnormal modeling of anterior portion of sella.

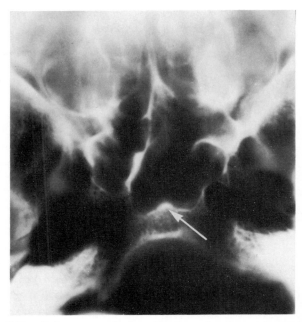

Fig 375.—Submentovertical projection showing sphenoid sinus pneumatization extending into basiocciput *(arrow).*

halves of the sphenoid bone, while the transverse septa represent fusion planes between the presphenoid and postsphenoid centers. The extent and the direction of the septa are variable. Partial septa are more common than complete septa. The extent of pneumatization of the postsphenoid below the sellar floor directly affects the thickness of the cortical bone (lamina dura) of the sellar floor. A septum inserting into the sellar floor modifies the configuration of the lamina dura in this region (Fig 376).

ANTERIOR CLINOID PROCESSES

The anterior clinoid processes are more laterally situated than the posterior clinoid processes and, in fact, do not actually contribute to the roof of the sella. They may vary in thickness and height from short, stubby structures to longer, slender struts. Occasionally, the anterior clinoid processes are asymmetric, e.g., one

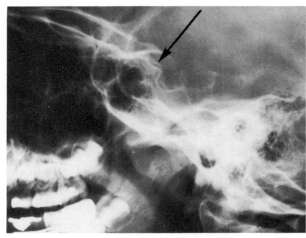

Fig 374.—Spurious high position of optic canal due to tilting of head *(arrow).*

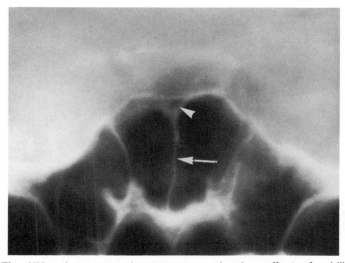

Fig 376.—Anteroposterior tomogram showing effect of midline sphenoidal septum *(arrow)* on sellar floor at site of insertion of septum *(arrowhead).*

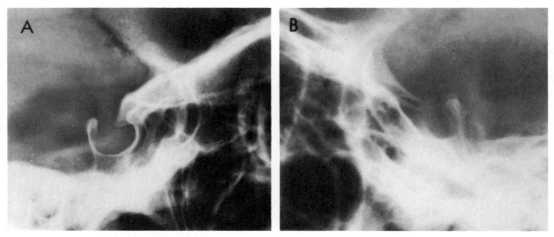

Fig 377.—A, normal stubby anterior clinoid processes. **B,** normal pointed anterior clinoid processes.

pointed and the other blunt. The well-defined, dense cortical outline of the normal anatomical variant distinguishes it from pathologic erosion due to a parasellar lesion (Figs 377 to 379). Occasionally, one or both anterior clinoid processes are pneumatized (Fig 380).

MIDDLE CLINOID PROCESSES

The middle clinoid process is a small, inconstant bony spur arising from the anterolateral margin of the sella turcica, behind the tuberculum sellae (Fig 381). Calcification or ossification of the ligamentous connection between the anterior and middle clinoid processes results in the formation of the caroticoclinoid canal (Fig

382). This may be unilateral or bilateral. Similarly, calcification or ossification of the ligament between the middle and posterior clinoid form a posterior pseudocanal on one or both sides (Fig 383).

POSTERIOR CLINOID PROCESSES

The posterior clinoid processes also vary in size, shape, and degree of pneumatization (Figs 384 and 385). The tips may be rounded or pointed and may incline anterolaterally or project superiorly. Pneumatization of the sphenoid bone may extend into the posterior clinoids. Rarely, one or both posterior clinoid processes may be absent. In the Towne projection, the normal

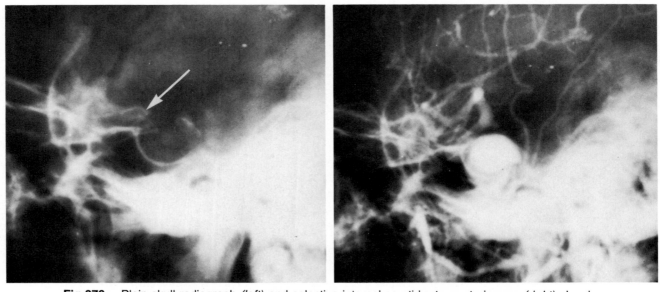

Fig 378.—Plain skull radiograph *(left)* and selective internal carotid artery arteriogram *(right)* showing an aneurysm elevating and sharpening the ipsilateral anterior clinoid process *(arrow).*

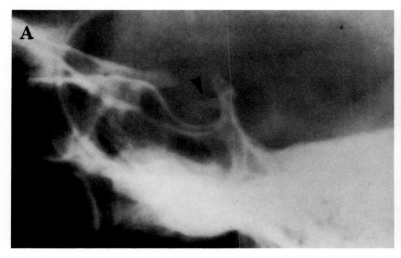

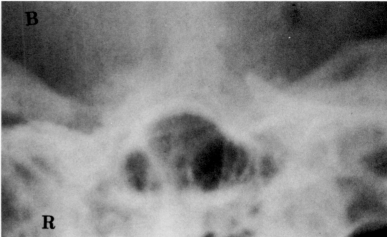

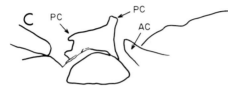

Fig 379.—Lateral **(A)** and Towne **(B)** views in a patient with asymmetry of anterior clinoid processes due to hypoplasia of right anterior clinoid. Note also bizarre appearance of short right posterior clinoid process *(arrowhead)* due to marked slope of dorsum. Line drawing of the Towne view **(C)** shows anterior clinoid process *(AC)* and posterior clinoid process *(PC)*.

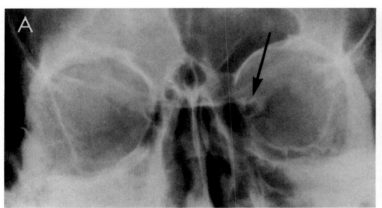

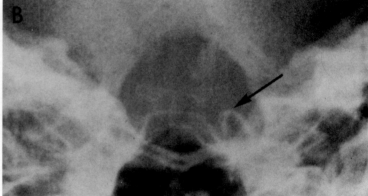

Fig 380.—Caldwell projection **(A)** and Towne view **(B)** showing pneumatized left anterior clinoid process *(arrow)*.

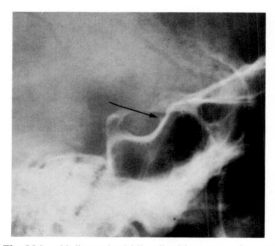

Fig 381.—Unilateral middle clinoid process *(arrow)*.

241

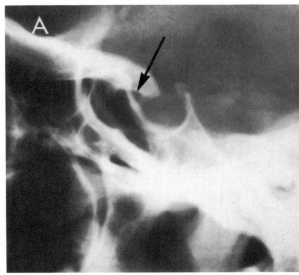
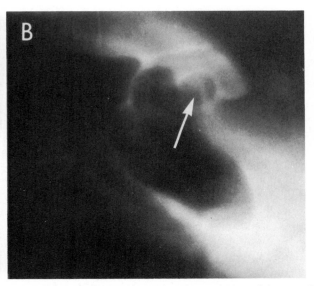

Fig 382.—A, calcification between middle and anterior clinoid processes forming small caroticoclinoid canal *(arrow).* **B,** lateral tomogram in another patient showing a larger right caroticoclinoid canal *(arrow).*

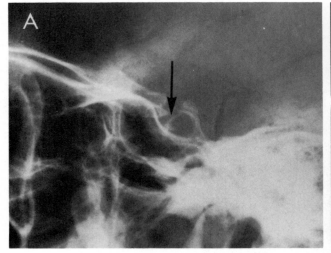
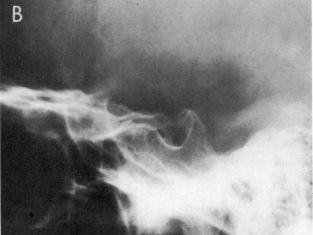

Fig 383.—A, calcification between middle and posterior clinoid processes *(arrow).* **B,** calcification between middle clinoid processes and anterior and posterior clinoid processes.

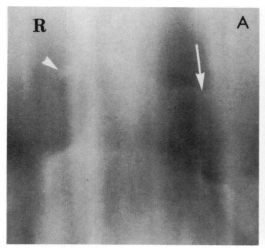

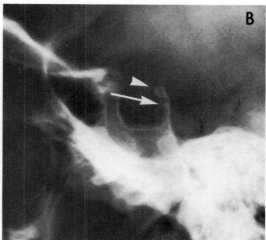

Fig 384.—Anteroposterior tomogram **(A)** and lateral radiograph **(B)** showing asymmetric posterior clinoid processes associated with lateral sloping of dorsum. Left posterior clinoid process *(arrow)* is considerably lower than the right *(arrowhead).*

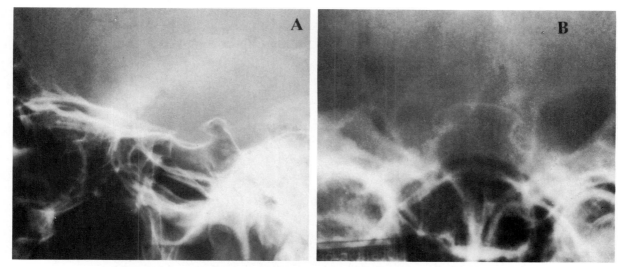

Fig 385.—Lateral **(A)** and Towne **(B)** views showing pneumatization of both posterior clinoid processes and the dorsum sellae in two different patients.

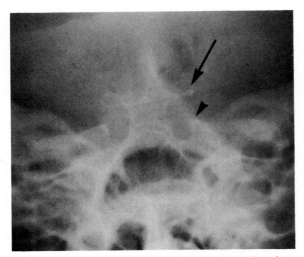

Fig 386.—Towne view showing symmetric anterior *(arrowhead)* and posterior *(arrow)* clinoid processes and dorsum sellae. Note that posterior clinoid processes have same well-defined cortical margins as the dorsum.

posterior clinoids have the same sharp outline as the dorsum sellae (Fig 386). The ligamentous connection between the anterior and posterior clinoid processes may calcify or ossify unilaterally or bilaterally (Fig 387).

DORSUM SELLAE

The dorsum sellae is the quadrilateral bony plate that marks the posterior boundary of the sella turcica. It consists of cancellous bone capped by an outer layer of cortical bone. The dorsum varies in size, shape, height, and thickness; it may be high or low, thick or thin, dense or pneumatized (Fig 388). Occasionally, it may have an asymmetric declivity best seen in the Towne

projection (Fig 389). The dorsum tends to have a thinner central concavity with thicker lateral margins. On the lateral roentgenogram, therefore, the anterior concave central cortex may be seen behind the anterior cortex on either side of the midline (Fig 390).

Although the anterior surface of the dorsum is usually smooth, the posterior surface may be somewhat irregular due to erosion by the basilar venous plexus (Fig 391). Rarely, a small bony spur projects from the posterior wall of the dorsum (Fig 392). The dorsum may be partially or completely pneumatized. The hallmark of the normal dorsum on the roentgenogram is the sharp, white, cortical outline (lamina dura) comparable to that of the sellar floor (Fig 393). The only areas where the lamina dura may normally be indistinct are the points of contact with the internal carotid artery, at the base of the dorsum in older persons (Fig 394).

SELLAR FLOOR

The floor of the sella is visualized on the lateral roentgenogram as a curved line, although its anterior wall may be fairly vertical (Figs 395 to 397). Occasionally, there is a small focal depression for the posterior lobe of the pituitary gland at the junction of the anterior surface of the dorsum with the floor. In the frontal projection, the horizontal portion of the floor may be slightly concave, flat or, less commonly, convex (Figs 398 and 399). This is best seen in the Caldwell projection or by anteroposterior tomography. When the floor slopes from side to side, it has a double or, less commonly, a triple contour (Fig 400).

In the lateral view, the floor has a sharply defined,

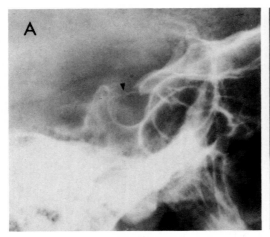 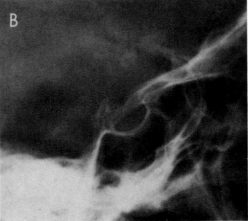

Fig 387.—**A,** unilateral calcification of ligament between anterior and posterior clinoid processes *(arrowhead)*.
B, bilateral ligamentous ossification between anterior and posterior clinoid processes.

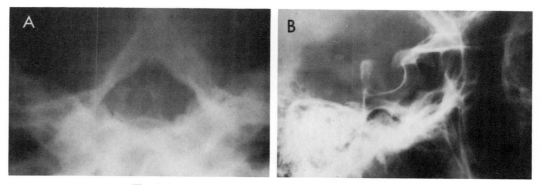

Fig 388.—Towne **(A)** and lateral **(B)** views showing
partial pneumatization of dorsum sellae.

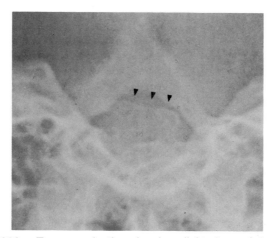

Fig 389.—Towne projection showing slight slope of dorsum
sellae from side to side *(arrowheads)*.

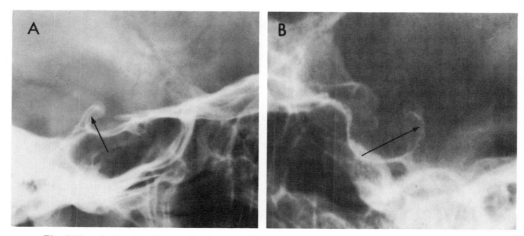

Fig 390.—Lateral radiographs in two different patients **(A** and **B)** showing the more
posterior location of thinner anterior central concavity of cortex of dorsum *(arrow)*.

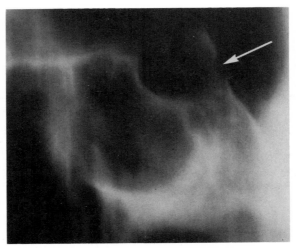

Fig 391.—Erosion of posterior surface of dorsum *(arrow),* i.e.,
upper clivus, by basilar venous plexus.

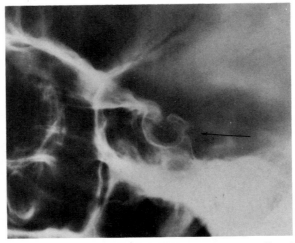

Fig 392.—Small spur on posterior aspect of dorsum sellae *(arrow).*

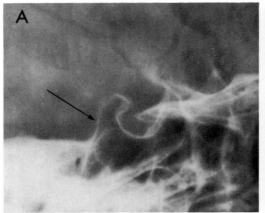
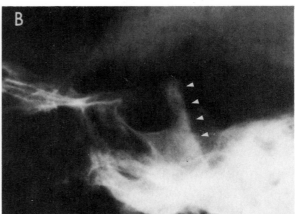

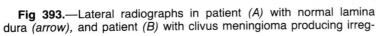

Fig 393.—Lateral radiographs in patient *(A)* with normal lamina
dura *(arrow),* and patient *(B)* with clivus meningioma producing irregular sclerosis of dorsum and loss of normal sharp lamina dura *(arrow-heads).*

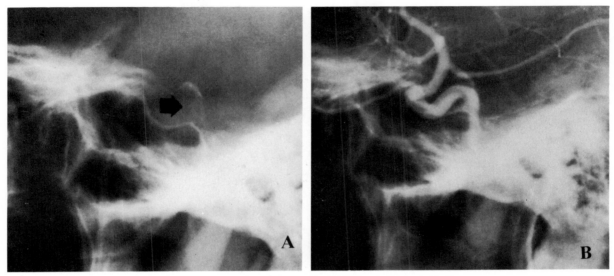

Fig 394.—Lateral plain film **(A)** and carotid arteriogram **(B)** in an elderly man showing loss of sharpness of lamina dura at base of dorsum *(arrow)* due to pulsations of tortuous internal carotid artery.

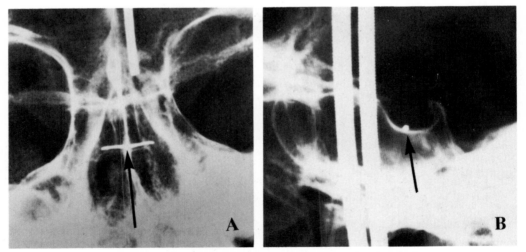

Fig 395.—Caldwell **(A)** and lateral **(B)** views of a dry skull with metallic marker on floor of sella *(arrow)*.

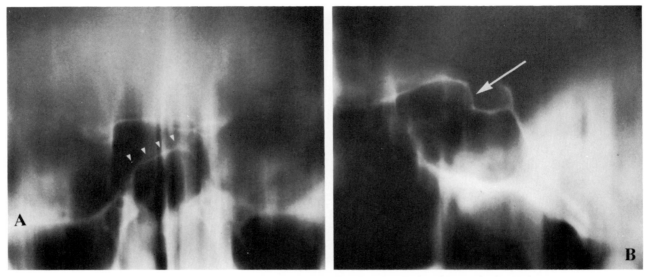

Fig 396.—Anteroposterior **(A)** and lateral **(B)** tomograms showing vertical anterior wall of sella *(arrow)*. Note also the sloping floor *(arrowheads)*.

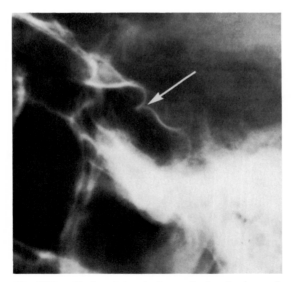

Fig 397.—Horizontal anterior wall of sella *(arrow)*.

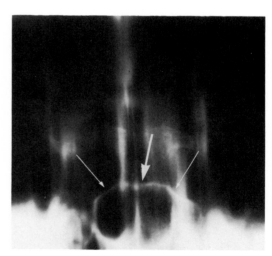

Fig 398.—Anteroposterior tomogram showing minimal concavity *(thick arrow)* in floor of sella and prominent lateral grooves for internal carotid artery *(thin arrow)*.

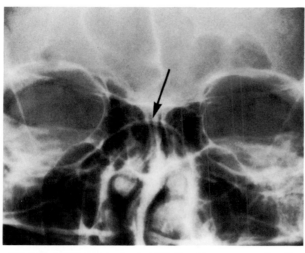

Fig 399.—Posteroanterior view in a patient with convex sellar floor *(arrow).*

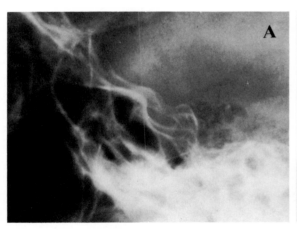

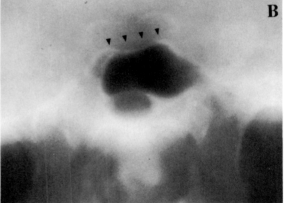

Fig 400.—Lateral radiograph **(A)** and anteroposterior tomogram **(B)** in a patient with normal sloping of sellar floor *(arrowheads),* presenting a double floor appearance in lateral projection. Diagram **(C)** shows mechanism of double floor formation.

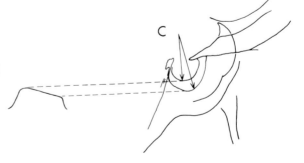

dense, cortical outline which continues onto the base of the anterior dorsum. When the body of the sphenoid is not significantly pneumatized, the cortex of the sellar floor rests on the cancellous sphenoid body. In the presence of a well-pneumatized sphenoid, however, the cortex of the sellar floor is contiguous with the fairly thick layer of compact bone which forms the roof of the sphenoid sinus. The sellar floor associated with a well-pneumatized sphenoid sinus is more resistant to erosive changes secondary to increased intracranial pressure.

SELLAR SIZE

For many years, the length and depth of the sellae were the only diameters used to determine sellar size. The length of the sella is represented by the distance between the tuberculum and the dorsum sellae on the lateral roentgenogram (top normal, 17 mm). The depth of the sella is determined on the same film by drawing a line from the tuberculum to the top of the dorsum. A perpendicular erected from this line to the lowest point in the sellar floor defines the depth of the sella (top normal, 14 mm) (Fig 401). In 1925, Haas suggested a method for measuring the area of the sella (top normal, 130 sq mm at 36 inches anode to film distance). Although this may be more accurate than two linear dimensions, it fails to consider the width of the sella. Volumetric measurements were introduced by Meldolesi and Pansadoro in 1937 and popularized by DiChiro and Nelson. The width of the sella can be measured on the Caldwell or the submentovertical projection or on an anteroposterior tomogram (normal, 10 to 15 mm).

The volume is calculated by multiplying one half × (length × depth × width). The normal volume varies considerably: 233 to 1,092 cu mm (DiChiro and Nelson) and 700 to 2,000 mm³ (Oon). Actually, most sellae that seem small on the lateral roentgenogram have a fairly generous width and a normal volume (Fig 402). The only small sella that has clinical significance is found in pituitary dwarfism.

Enlargement of the sella without bone destruction may occur in a variety of intracranial lesions, or secondary to hormonal deficiency, i.e., cretinism and untreated hypogonadism. In the latter instances, the ab-

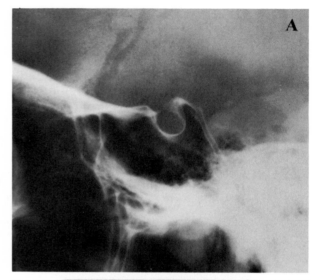

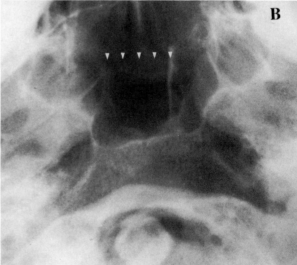

Fig 402.—Lateral view (A) in a normal adult showing relatively small anteroposterior and craniocaudad sellar diameters. Base view (B), however, shows a relatively wide transverse diameter *(arrowheads)* and a normal sellar volume.

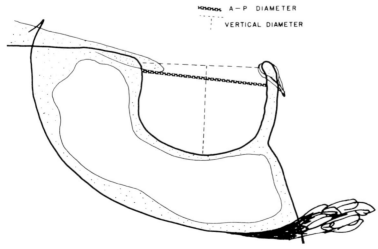

Fig 401.—Measurements of anteroposterior and vertical diameters of sella turcica.

sence of thyroxine and testosterone, respectively, produces a negative feedback mechanism, resulting in hyperplasia and unrestrained secretion of thyrotropic hormone in cretinism and of gonadotropic hormone in hypogonadism. This can enlarge the sella turcica without disrupting its bony outline—the so-called primary sella. Unfortunately, the gamut of the normal sellar volume is so broad that the pathologic sometimes overlaps the normal. Hence, in borderline cases, the volume of the sella per se, in the absence of other findings, is of limited value.

Most often, uniform sellar enlargement with a normal lamina dura is due to a pituitary tumor (Figs 403 and 404). However, it can also be produced by an empty sella (Fig 405), craniopharyngioma (Fig 406), or intra-

sellar aneurysm. Although the lamina dura may appear to be intact by conventional radiography, pluridirectional tomography at 1-mm intervals may demonstrate thinning or subtle erosion. Sellar enlargement in these patients is associated with depression of the floor, and posterior displacement and thinning of the dorsum. The sella appears "ballooned," with its walls molded around the expanding intrasellar mass. The posterior clinoid processes are usually intact. At times, the enlargement involves one side more extensively, resulting in asymmetric depression of the floor. In the frontal projection, the floor slopes to one side; this gives the appearance of a double floor in the lateral view. The normal frontal tomogram commonly demonstrates a flat or smooth, shallow central depression (< 2 mm) in the

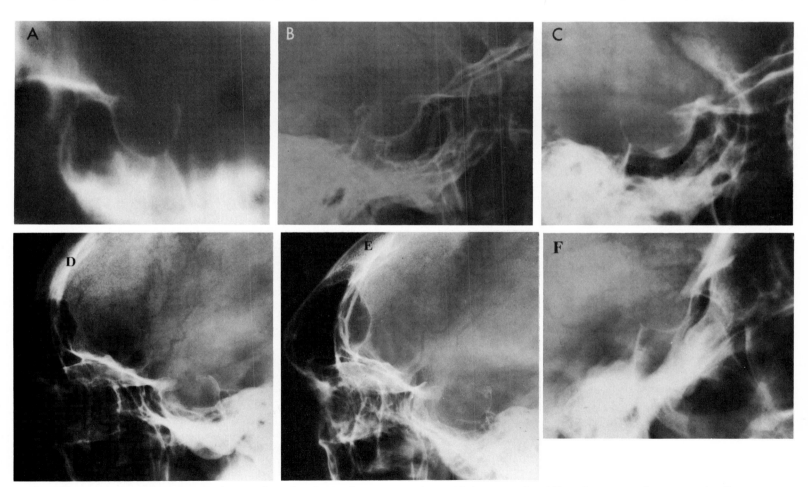

Fig 403.—Lateral roentgenograms in a series of patients demonstrating variations of primary sellar enlargement. **A,** chromophobe adenoma particularly affecting the floor and dorsum. **B,** double floor due to small chromophobe adenoma. **C,** depression of the floor and posterior displacement of thinned, intact dorsum in a patient with large chromophobe adenoma. **D,** generalized enlargement of sella in a patient with large eosinophilic adenoma and acromegaly. **E,** same patient 10 years later with progressive enlargement of sella with intact walls. Note growth of frontal sinuses over the 10-year period. **F,** chromophobe adenoma producing appearance of secondary sella. Close inspection of original films revealed an intact, markedly thinned, posteriorly displaced dorsum sellae.

ues, the bone resorption extends anteriorly into the lamina dura overlying a pneumatized sphenoid sinus. The double layer of cortical bone overlying a pneumatized sinus tends to be more resistant to the effects of increased intracranial pressure than does the single cortical layer overlying a nonpneumatized sinus. The erosive changes may ultimately involve the entire sella, the planum sphenoidale, the sulcus chiasmatis, and the

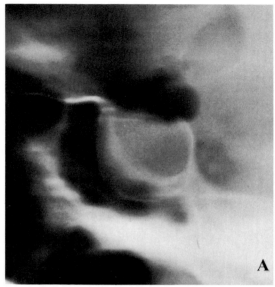

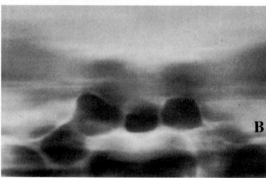

Fig 404.—Lateral **(A)** and anteroposterior **(B)** tomograms in a patient with a double floor due to asymmetric growth of large chromophobe adenoma. Lateral pneumoencephalogram shows no evidence of suprasellar extension.

floor, with rounded lateral margins. Uncommonly, the concavity may be deeper than 2 mm, and the rounded lateral margins of the sellar floor may be sharpened. This normal variant cannot be distinguished radiographically from a small intrasellar tumor. Progressive growth of an intrasellar lesion may ultimately produce loss of the lamina dura, and elevation and undercutting of the anterior clinoid processes on one or both sides.

Sellar changes also occur in patients with increased intracranial pressure (Fig 407) and hydrocephalus (Fig 408)—so-called secondary sella. The first demonstrable abnormality is loss of the lamina dura along the floor over the nonpneumatized portion of the sphenoid. The crisp, thin cortical bone becomes mottled and ill-defined, and the normally sharp lamina dura becomes discontinuous. If increased intracranial pressure contin-

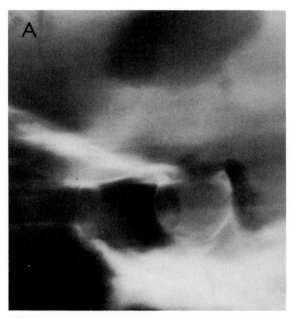

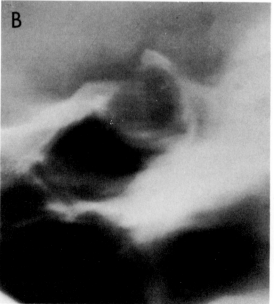

Fig 405.—Primary sella in a patient with arachnoidal diverticulum, i.e., empty sella, demonstrated by pneumoencephalography. **A,** brow up; **B,** brow down.

REFERENCES

Acheson R. M.: Radiographic determination of the growth of the pituitary fossa in preschool children. *Br. J. Radiol.* 27:298–300, 1954.

Acheson R. M.: Measuring the pituitary fossa from radiographs. *Br. J. Radiol.* 29:76–80, 1956.

Albert M., LeMay M.: Demineralization of the dorsum sellae associated with alcoholism. *Br. J. Radiol.* 41:331–332, 1968.

Anderson R. D.: Tortuosity of the cavernous carotid arteries causing sellar expansion simulating pituitary adenoma. *Am. J. Roentgenol.* 126:1203–1210, 1976.

Bar R. S., Mazzaferr E. L., Malarkey W. B.: Primary empty sella, galactorrhea, hyperprolactinemia, and renal tubular acidosis. *Am. J. Med.* 59:863–866, 1975.

Barnett D. J.: Radiologic aspects of craniopharyngiomas. *Radiology* 72:14–18, 1959.

Batson O. V.: Personal communication.

Bergland R. M., Ray B. S., Torack R. M.: Anatomical variations in the pituitary gland and adjacent structures in 225 human autopsy cases. *J. Neurosurg.* 28:93–99, 1968.

Besser G. M.: The pituitary fossa—normal or abnormal? *Br. J. Radiol.* 49:652–653, 1976.

Bower B. F.: Pituitary enlargement secondary to untreated primary hypogonadism. *Ann. Intern. Med.* 69:107–109, 1968.

Bruneton J. N., Drouillard J. P., Sabatier J. C., et al.: Normal variants of the sella turcica. *Radiology* 131:99–104, 1979.

Burrows E. H.: So-called J-sella. *Br. J. Radiol.* 37:661–669, 1964.

Burrows H., Cave A. J. E., Parbury K.: A radiological comparison of the pituitary fossa in male and female whites and negroes. *Br. J. Radiol.* 16:87–89, 1943.

Camp J. D.: The normal and pathologic anatomy of the sella turcica as revealed at necropsy. *Radiology* 1:65–73, 1925.

Camp J. D.: Normal and pathological anatomy of sella turcica as revealed by roentgenograms. *Am. J. Roentgenol.* 12:143–156, 1924.

Camp J. D.: Roentgenologic observations concerning erosion of sella turcica. *Radiology* 53:666–674, 1949.

Cushing H.: *The Pituitary Body and Its Disorders.* Philadelphia, J. B. Lippincott Co., 1912.

Cushing H.: Basophile adenomas of pituitary body: Their clinical manifestations (pituitary basophilism). *Bull. Johns Hopkins Hosp.* 50:137–195, 1932.

Cushing H.: *Papers Relating to the Pituitary Body, Hypothalamus and Parasympathetic Nervous System.* Springfield, Ill., Charles C Thomas, Publisher, 1932.

Danziger J., Wallace S., Handel S., et al.: The sella turcica in primary end organ failure. *Radiology* 131:111–115, 1979.

Deery E. M.: Calcification in pituitary adenomas. *Endocrinology* 13:455–458, 1929.

DiChiro G., Lindgren E.: Bone changes in cases of suprasellar meningioma. *Acta Radiol.* 38:133–138, 1952.

DiChiro G.: The width (third dimension) of the sella turcica. *Am. J. Roentgenol.* 84:26–37, 1960.

DiChiro G., Nelson K. B.: The volume of the sella turcica. *Am. J. Roentgenol.* 87:989–1008, 1962.

Dott N. M., Bailey P., Cushing H.: A consideration of hypophyseal adenomata. *Br. J. Surg.* 13:314–366, 1925–1926.

DuBois P. J., Orr D. P., Hoy R. J., et al.: Normal sellar variations in frontal tomograms. *Radiology* 131:105–110, 1979.

duBoulay G. H., El Gammal T.: The classification, clinical value and mechanism of sella turcica changes in raised intracranial pressure. *Br. J. Radiol.* 39:421–442, 1966.

duBoulay G. H., Trickey S. E.: The choice of radiological investigation in the management of tumors around the sella. *Clin. Radiol.* 18:349–365, 1967.

duBoulay G. H., Trickey S. E.: The sella in aqueduct stenosis and communicating hydrocephalus. *Br. J. Radiol.* 43:319–326, 1970.

Dussault J., Plamondon C., Volpe R.: Aneurysms of the internal carotid artery simulating pituitary tumours. *Can. Med. Assoc. J.* 101:785–790, 1969.

Enfield C. D.: The normal sella. *J.A.M.A.* 79:934–935, 1922.

Engels E.: The roentgen appearance of the carotid sulcus of the sphenoid bone. *Acta Radiol.* 49:113–116, 1958.

Epstein B. S.: Shortening of the posterior wall of the sella turcica caused by dilatation of the third ventricle or certain suprasellar tumors. *Am. J. Roentgenol.* 65:49–55, 1951.

Farinas P. L.: Value of x-ray examination of sella turcica in sagittal position. *Radiology* 32:411–415, 1939.

Ferrier P. E., Stone E. F. Jr.: Familial pituitary dwarfism associated with an abnormal sella turcica. *Pediatrics* 43:858–865, 1969.

Finby N., Kraft E.: The aging skull: Comparative roentgen study, 25 to 34 year interval. *Clin. Radiol.* 49:113–116, 1972.

Fisher R. L., DiChiro G. H.: The small sella turcica. *Am. J. Roentgenol.* 91:996–1008, 1964.

Fry K. I., duBoulay G. H.: Some observations on the sella in old age and arterial hypertension. *Br. J. Radiol.* 38:16–22, 1965.

Gabriele O. F.: The empty sella syndrome. *Am. J. Roentgenol.* 104:168–170, 1968.

Geehr R. B., Allen W. E. III, Rothman S. L. G., et al.: Pluridirectional tomography in the evaluation of pituitary tumors. *A. J. R.* 130:105–109, 1978.

Goldhamer K., Schüller A.: Die Varietaten der Sella Turcica. *Fortschr. Geb. Röntgenstrahlen* 33:894–900, 1925.

Gordon M. B., Bell A. L.: A roentgenographic study of the sella turcica in normal children. *N. Y. State J. Med.* 22:54–58, 1922.

Gordon M. B., Bell A. L.: Further roentgenographic studies of the sella turcica in abnormal children. *J. Pediatr.* 9:781–790, 1936.

Harlin R. S., Givens J. R.: Sheehan's syndrome associated with eclampsia and a small sella turcica. *South. Med. J.* 61:909–911, 1968.

Haas L. L.: Erfahrungen auf dem Gebiete der radiologischen Selladiagnostik. *Fortschr. Geb. Röntgenstrahlen* 33:419–422, 1925; 33:469–494, 1925.

Haas L. L.: Einzelheiten aus der Röntgendiagnostik der Sella turcica. *Fortschr. Geb. Röntgenstrahlen* 50:465–649, 1934; 51:147–152, 1935; 52:186–188, 1935.

Haas L. L.: The size of the sella turcica by age and sex. *Am. J. Roentgenol.* 72:754–761, 1954.

Hare H. F., Silveus E., Smedal M. I.: Roentgenologic diagnosis of pituitary tumors. *Radiology* 52:193–198, 1949.

Heublein G. W.: Some observations concerning the hypophyseal fossa. *Am. J. Roentgenol.* 56:299–319, 1946.

Hrdlicka A.: Dimensions of normal pituitary fossa or sella turcica in white and negro races. *Arch. Neurol. Psychopath.* 1:679–698, 1898.

Hsu T., Shapiro J. R., Tyson J. E., et al.: Hyperprolactinemia associated with empty sella syndrome. *J.A.M.A.* 235:2002–2004, 1976.

Israel H.: Continuing growth in sella turcica with age. *Am. J. Roentgenol.* 108:516–527, 1970.

Janicki P. C., Limbacher J. P., Guinto F. C. Jr.: Agenesis of the internal carotid artery with a primitive transsellar communicating artery. *Am. J. Roentgenol.* 132:130–132, 1979.

Jewett C. H.: Teleoroentgenography of the sella turcica with observations in one hundred cases. *Am. J. Roentgenol.* 7:352–355, 1920.

Johnston G. E.: Radiography of the sella turcica and pituitary body. *N. Y. State J. Med.* 16:559–561, 1916.

Jones J. R., Kemmann E.: Sella turcica abnormalities in an anovulatory population. *Obstet. Gynecol.* 48:76–78, 1976.

Kaufman B.: The "empty" sella turcica: Manifestation of the intrasellar subarachnoid space. *Radiology* 90:931–941, 1968.

Kaufman B., Sandstrom P. H., Young H. F.: Alteration in size and configuration of the sella turcica as the result of prolonged cerebrospinal fluid shunting. *Radiology* 97:537–542, 1970.

Kier E. L.: The infantile sella turcica: New roentgenologic and anatomic concepts based on a developmental study of the sphenoid bone. *Am. J. Roentgenol.* 102:747–767, 1968.

Kier E. L.: "J" and "omega" shape of sella turcica: Anatomic clarification of radiologic misconceptions. *Acta Radiol.* 9:91–94, 1969.

Kier E. L., Rothman S. L. G.: Radiologically significant anatomic variations of the developing sphenoid in humans, in Bosma J. F. (ed.): *Development of the Basicranium.* NIH 76–989. U.S. Dept. of Health, Education, and Welfare, 1976, 107–140.

Kishore P. R. S., Kaufman A. B., Melichar F. A.: Intrasellar carotid anastomosis simulating pituitary microadenoma. *Radiology* 132:381–383, 1979.

Kleinberg D. L., Noel G. L., Frantz A. G.: Galactorrhia: A study of 235 cases, including 48 with pituitary tumors. *N. Engl. J. Med.* 296:289–600, 1977.

Kornblum K.: Alterations in structure of sella turcica as revealed by roentgen ray. *Arch. Neurol. Psychiat.* 27:305–320, 1932.

Kornblum K.: Deformation of the sella turcica in tumors of the middle cranial fossa. *Am. J. Roentgenol.* 31:23–30, 1934.

Kornblum K., Osmond L. H.: Deformation of sella turcica by tumors in the pituitary fossa. *Ann. Surg.* 101:201–211, 1935.

Kovacs A.: Untersuchungen uber die Sellagrosse nach Haas Bei Kindern und bei Erwachsenen. *Fortschr. Geb. Röntgenstrahlen* 50:469–482, 1934.

Lee W. M., Adams J. E.: The empty sella syndrome. *J. Neurosurg.* 28:351–356, 1968.

Lowman R. M., Robinson F., McAllister W. B.: Craniopharyngeal canal. *Acta Radiol. (Diag.)* 5:41–54, 1966.

Mahmoud M. E. S.: The sella in health and disease. *Br. J. Radiol,* suppl. 8, 1958, pp. 1–100.

McLachlan M. S. F., Wright A. D., Doyle F. H.: Plain film and tomographic assessment of the pituitary fossa in 140 acromegalic patients. *Br. J. Radiol.* 43:360–369, 1970.

McLachlan M. S. F., Banna M.: Observer variation in interpreting radiographs of the pituitary fossa. *Invest. Radiol.* 14:23–26, 1979.

Mortara R., Norrell H.: Consequences of a deficient sellar diaphragm. *J. Neurosurg.* 32:565–573, 1970.

Oon C. L.: The size of the pituitary fossa in adults. *Br. J. Radiol.* 36:294–299, 1963.

Oon C. K., Lavender J. P., Joplin G. F.: The width of the normal pituitary gland: A comparison of two radiological methods of measurement. *Br. J. Radiol.* 35:418–422, 1962.

Pancoast H. K.: Interpretation of roentgenograms of pituitary tumors. *Am. J. Roentgenol.* 27:697–716, 1932.

Pancoast H. K., Pendergrass E. P., Schaeffer J. P.: *The Head and Neck in Roentgen Diagnosis.* Springfield, Ill., Charles C Thomas, Publisher, 1940.

Penkrot R. J., Bures C.: The apparently eroded dorsum sella: A new anomaly. *A. J. R.* 132:1005–1006, 1979.

Post K. D., et al.: Selective transsphenoidal adenomectomy in women with galactorrhea-amenorrhea. *J.A.M.A.* 242:158–162, 1979.

Pruett B. S.: Dimensions of hypophyseal fossa in man. *Am. J. Phys. Anthropol.* 11:205–222, 1928.

Radberg C.: Some aspects of the asymmetric enlargement of the sella turcica. *Acta Radiol. (Diag.)* 1:152–163, 1963.

Rasmussen A. T.: A quantitative study of the human hypophysis cerebri or pituitary body. *Endocrinology* 8:509–524, 1924.

Renn W. H., Rhoton A. L. Jr.: Microsurgical anatomy of the sellar region. *J. Neurosurg.* 43:288–298, 1975.

Riach I. C. F.: The pituitary fossa in childhood with particular reference to hypopituitarism. *Br. J. Radiol.* 39:241–248, 1966.

Rogol A. D., Eastman R. C.: Prolactin and pituitary tumors. *Am. J. Med.* 66:547–548, 1979.

Rothman S. L. G., Kier E. L., Allen W. E. III: The radiology of transsphenoidal hypophysectomy: A review of 100 cases. *Am. J. Roentgenol.* 127:601–606, 1976.

Royster L. T., Rodman N. F.: The size of the sella turcica in relation to body measurements. *Trans. Am. Pediatr. Soc.* 84:246–266, 1922.

Schaeffer J. P.: Some points in the regional anatomy of the optic pathway with special reference to tumors of the hypophysis cerebri and resulting ocular changes. *Anat. Rec.* 28:243–279, 1924.

Scheuermann H.: The roentgenological picture of the normal and the pathological sella turcica. *Acta Radiol.* 13:404–432, 1932.

Schüller A.: *Roentgen Diagnosis of Diseases of the Head.* St. Louis, C. V. Mosby Co., 1918.

Schüller A.: The sella turcica. *Am. J. Roentgenol.* 16:336–340, 1926.

Silverman F. N.: Roentgen standards for size of the pituitary fossa from infancy through adolescence. *Am. J. Roentgenol.* 78:451–460, 1957.

Smith T. R., Kier E. L.: Unfused planum sphenoidale: Differentiation from fracture. *Radiology* 98:305–509, 1971.

Steinbach H. L., Feldman R., Goldberg M. B.: Acromegaly. *Radiology* 72:535–549, 1959.

Swanson H. A., duBoulay G.: Borderline variants of the normal pituitary fossa. *Br. J. Radiol.* 48:366–369, 1975.

Syvertson A., Haughton V. M., Williams, A. L., et al.: The computed tomographic appearance of the normal pituitary gland and pituitary microadenomas. *Radiology* 133:385–391, 1979.

Thomson J. L. G.: Enlargement of the sella turcica: A report on 27 cases. *Br. J. Radiol.* 28:454–461, 1955.

Vezina J. L., Sutton T. J.: Prolactin-secreting pituitary microadenomas. *Am. J. Roentgenol.* 120:46–54, 1974.

Vezina J. L., Sutton T. J., Maltais R., et al.: Prolactin-secreting pituitary microadenomas. *Acta Radiol.*, suppl. 347, 1975, pp. 561–566.

Vezina J. L.: Prolactin-secreting pituitary adenomas: Radiologic diagnosis, in Robyn, C. and Harter, M. (eds.), *Progress in Prolactin Physiology and Pathology.* New York, Elsevier North-Holland, Inc., 1978.

White J., Ballatine H. T. Jr.: Intrasellar aneurysms simulating hypophyseal tumors. *J. Neurosurg.* 18:34–50, 1961.

Zatz L. M., Janon E. A., Newton T. H.: The enlarged sella and the intrasellar cistern. *Radiology* 93:1085–1091, 1969.

13

Cranial Mensuration

SHAPE OF SKULL

Retzius devised a cephalic index to classify the many varied skull shapes. The formula to obtain this index is as follows:

$$I = \frac{B \times 100}{L},$$

where I = cephalic index, B = maximal internal breadth of skull, and L = maximal internal length of skull.

Although skulls differ markedly in shape, they may be conveniently classified into three major types:

1. The dolichocephalic (Gr. *dolichos*, long + *kephalē*, head) skull, with a cephalic index less than 70, is common among Australians, Eskimos, Fiji islanders, Zulus, and Kaffirs (Fig 414, A).

2. The mesocephalic (Gr. *mesos*, middle) skull, with a cephalic index ranging between 70 and 80, is commonly found in Europeans.

3. The brachycephalic (Gr. *brachys*, short) skull, with a cephalic index greater than 80, is found among the American Indians, Burmese, and Malayans (Fig 414, B).

There are minor variations within these principal groups. One striking configuration, bathrocephaly (Gr. *bathron*, base or pedestal), characterized by overriding of the parietal and occipital bones, has no known pathologic significance (Figs 415 and 416). Similarly, excessively long or wide skulls are not necessarily pathologic. On the other hand, various forms of premature sutural synostosis (craniostenosis) may produce similar exaggerated shapes. Since the skull is held rigid at the site of premature sutural closure, there is little or no growth perpendicular to the long axis of the obliterated suture. At the same time, there is compensatory overgrowth in other directions.

Premature craniosynostosis is best classified by the shape of the skull resulting from obliteration of specific sutures. Thus, premature closure of the coronal suture produces a skull with a short anteroposterior diameter and compensatory overgrowth in the vertical and lateral directions. The result is the brachycephalic type of craniosynostosis. On the other hand, premature synostosis of the sagittal suture interferes with lateral growth of the skull. Simultaneously, there is increased growth of the vertical and anteroposterior diameters, producing the dolichocephalic or scaphocephalic (Gr. *skaphe*, boat) type of craniosynostosis. Premature closure of both the coronal and sagittal sutures results in the oxycephalic (Gr. *oxys*, sharp) or turricephalic (L. *turris*, tower) form of brachycephaly (see Fig 293). Unilateral premature closure of one or more transverse sutures produces an asymmetry termed plagiocephaly (Gr. *plagios*, oblique) (see Figs 290 and 291).

Pendergrass and Hodes have called attention to a mimicry of the turricephalic skull in children confined to bed for long periods with the occiput in a dependent position. Another unusual configuration known as hypertelorism was described by Greig in 1924 (Fig 417). This is a condition characterized by deep, circular orbits widely separated from each other. A metopic suture is frequently present. According to Greig, hypertelorism is due to disproportionate overgrowth of the lesser sphenoidal wings. Welcker, however, believed that overgrowth of the frontal bone in the presence of a patent metopic suture, pushes the orbits apart. Not infrequently, an increased interorbital distance may be noted clinically without corresponding roentgenographic findings. Although mental deficiency may accompany severe hypertelorism, minor forms of this deformity occur as a normal variant without associated mental or other disturbances.

Surface Landmarks

The following list comprises the more important points of orientation on the surface of the skull (Fig 418).

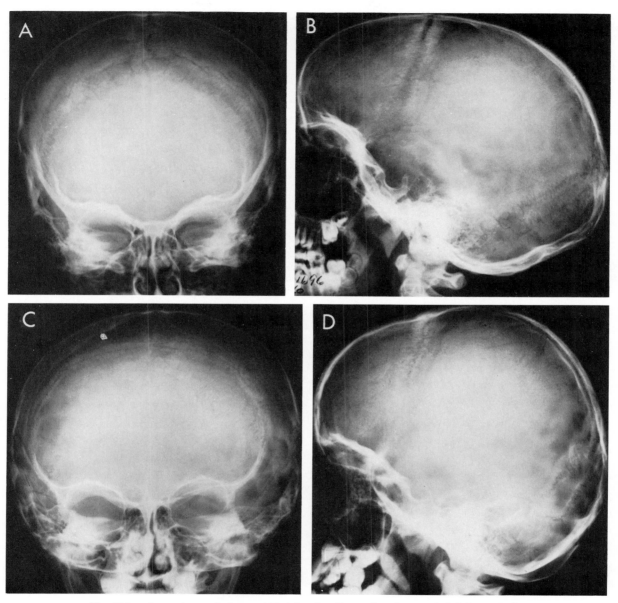

Fig 414.—A, posteroanterior and **B,** lateral radiographs of normal dolichocephalic skull. **C,** posteroanterior and **D,** lateral views of normal brachycephalic skull.

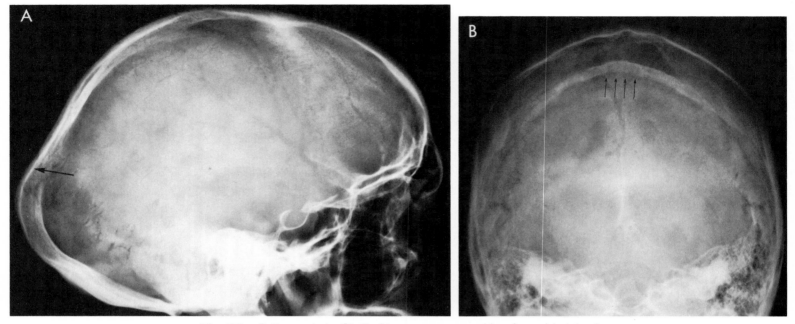

Fig 415.—Bathrocephaly. Shelf of bone appears as ridge *(arrow)* in lateral
view **(A)**, and as an overlay density in Towne projection **(B)**.

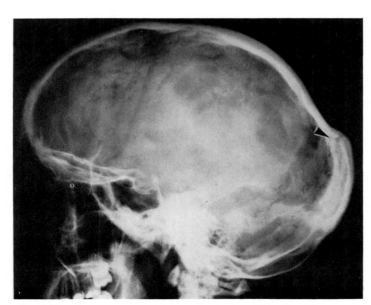

Fig 416.—Pronounced bathrocephaly with significant stepoff between parietal and occipital bones *(arrowhead)*.

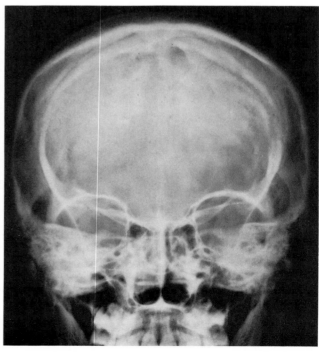

Fig 417.—Hypertelorism in an otherwise normal person. Note the wide interorbital distance.

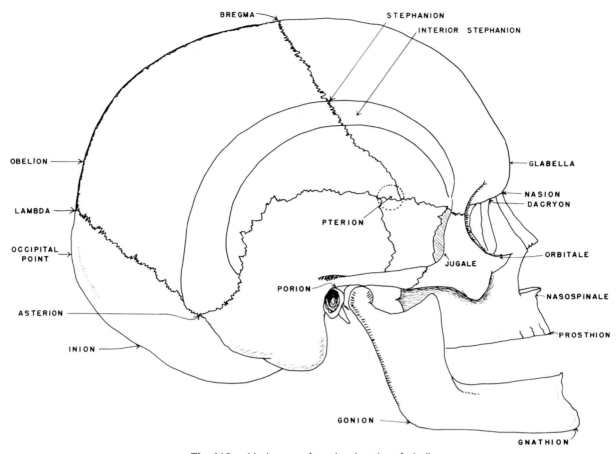

Fig 418.—Various surface landmarks of skull.

Nasion (L. *nasus*, nose): The middle of the nasofrontal suture.

Glabella (L. *glaber*, smooth): A point midway between the superciliary ridges just above the nose.

Bregma (Gr. *bregma*, front part of the head): The point of junction of the coronal and sagittal sutures.

Obelion (Gr. *obelos*, a spit): A point on the sagittal suture between the parietal foramina.

Vertex: The summit of the cranial vault.

Lambda (Gr. letter *lambda*, λ): The junction of the lambdoidal and sagittal sutures.

Inion (Gr. *inion*, nape of neck): The external occipital protuberance.

Asterion (Gr. *aster*, star): The region of the posterolateral fontanelle where the lambdoid, parietomastoid, and occipitomastoid sutures meet.

Basion (Gr. *basis*, base): The middle of the anterior margin of the foramen magnum.

Opisthion (Gr. *opisthios*, posterior): The middle of the posterior margin of the foramen magnum.

Pterion (Gr. *pteron*, wing): The region of the anterolateral fontanelle where the angles of the frontal, parietal, greater wing of the sphenoid, and squamous portion of the temporal bones articulate with one another. These sutures may be arranged like the letter H, with the parietal bone and greater sphenoidal wing separating the frontal bone from the squamous portion of the temporal bone. In other cases, the sutures may take the form of an X. Occasionally, the frontal bone and the squamosal portion of the temporal bone articulate with each other, thus separating the greater sphenoidal wing from the parietal bone.

Auricular Point: The center of the external auditory meatus.

Dacryon (Gr. *dacryon*, a tear): The point of articulation of the frontal, lacrimal, and maxillary bones.

Stephanion (Gr. *stephanos*, circle or crown): The point where the coronal suture crosses the temporal line.

Gonion (Gr. *gonia*, angle): The lateral margin of the angle of the mandible.

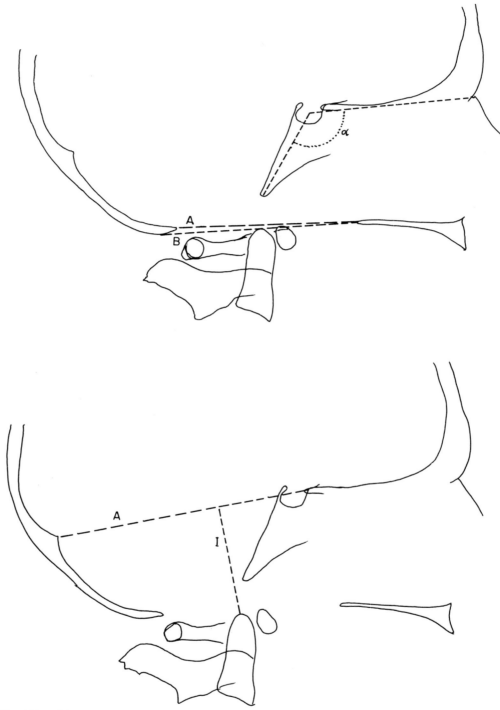

Fig 419.—Diagram illustrating *(top)* the basal angle (γ), Chamberlain's line *(A)*, and McGregor's modification of the latter *(B); (bottom)* tuberculocruciate line *(A)* and Klaus' height index *(I)*.

Gnathion (Gr. *gnathos*, jaw): The most prominent anterior point of the chin in the midline.

Occipital Point: The most posterior median point above the external occipital protuberance.

OTHER MEASUREMENTS

In addition to the cephalic index, there are several other measurements worthy of mention: (1) the basal angle, (2) Chamberlain's line and its modifications, and (3) the digastric line.

Basal Angle

The basal angle is the angle between the plane of the midbase of the anterior fossa and the plane of the clivus. The basal angle is measured by drawing a line on the lateral skull roentgenogram from the nasion to the center of the sella turcica. A second line is drawn from the latter point to the anterior lip of the foramen magnum. The inferior angle subtended by these lines is called the basal angle (Figs 419 and 420). Some prefer to use the tuberculum sellae as a reference point instead of the middle of the sella. In either case, the difference in measuring the angle is only a few degrees. The normal basal angle is usually in the range of 120 to 140 degrees. Skulls with a basal angle less than 120 degrees are considered to have a kyphotic base (Fig 421). Skulls with a basal angle greater than 145 degrees are said to have platybasia (Fig 422). Platybasia merely signifies an obtuseness or flatness of the base of the skull and has no clinical significance per se. Unfortunately, platybasia has been confused with basilar invagination, with which it may be associated. Thus, Chamberlain in his classic paper did not differentiate between the two conditions, and this confusion has unfortunately persisted.

Phylogenetic studies demonstrate a decreasing basal angle ascending from the lowest vertebrate forms to man. Thus, the reptile has the largest basal angle (180 degrees), with the floor of the anterior fossa, the clivus, and the spinal canal aligned in a straight line. Early in embryogenesis the human fetus also has a relatively straight base. As fetal development proceeds, flexion of the cranial base occurs at the spheno-occipital junction, and the face assumes a position below the cranium. The ventral aspect of the developing brain stem also becomes flexed at the sella turcica, so that the spinal cord and the foramen magnum change their straight posterior relationship to the brain to a more vertical one (Figs 423 and 424). The resulting increased

flexure of the skull base enlarges the volume of the cranial cavity to accommodate the marked brain growth that occurs in early childhood. Man has the smallest basal angle of all the primates: 120 to 140 degrees. Most mammals below the primate level have basal angles somewhat less than 180 degrees, while the subhuman primates tend to have basal angles greater than 150 degrees and less than 180 degrees.

Laitman, Heimbach, and Crelin have shown that there is an important relationship between the position of the tongue and larynx, the orientation of the pharyngeal constrictors, and the basal angle.

Newborn human infants and subhuman primates have a larger basal angle (145 to 150 degrees) than the older child and adult. This corresponds to the relatively high position of the tongue, epiglottis, and larynx. The resting tongue is entirely in the oral cavity, the larynx has a fairly high position, and the epiglottis is intranarial. This makes it possible for the epiglottis to slide up behind the soft palate and lock the larynx into the nasopharynx. The result is a one-tube airway between the external nares and the lungs. Because nonhuman primates and newborn humans are obligate nose breathers, they are able to breathe and swallow liquids at the same time. The high position of the larynx severely reduces the supralaryngeal air-containing pharynx, which modifies laryngeal sounds in older humans. The sounds produced are limited to those created at the vocal cords, with minimal modification in the oral cavity.

By age 4, the posterior third of the tongue has descended into the neck to form the vertical upper anterior wall of the pharynx. The epiglottis has also lost its intimate contact with the uvula. The larynx has descended farther down into the neck to open into the distal pharynx. This produces a prominent supralaryngeal pharynx that can modulate sounds originating at the vocal cords, an important aspect of the production of articular speech. These geographic changes in the position of the tongue, epiglottis, and larynx coincide with a reduction of the basal angle (135 degrees) (Figs 425 to 427), development of the pharyngeal musculature, and loss of the ability to breathe and swallow liquids simultaneously. The basal angle remains fairly constant after age 3 to 4, probably because of its nexus to bones derived from the primitive chondrocranium.

Kosowicz and Rzymski have pointed out an interesting relationship between the development of the skull base and various abnormalities of the sex chromosomes. A reduced number of sex chromosomes, e.g., Turner's

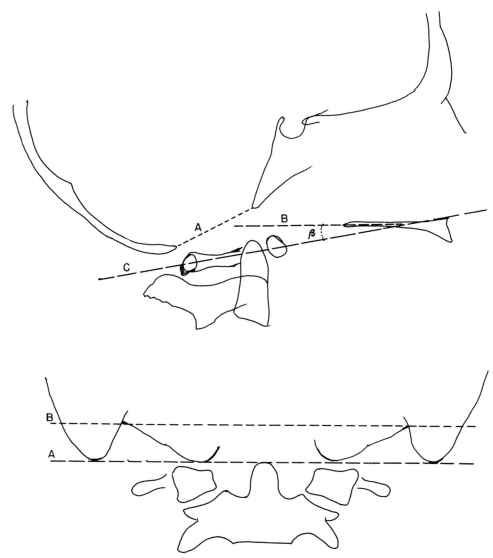

Fig 420.—Additional measurements used to diagnose basilar impression are *(top)* Boogard's line *(A)*, and Bull's angle (β) included between lines *B* and *C*; *(bottom)* Fischgold and Metzger's bimastoid line *(A)*, and digastric (biventer) line *(B)*.

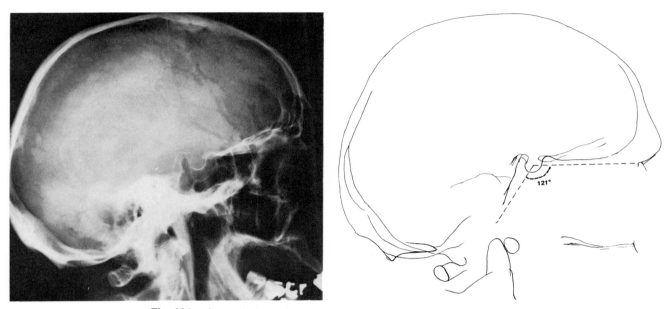

Fig 421.—Lateral view of normal skull with a relatively kyphotic base (121 degrees).

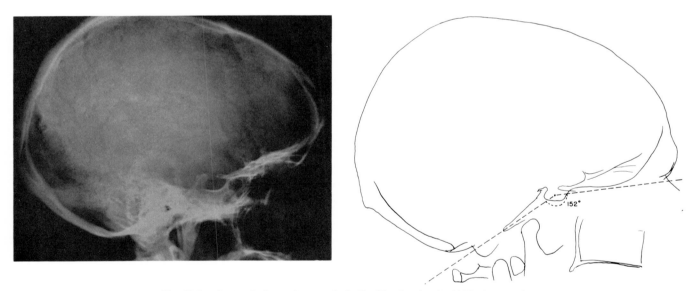

Fig 422.—Lateral view of normal skull with platybasia (152 degrees).

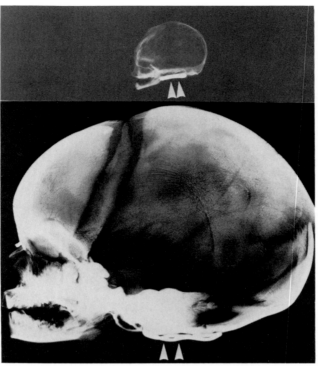

Fig 423.—Lateral radiographs of skull of stillborn fetus of 9 weeks gestation *(top)* and 40 weeks, i.e., term *(bottom)*, showing basal an-gle approaching 180 degrees early in fetal life and 150 degrees at birth. Note region of the foramen magnum *(arrowheads)*.

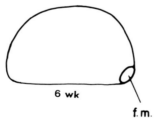

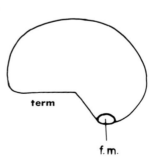

Fig 424.—Diagram (after Sperber) showing progressive flexure of cranial base during fetal development. Note dramatic change in direc-tion of foramen magnum from the horizontal (6 weeks) to the vertical (at term).

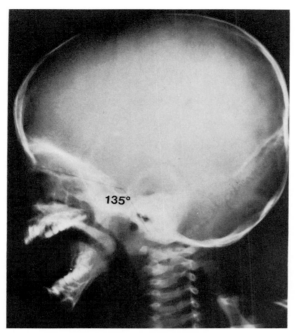

Fig 425.—Lateral view of normal skull in a 1-year-old boy with a basal angle of 135 degrees.

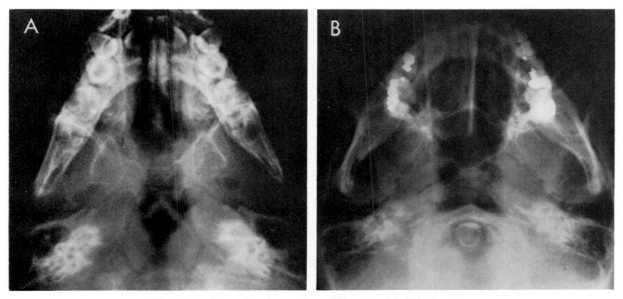

Fig 426.—Base view in newborn **(A)** and adult **(B)** showing enlargement of skull base and caudal migration of larynx.

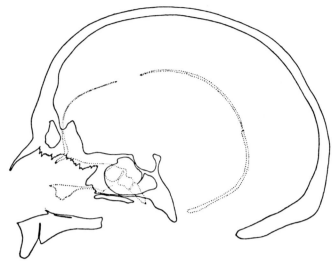

Fig 427.—Diagram of a sagittal section through the neonatal skull (····) and the adult skull(—) superimposed on the basal line (after Welcker).

syndrome with 45 X constitution, is associated with an increased basal angle. An excess of sex chromosomes, e.g., Klinefelter's syndrome (47 XXY), the 47 XYY syndrome, and the 47 XXX constitution, is associated with a decreased basal angle.

Kosowicz and Rzymski also reported that patients with various hormonal disorders do not have a primary change in the basal angle. Thus, the basal angle is normal in patients with pituitary dwarfism, eunuchism, pseudohermaphroditism, the congenital adrenogenital syndrome, deficiency of growth hormone, deficiency or excess of androgens, and isolated abnormal gonadal development without sex chromosome abnormalities. Some patients with acromegaly have an increased basal angle because of displacement of the tuberculum sella, but this is a secondary change.

In contradistinction to platybasia, basilar invagination refers to upward displacement of that part of the occipital bone forming the posterior half of the foramen magnum. In addition, the normal oval outline of the foramen magnum may be contracted and distorted, the slope of the clivus diminished, the petrous portion of the temporal bone pushed upward, and variable degrees of atlantoaxial fusion present. In effect, the cervical spine appears to have been pushed cephalad. Basilar impression and platybasia may exist together or separately.

While isolated platybasia is always asymptomatic, basilar invagination may either be asymptomatic or pro-

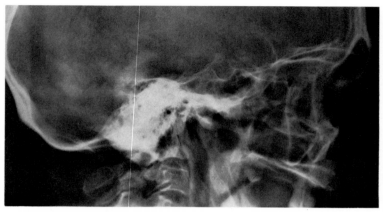

Fig 428.—Basilar impression in a patient with complete atlanto-occipital assimilation.

duce compression of the medulla and upper cervical cord, with resulting symptoms that can simulate degenerative neuropathies, cerebellar and high cervical tumors, and the Arnold-Chiari syndrome. Basilar impression may be congenital (primary) (Figs 428 and 429) or acquired (secondary to generalized skeletal demineralization or abnormal cranial ossification, e.g., Paget's disease) (Fig 430).

Chamberlain's Line

In 1938 Chamberlain described an arbitrary line (see Fig 419) on the lateral skull film drawn from the poste-

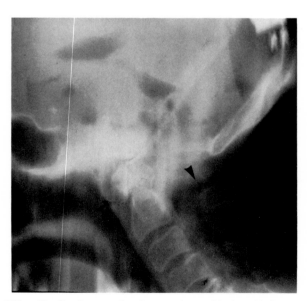

Fig 429.—Basilar impression in a patient with Arnold-Chiari malformation. Lateral pneumoencephalogram clearly shows cerebellar tonsils *(arrowhead)* displaced caudally into upper cervical canal.

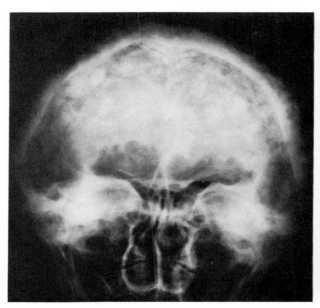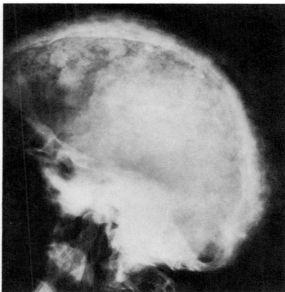

Fig 430.—Posteroanterior *(left)* and lateral *(right)* radiographs in a patient with acquired basilar impression due to advanced Paget's disease. Note upward displacement of the dens.

rior margin of the hard palate to the posterior margin of the foramen magnum. Body-section radiography may be helpful in defining the posterior rim of the foramen magnum when it is not clearly seen in the conventional lateral roentgenogram. Chamberlain originally stated that the normal odontoid tip lay below this line. However, Saunders measured the position of the tip of the dens with respect to Chamberlain's line in 100 normal skulls and found a significant normal variation: the arithmetic mean position of the tip of the dens was approximately 1 mm below the reference line. From the graph shown in Figure 431 it is obvious that even large deviations above the line may be normal.

Several modifications of Chamberlain's line have been suggested because of occasional difficulty in accurately localizing the posterior lip of the foramen magnum. Thus, McGregor draws a line from the dorsal surface of the posterior margin of the hard palate to the most caudal point of the occipital curve, a point easier to identify than the posterior lip of the foramen magnum. McCrae draws a line connecting the anterior and posterior margins of the foramen magnum, while Bull measures the angle between the plane of the atlas and the hard palate (< β). (The plane of the atlas is obtained by drawing a line joining the midpoints of the anterior and posterior atlantal arches on the lateral radiograph.) According to Bull, the normal range for < β should not exceed 10 to 13 degrees. Boogard measured the angle between the

clivus and the plane of the foramen magnum (normally 119 to 136 degrees) and considered values greater than 136 degrees to be diagnostic of basilar impression.

Another method utilizing the lateral projection is Klaus's height-height index, which measures the distance from the tip of the dens to a line joining the tuberculum sellae and the internal occipital protuberance (tuberculocruciate line). According to Klaus, the normal measurements are 40 to 41 mm, the index being less than 30 mm in basilar impression and 30 to 36 mm in platybasia.

On the other hand, Fischgold and Metzger employ an anteroposterior projection (tomogram) to measure the distance between the tip of the dens and a line drawn through the mastoid tips and to a second line joining the digastric grooves. (The grooves lie at the junction of the medial aspect of the mastoid processes with the base of the skull.) Although the bimastoid line is unreliable because of its inconstant relationship to the skull base, the digastric (biventer) line is helpful. Normally, the digastric line lies above the dens and approximately 10 mm above the middle of the atlanto-occipital joints.

It must be evident from the great number of methods that no single measurement is absolute or foolproof. Both Chamberlain's line and McGregor's line use the hard palate as a landmark, a point of variable position that is not part of the base of the skull. Obviously, the

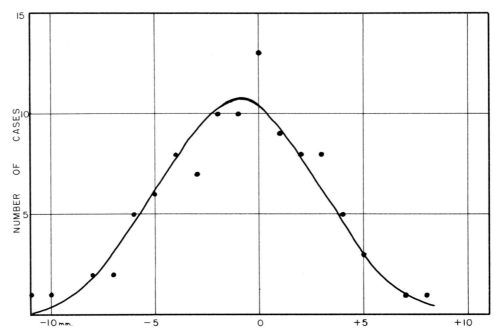

Fig 431.—Normal variations in relationship of tip of the dens to Chamberlain's line. (After Saunders). Minus values recorded refer to distance below and plus values to distance above Chamberlain's line.

position of the palate is intimately related to the development of the facial bones. A low palate may result in an erroneous diagnosis of basilar impression, while a high palate may cause the diagnosis to be missed. An occasional normal variant in the form of an elongated dens may also give rise to an erroneous diagnosis of basilar impression. In contradistinction to the disadvantages of the lateral projection, anteroposterior tomograms of the base of the skull do delineate the outline of the foramen magnum, thus making accurate diagnosis possible.

In my opinion, any of the above methods is satisfactory if it is intelligently applied and not interpreted too literally. I tend to use Chamberlain's or McGregor's line and the digastric line. If half of the dens lies above Chamberlain's or McGregor's line, basilar impression is present. Basilar impression is also present if the digastric line is at or below the level of the atlanto-occipital joints. It is important to remember that the normal relationship between the cervical spine and the base of the skull may vary considerably. The degree of flexion of the head does not significantly modify these measurements.

REFERENCES

Boogard J. A.: Basilar impression: Its causes and consequences. *Ned. Tijdschr. Geneeskd.* 2:81–108, 1865.

Bull G. W. D., Nixon W. L. B., Pratt R. T. C.: The radiolog-

ical criteria and familial occurrence of primary basilar impression. *Brain* 78:229–247, 1955.

Chamberlain W. E.: Basilar impression (platybasia). *Yale J. Biol. Med.* 11:487–496, 1939.

Craig W. M., Walsh M. N., Camp J. D.: Basilar invagination of the skull—so-called platybasia: Report of three cases. *Surg. Gynecol. Obstet.* 74:751–754, 1942.

Gladstone R. J., Erichsen-Powell W.: Manifestations of occipital vertebrae and fusion of the atlas with the occipital bone. *J. Anat. Physiol.* 49:190–209, 1915.

Goozdanovic V., Dogan S.: The use of tomography in diagnosis of basilar impression. *Acta Radiol.* 35:124–132, 1951.

Haas L. L.: Roentgenological skull measurements and their diagnostic applications. *Am. J. Roentgenol.* 67:197–209, 1952.

Klaus E.: X-ray diagnosis of platybasia and basilar impression: Further experiences with new diagnostic method. *Fortschr. Geb. Röntgenstrahlen* 86:460–469, 1957.

Kosowicz J., Rzymski K.: Radiological features of the skull in Klinefelter's syndrome and male hypogonadism. *Clin. Radiol.* 26:371–378, 1975.

Laitman J. T., Crelin E. S.: Postnatal development of the basicranium and vocal tract region in man, in Bosma J. F. (ed): *Development of the Basicranium.* NIH 76–989. U.S. Dept. of Health, Education and Welfare, 1976, pp. 206–219.

Laube P. J., Turner O.: Platybasia. *Yale J. Biol. Med.* 13:644–648, 1941.

Lindgren E.: Roentgenologic views on basilar impression. *Acta Radiol.* 22:297–302, 1941.

Lombardi G.: The occipital vertebra. *Am. J. Roentgenol.* 86:260–269, 1961.

McGregor M.: Significance of certain measurements of the

skull in the diagnosis of basilar impression. *Br. J. Radiol.* 21:171–181, 1948.

McRae D. L.: Bony abnormalities in the region of the foramen magnum: Correlation of the anatomic and neurologic findings. *Acta Radiol.* 40:335–354, 1953.

McRae D. L., Barnum A. S.: Occipitalization of the atlas. *Am. J. Roentgenol.* 70:23–46, 1953.

McRae D. L.: The significance of abnormalities of the cervical spine. *Am. J. Roentgenol.* 84:3–25, 1960.

McRae D. L.: Craniovertebral junction, in Newton T. H., Potts D. G. (eds.): *The Skull.* Book 1: *Radiology of the Skull and Brain,* vol. 1. St. Louis, C. V. Mosby Co., 1971.

Peyton W. T., Peterson H. O.: Congenital deformities in region of foramen magnum: Basilar impression. *Radiology* 38:131–144, 1942.

Poppel M. H. Jacobsen H. G., Duff B. K., et al.: Basilar impression and platybasia in Paget's disease. *Radiology* 61:639–644, 1953.

Saunders W. W.: Basilar impression: The position of the normal odontoid. *Radiology* 41:589–590, 1943.

Schüller A.: Zur Röntgen-Diagnose der Basalen Impression des Schädels. *Wien. Med. Wochenschr.* 61:2594–2599, 1911.

Schüller A.: The diagnosis of basilar impression. *Radiology* 34:214–216, 1940.

Shapiro R., Robinson F.: Anomalies of the craniovertebral border. *Am. J. Roentgenol.* 127:281–287, 1976.

Sperber G. H.: *Craniofacial Embryology.* Bristol, England, John Wright & Sons, 1973.

Spillane J. D., Pallis C., Jones A. M.: Developmental abnormalities in the region of the foramen magnum. *Brain* 80:11–48, 1958.

Welcker, H.: Untersuchungen über Wachstum und Bau des menschlichen Schädels. Leipzig, W. Engelmann, 1862.

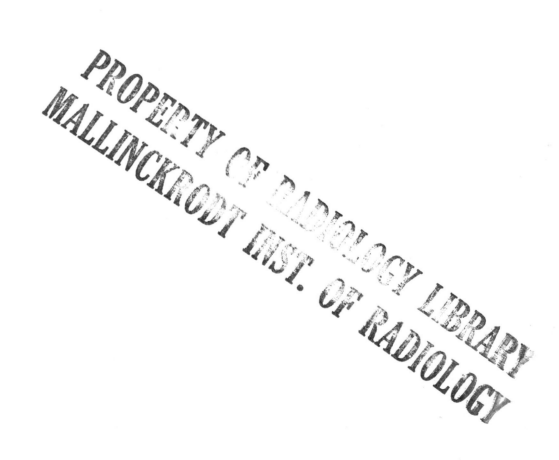

14

The Clivus, Foramen Magnum, and Craniovertebral Border

THE CLIVUS

The clivus is the bony slope on the endocranial aspect of the skull base extending from the dorsum sellae superiorly to the anterior margin of the foramen magnum (basion) inferiorly (Fig 432). Laterally on each side it is bounded by the petro-occipital fissure, which houses the inferior petrosal sinus (Figs 433 and 434). The smooth endocranial surface of the clivus usually has a slight concavity somewhat more pronounced at the level of the jugular tubercles, which mark the inferolateral margins of the clivus (Figs 435 and 436). The exocranial surface is rough at the sites of attachment of the pharyngeal muscles and fibrous raphe. Occasionally, the endocranial surface is also somewhat irregular because of erosion produced by pulsations of the basilar venous plexus (Fig 437). The ventral aspect of the pons and medulla are intimately related to the clivus, separated only by the pontine and medullary subarachnoid cisterns.

The clivus is composed of an anterosuperior sphenoid segment and an inferoposterior occipital portion. The spheno-occipital synchondrosis between these two components is usually fused by age 20. Although the clivus can be visualized by conventional radiography in the lateral projection, significant pneumatization of the mastoid interferes with good detail. The clivus is best demonstrated by lateral tomography in the midsagittal plane and by frontal tomography in a plane parallel to the slope of the clivus. In the lateral view, the clivus is portrayed as a triangle, with its apex at basion and its base on the dorsum sellae. The hallmark of a normal clivus is the sharp, white, cortical line along its dorsal and ventral surfaces produced by compact cortical bone. The central cancellous portion is pneumatized by the sphenoid sinus to a varying degree.

Increased concavity of the clivus (> 4 mm) is usually due to chronic increased intracranial pressure from a variety of supratentorial and infratentorial lesions. Similarly, an increased interjugular distance, according to Kruyff and Munn, may be indicative of chronic increased intracranial pressure. However, the measurement of interjugular distance is not helpful too often because of difficulty in visualizing the jugular tubercles. The' clivus is foreshortened and vertically oriented in achondroplasia because of the inherent disturbed growth of the chondrocranium.

THE FORAMEN MAGNUM

The foramen magnum is the large opening in the occipital bone through which the cranial cavity communicates with the vertebral canal. It transmits the medulla oblongata, the spinal portion of the accessory nerves, the vertebral arteries, the anterior and posterior spinal arteries, and veins communicating with the internal vertebral venous plexus. The apical dental ligament and the ascending slip of the cruciate ligament are attached to the inner aspect of the anterior rim of the foramen magnum. The alar ligaments, or check ligaments of the axis, are attached to the medial aspect of the occipital condyles. The midpoints on the anterior and posterior margins of the foramen magnum are respectively called basion and opisthion.

The foramen magnum is best visualized in the routine Chamberlain-Towne view. It is also well seen in tomographic cuts in the submentoventral projection. In the lateral view, especially with tomography, the anterior and posterior margins of the foramen magnum can be defined. The foramen magnum is usually round or oval in shape, with the long diameter oriented anteroposteriorly. Uncommonly, there are minor congenital anomalies present, e.g., a keyhole- or delta-shaped defect anteriorly or a midline notch posteriorly.

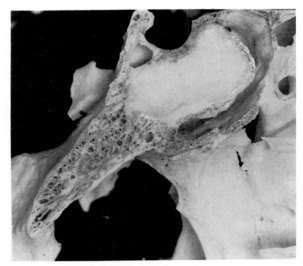

Fig 432.—Midline sagittal section of clivus and portion of sphenoid bone.

The foramen is small in patients with achondroplasia (Fig 438), occipital dysplasias, or various craniovertebral anomalies associated with abnormal segmentation (Fig 439). The foramen can also be reduced in size in patients with various productive bone diseases, e.g., osteopetrosis and Paget's disease. Enlargement of the foramen magnum with intact bony margins may be due either to chronic increased intracranial pressure or to di-

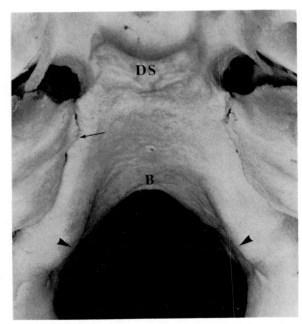

Fig 433.—Clivus from above. Jugular tubercles *(arrowhead)*, dorsum sellae *(DS)*, basion *(B)*, and petro-occipital fissure *(arrow)* are identified.

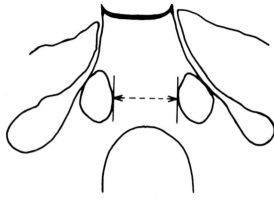

Fig 434.—Line drawing traced from radiograph showing interjugular diameter *(arrows)*, indicative of width of inferior portion of clivus.

rect pressure from an expanding intraforaminal mass, e.g., syringomyelia and neoplasms. Localized destruction of one of the margins of the foramen is usually due to a malignant tumor, e.g., metastatic carcinoma and chordoma. In children, a destructive focus may be produced by histiocytosis.

THE CRANIOVERTEBRAL JUNCTION

Embryology

The occipital bone develops from the union of at least four primary somites, which correspond to the primary roots of the hypoglossal nerve. The first somite disappears by the end of the third week of gestation. The other three somites fuse into a single mass.

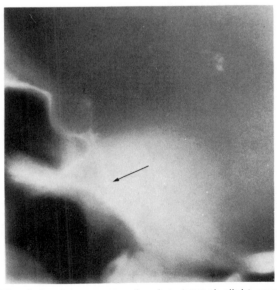

Fig 435.—Lateral tomogram showing normal slight concavity of lower clivus *(arrow)*.

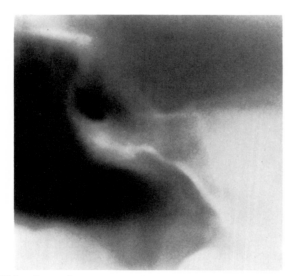

Fig 436.—Lateral tomogram showing relatively vertical, flat clivus and no concavity in a 78-year-old woman.

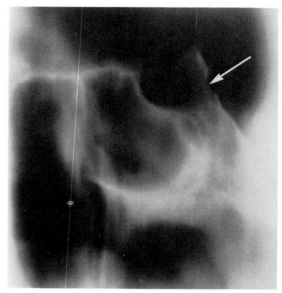

Fig 437.—Lateral tomogram showing erosion of endocranial aspect of clivus by basilar venous plexus *(arrow)*.

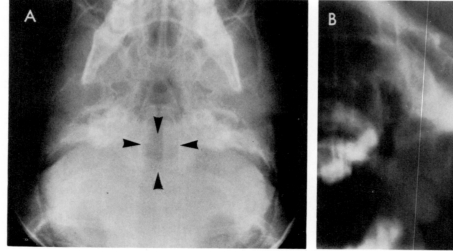

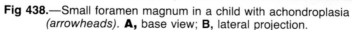

Fig 438.—Small foramen magnum in a child with achondroplasia *(arrowheads)*. **A,** base view; **B,** lateral projection.

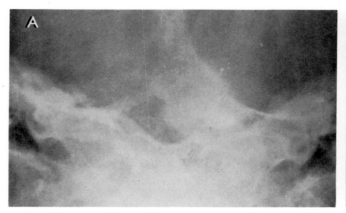 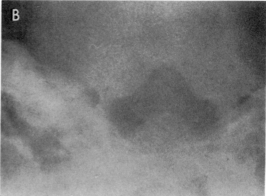

Fig 439.—A, asymmetric coarctation of foramen magnum in a patient with atlanto-occipital assimilation. **B,** cloverleaf deformity of foramen magnum in a young male with multiple occipitovertebral anomalies.

In some lower vertebrates, e.g., reptiles, the cranial half of the first cervical sclerotome persists as a separate bone, the proatlas, between the occiput and C-1. In man, however, it normally is assimilated into the occipital condyles and also forms the tip of the dens. The anlage for the body of C-1 separates from its arches and gives rise to the remainder of the dens. Thus, the dens has a dual origin from the body of C-1 and from the cranial half of the first cervical sclerotome.

The caudal half of the first cervical sclerotome gives rise to the anterior and posterior arches of the atlas as well as its lateral masses. The body, posterior arch, and transverse processes of C-2 are derived from the second cervical sclerotome (Fig 440).

On the evolutionary scale, the craniovertebral junction moves caudally as various vertebral segments are assimilated into the postotic calvaria. It is helpful to think of the craniovertebral border as an embryologically unstable zone subject to variation, much like the lumbosacral junction, where lumbarization of S-1 and sacralization of L-5 are common.

If the distal occipital sclerotomes and the cranial end of the first cervical sclerotome are incompletely assimilated into the occiput, various expressions of an occipital vertebra occur. On the other hand, if normal segmentation fails to occur, atlantoaxial fusion results. Thus, an occipital vertebra and atlanto-occipital fusion represent opposite ends of a continuous spectrum.

Incomplete Assimilation

TRANSVERSE BASIOCCIPITAL FISSURE

The simplest form of incomplete assimilation of the primitive occipital somites is a transverse cleft in the basiocciput. The fissure may be unilateral or bilateral, partial or complete (Fig 441).

THIRD OCCIPITAL CONDYLE

This anomaly is characterized by a single midline bony knob either attached to the anterior margin of the foramen magnum or separated therefrom by a few millimeters (Fig 442). The third occipital condyle may have a facet for articulation with the dens or with the anterior arch of C-1, especially in the presence of atlanto-occipital synostosis.

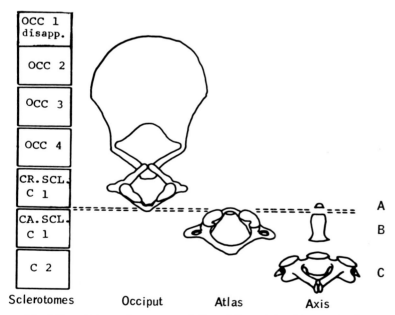

Fig 440.—Schematic representation of the origin of bony structures of craniovertebral region. (Modified from List.) (From Shapiro, R., and Robinson, F.: *Am. J. Roentgenol.* 127:281–287, 1976.)

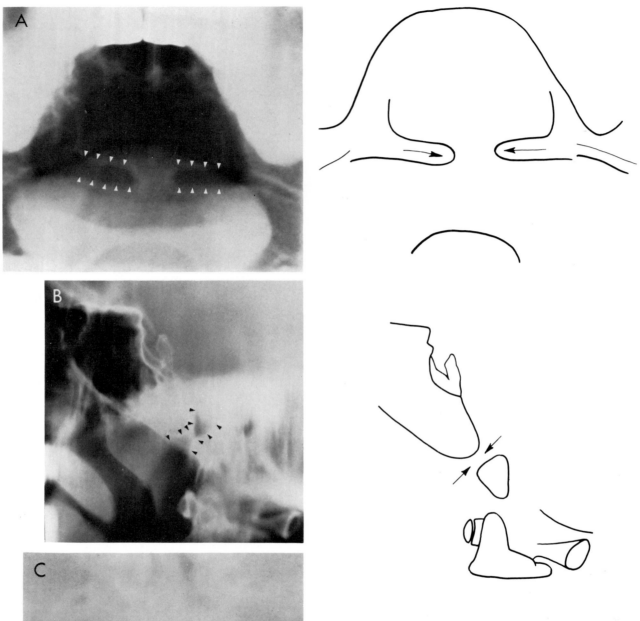

Fig 441.—Radiograph and line drawing in modified open mouth Waters projection **(A)** and in lateral projection **(B)** showing bilateral clefts in basiocciput *(arrowheads)* of a 15-year-old boy. Modified Waters projection **(C)** in a neonate showing similar bilateral cleft defect in basiocciput *(arrowheads)*. (From Johnson, G. F., and Israel, H.: *Radiology* 133:101–103, 1979.)

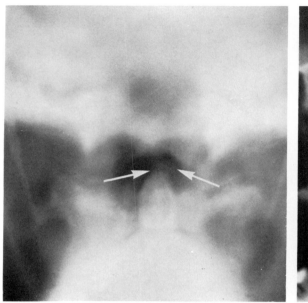
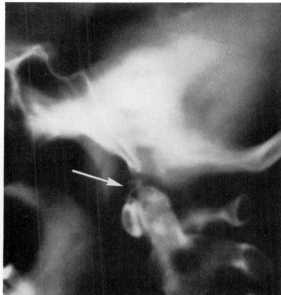

Fig 442.—Anteroposterior *(left)* and lateral *(right)* tomograms of a patient with third occipital condyle *(arrow)*.

BASILAR PROCESSES

Separate or attached dual paramedian tubercles along the anterior margin of the foramen magnum are a rare finding (Fig 443). These processes may have articular facets for the anterior rim of C-1.

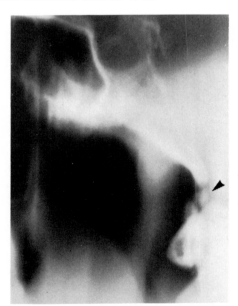

Fig 443.—Lateral tomogram demonstrating basilar process *(arrowhead)* articulating with superior rim of anterior arch of C-1 by a pseudoarthrosis. The base view, which is not reproducible, showed two paramedian ossicles, one on either side of anterior rim of foramen magnum.

OS ODONTOIDEUM

The os odontoideum is usually a congenital anomaly, but rarely a similar appearance can be a sequel of trauma. The abnormality is characterized by a separate bone associated with a cupola-shaped, hypoplastic dens (Fig 444). The discrete ossicle may be directly above the hypoplastic dens or anterior and superior to the dens closer to the basiocciput. It may be attached to the anterior arch of C-1 in the midline or slightly lateral thereto. Occasionally, the os odontoideum articulates with the basiocciput by a pseudarthrosis.

BILATERAL ATLANTAL FACETS

These facets are a vestige of the cranial half of the first cervical sclerotome, which normally forms the dorsal portion of the lateral atlantal masses (Fig 445).

Atlanto-Occipital Fusion

ATLANTO-OCCIPITAL SYNOSTOSIS

Fusion of C-1 with the basiocciput may be unilateral (Fig 446) or bilateral (Fig 447). When bilateral, the fusion is not necessarily symmetric. The bony fusion may involve the posterior atlantal arch or more commonly, the anterior atlantal arch, or both. It may occur as an isolated anomaly or together with other vertebral abnor-

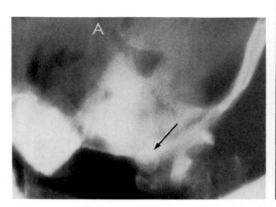
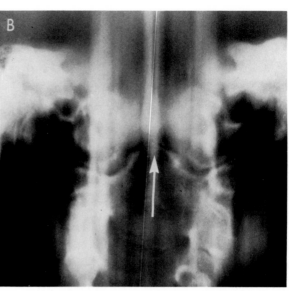

Fig 444.—**A,** lateral pneumotomogram in a 1-year-old girl with Down's syndrome showing os odontoideum *(arrow)*. **B,** anteroposterior tomogram showing deformed, hillock-shaped, hypoplastic dens in an adult with os odontoideum *(arrow)*. (From Shapiro, R., and Robinson, F.: *Am. J. Roentgenol.* 127:281–287, 1976.)

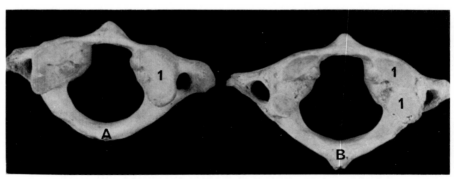

Fig 445.—Normal single atlantal articulation (**A,***1*) and bipartite atlantal articulations (**B,** *1,1*).

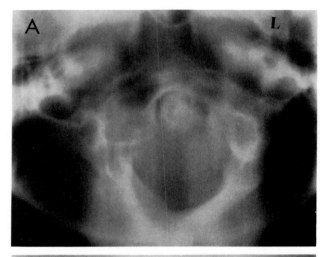

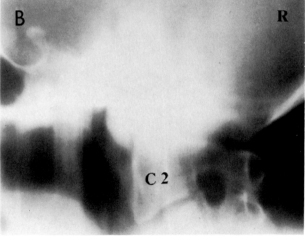

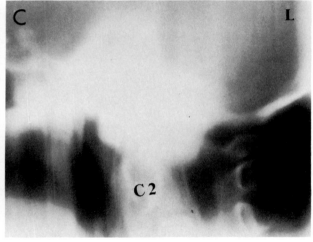

Fig 446.—Tomograms in base view **(A)**, and right **(B)** and left **(C)** lateral views showing unilateral assimilation of C-1 on the right. Note normal relationship on left side.

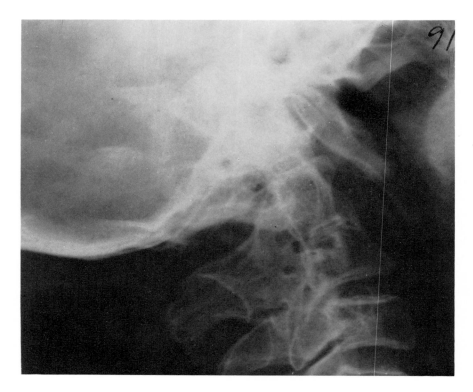

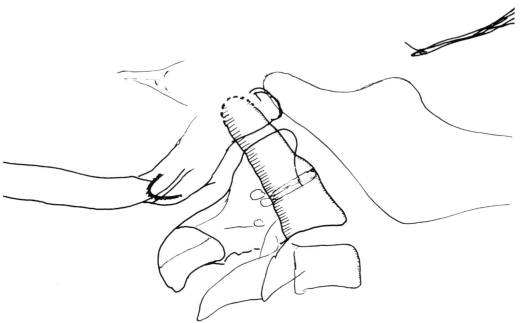

Fig 447.—Lateral radiograph and line drawing showing bilateral atlanto-occipital assimilation. Note also segmentation abnormality at C2–3, a common associated finding.

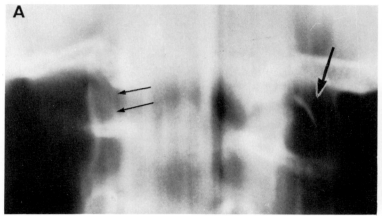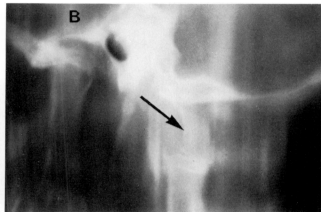

Fig 448.—Anteroposterior **(A)** and oblique **(B)** tomograms in a 32-year-old woman showing right epitransverse process *(small arrows)* and left paracondylar process *(large arrow)*. (From Shapiro, R., and Robinson, F.: *Am. J. Roentgenol.* 127:281–287, 1976.)

malities, e.g., failure of segmentation, particularly at C-2 and C-3. Lateral radiographs in flexion and extension demonstrate absence of motion between C-1 and the occiput.

According to McCrae, only 25 to 33% of patients with atlanto-occipital synostosis have neurologic involvement. In my experience, neurologic involvement is usually secondary to the presence of one or more of the following associated abnormalities: (1) constriction of the foramen magnum, (2) basilar impression, or (3) hydrocephalus due to adhesions, the Arnold-Chiari malformation, the Dandy-Walker syndrome, or syringohydromyelia.

ATLANTO-OCCIPITAL OSSIFICATION

The paracondylar process is a broad-based, cone-shaped, bony mass projecting down from the lateral aspect of the occipital condyle toward the transverse process of C-1. The term "paramastoid process" is inappropriate in man, since the bony process is not connected to the mastoid tip.

The epitransverse process is a thinner strut of bone arising from the transverse process of the atlas and projecting craniad toward the occipital condyle. In a sense, the epitransverse process is a mirror image of the paracondylar process.

The paracondylar and the epitransverse processes may exist singly or together; they may be unilateral or bilateral (Fig 448). They may occur as isolated anomalies or as part of a complex of craniovertebral junction abnormalities, e.g., atlanto-occipital synostosis. These bony projections represent vestiges of the cranial half of the first cervical sclerotome.

REFERENCES

Cohen L., Macrae D.: Tumors in the region of the foramen magnum. *J. Neurosurg.* 19:462–469, 1962.

Cohen M., Rosenthal A. D., Matson D. D.: Neurological abnormalities in achondroplastic children. *J. Pediatr.* 71:367–376, 1967.

Coin C. G., Malkasian D. R.: Foramen magnum, in Newton T. H., Potts, D. G. (eds.): *The Skull.* Book 1: *Radiology of the Skull and Brain,* vol. 1. St. Louis, C. V. Mosby Co., 1971.

Coin C. G., Malkasian D. R.: Clivus, in Newton T. H., Potts D. G. (eds.): *The Skull.* Book 1: *Radiology of the Skull and Brain,* vol. 1. St. Louis, C. V. Mosby Co., 1971.

DiChiro G., Anderson W. B.: Clivus. *Clin. Radiol.* 16:211–223, 1965.

Fischer E.: Neue Befunde am Vorderrand des Foramen occipitale magnum. *Fortschr. Roentgenstr.* 99:805–808, 1963.

Kruyff E.: Occipital dysplasia in infancy. *Radiology* 85:501–506, 1965.

Kruyff E., Munn J. D.: Posterior fossa tumors in children. *Am. J. Roentgenol.* 89:951–965, 1963.

McRae D. L.: Bony abnormalities in the region of the foramen magnum: Correlation of the anatomic and neurologic findings. *Acta Radiol.* 4:335–354, 1953.

15

The Paranasal Sinuses

The air-containing paranasal sinuses normally consist of paired frontal, maxillary, and sphenoidal sinuses, and the various ethmoidal cells. All of the sinuses develop as outpouchings of the nasal mucous membrane during the fourth month of fetal life. Since many of the cells migrate some distance from their site of origin, marked variations in morphology and geographic extent of the sinuses are common. Failure to appreciate this may result in unsuccessful treatment of persistent sinus disease (Fig 449).

FRONTAL SINUSES

The frontal sinus and various anterior ethmoidal cells have a common anlage in the frontal recess of the middle meatus of the nose. The frontal recess can be clearly recognized as a superior extension of the middle meatus during the fourth fetal month (Fig 450). In the next few months, the mucosa of the lateral wall of the frontal recess is thrown into a series of folds, and the furrows between the folds evaginate. Like all sinus development, continued extension takes place by progressive pseudopod-like advancement of the mucosa and simultaneous resorption of the overlying cancellous bone.

Pneumatization first occurs in the horizontal (orbital) plate of the frontal bone during the first year of life. Pneumatization of the vertical plate begins during the latter half of the second postnatal year and progresses slowly to reach the level of nasion by age 4. Moss and Young have shown that the frontal bone is not a single functional unit. The inner table is actually part of the cerebral capsule, since its periosteum is the outer layer of the dura. Hence, growth of the inner table is governed by the development and configuration of the frontal lobes.

On the other hand, the outer table is functionally independent of the inner table. During the first few years of life, as the frontal lobes grow, the inner table drifts anteriorly, carrying the outer table with it in the ab-

sence of a significant diploe (see Fig 88). By age 6 to 7, after major development of the frontal lobes has occurred, growth of the inner table becomes arrested. However, the functionally independent outer table continues to drift anteriorly in response to the growing nasomaxillary facial complex. This brings about progressive separation of the inner and outer tables. The intervening spacial gap is filled by the frontal sinuses.

The anteroposterior extent of the frontal sinuses is best shown in the lateral and overextended base views (Fig 451). These projections readily differentiate the density of unilateral poor pneumatization of the vertical plate of the frontal bone from chronic osteitis.

When the septum frontale is not in the midline, the sinuses are asymmetric (Fig 452). Another cause of asymmetric frontal sinuses is partial or complete failure of pneumatization of one vertical plate of the frontal bone (Fig 453). If the septum is midline in position, the sinuses tend to be symmetric (Fig 454). In this regard, a persistent metopic suture is commonly associated with relatively small, symmetric frontal sinuses (Fig 455). Rarely, the frontal sinuses have no septum separating the two sides (Fig 456). The adult frontal sinuses are seldom simple chambers (Fig 457), being frequently compartmented by incomplete bony septa; uncommonly, the septation is complex (Fig 458).

Occasionally, there is a congenital or acquired opening in the septum frontale. MacMillan has reported herniation of the diseased sinus mucosa through such a defect into the adjacent normal sinus. Occasionally, supernumerary sinuses are present. Rarely, pneumatization is so profuse that it extends beyond the frontal bones into the lesser and greater sphenoidal wings, the parietal, temporal, and nasal bones, and the frontal processes of the maxilla (Fig 459). Hypersecretion of the growth factor of the anterior lobe of the pituitary gland, i.e., acromegaly, is commonly associated with marked pneumatization of the frontal sinuses (Fig 460). Conversely, the true pituitary dwarf who lacks growth hor-

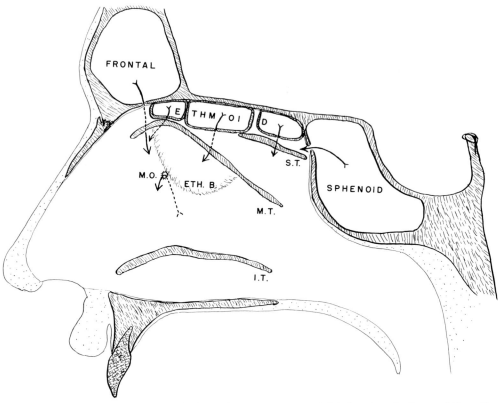

Fig 449.—Schematic lateral view of right side sectioned through right paramedian sagittal plane, showing drainage of paranasal sinuses. (After Caffey.) Note usual channels and openings of sinuses *(arrows)* as described in the text. Distribution of ethmoidal groups of cells and their drainage ostia are particularly variable. Maxillary sinus ostium *(M.O.)* lies just in front of the ethmoid bulla *(ETH. B.)*. Note superior *(S.T.)*, middle *(M.T.)*, and inferior turbinates *(I.T.)*. Corresponding meatuses lie beneath each turbinate. Superior meatus lies above and posterior to superior turbinate.

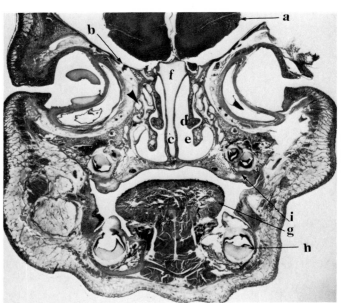

Fig 450.—Coronal section through region of fronto-ethmoidal recess *(arrowhead)* in a 32-week-old fetus. Hematoxylin eosin. Any of these cells may develop into the frontal sinus. Note frontal lobe *(a)*, floor of anterior fossa *(b)*, nasal septum *(c)*, middle turbinate *(d)*, inferior turbinate *(e)*, body of vomer *(f)*, tongue *(g)*, deciduous first molar *(h)*, and alveolar process of maxilla *(i)*. (From Shapiro, R., and Schorr, S.: *Invest. Radiol.* 15:191, 1980.)

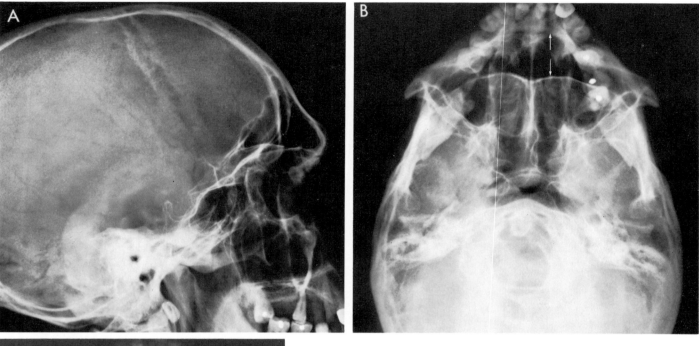

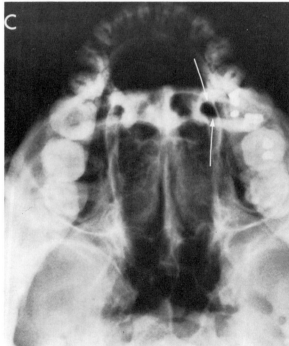

Fig 451.—Large normal frontal sinuses extending into orbital roofs **(A)**. Overextended base view **(B)** demonstrates anterior and posterior walls of frontal sinuses *(arrows)*. Overextended base view **(C)** in a patient with shallow frontal sinuses *(arrows)*.

mone has no pneumatization of the frontal sinuses (Fig 461). The roentgenologic differential diagnosis between the small sella characteristic of the pituitary dwarf and any other small sella with no clinical significance rests upon the presence of normally pneumatized frontal sinuses in the latter (Fig 462).

The normal paranasal sinus has a thin, sharp, dense, white line bordering its margins (Figs 463 to 466). This line, which represents the mucoperiosteal interface, may be modified by disease in several ways:

1. Thickening of the mucous membrane by edema, chronic inflammation, fibrosis, or tumor diminishes the contrast of the bone-air interface (Figs 467 and 468). This is the earliest roentgenologic finding in inflammatory or allergic disease involving a paranasal sinus.

2. Opacification of a sinus may be due to diffuse mucosal thickening, chronic osteitis, a soft tissue mass, or fluid. If fluid completely fills a sinus, it cannot be differentiated from other causes of sinus opacification. If, however, it partially fills the sinus, it can be recognized by demonstrating an air-fluid level (Figs 469 and 470). This requires the use of a horizontal beam.

3. Increased bone density accompanied by loss of definition of the mucoperiosteal line indicates chronic sinusitis that has extended into, and involved, the bone in a chronic inflammatory process, i.e., osteitis (Fig 471). In the absence of clinical and other evidence of chronic

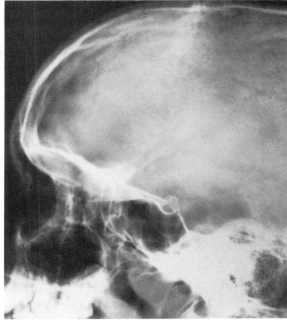

Fig 462.—Small sella in asymptomatic, normal 10-year-old girl with pneumatization of vertical plate of frontal bone. (From Shapiro, R., and Schorr, S.: Invest. Radiol. 15:191, 1980.)

inflammation, localized bony sclerosis should raise the question of a primary or secondary osteoblastic tumor.

4. Loss of the mucoperiosteal line associated with relative radiolucency of a sinus is usually due to destruction of the overlying bone by an expanding mucocele (Fig 472). The diagnosis of a mucocele, most common in the frontal sinus, may be missed in the presence of an opaque contralateral sinus because the mucocele may simulate the radiolucent appearance of a normal sinus. The distinguishing feature is the absence of a sharply defined mucoperiosteal line.

Thinning and expansion of the intact bony margins of a sinus are generally due to pressure from a slow-growing neoplasm that is usually, though not always, benign. Contrariwise, bone destruction usually, but not always, indicates malignancy. Some benign neoplasms, e.g., inverted papilloma, and various granulomas, e.g., Wegener's granuloma, may destroy the adjacent bone.

ETHMOID CELLS

The ethmoidal sinuses develop in the nasal cavity by the fourth fetal month. They are primarily evaginations of the nasal mucosa from the middle, superior, and first supreme nasal meatuses. Histologic sections of the

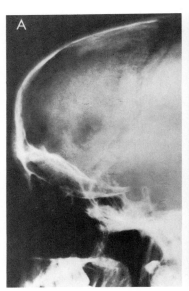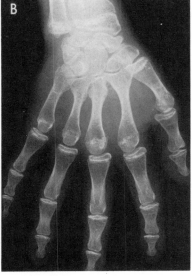

Fig 461.—Lateral skull film (A) in a 60-year-old pituitary dwarf. Note failure of pneumatization of vertical plate of frontal bone and small sella turcica. Film of the hand (B) shows incomplete epiphyseal fusion. (From Shapiro, R., and Schorr, S.: Invest. Radiol. 15:191, 1980.)

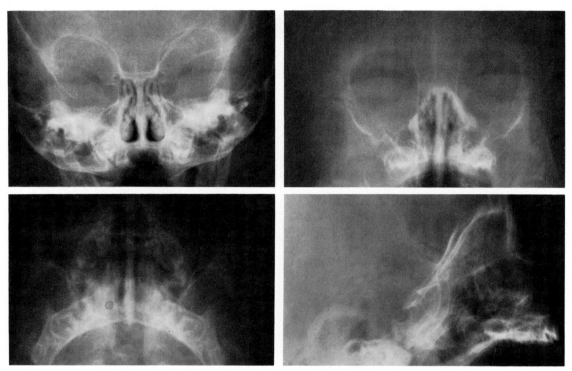

Fig 463.—Normal paranasal sinuses at age 6 months.
Small maxillary and ethmoidal sinuses are readily apparent.

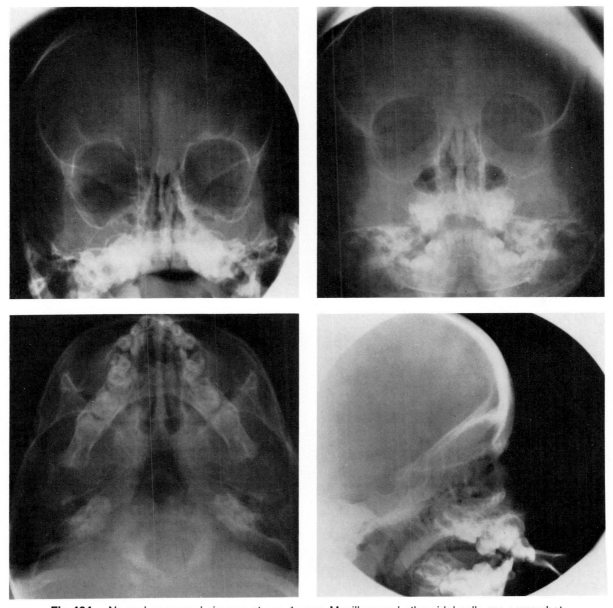

Fig 464.—Normal paranasal sinuses at age 1 year. Maxillary and ethmoidal cells are somewhat better developed than at age 6 months, but frontals and sphenoids are not pneumatized.

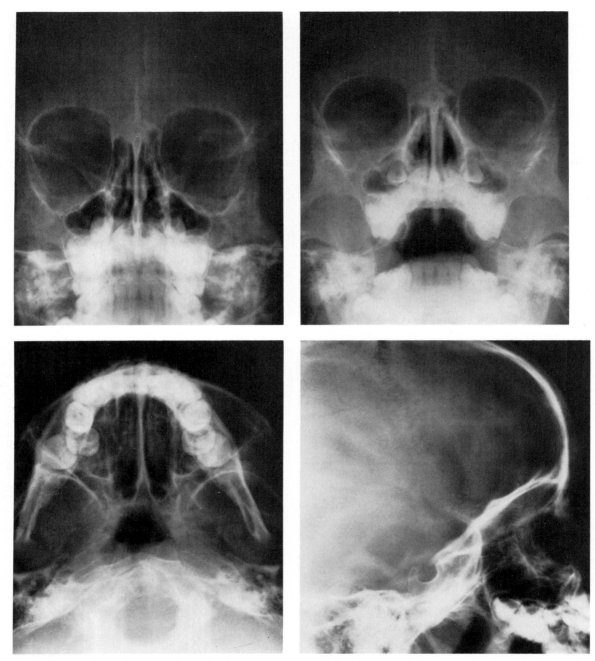

Fig 465.—Paranasal sinuses at age 5 years. Beginning invasion of frontal bone by air cells is seen, but origin of these cells cannot be distinguished. Similarly, base view shows early pneumatization of sphenoid bone.

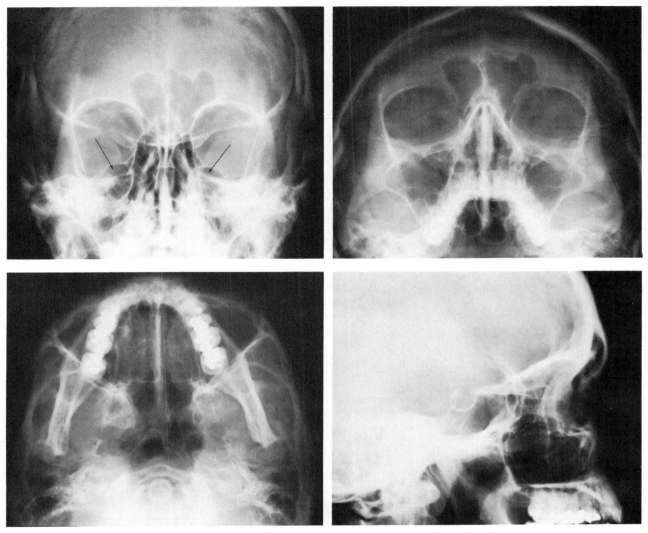

Fig 466.—Normal paranasal sinuses in a young adult. Note marked bilateral pneumatization of pterygoid processes *(arrows)*.

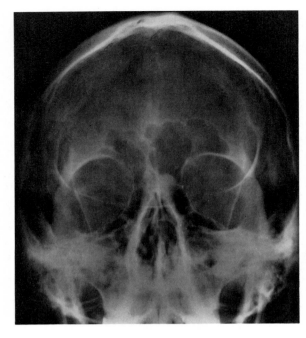

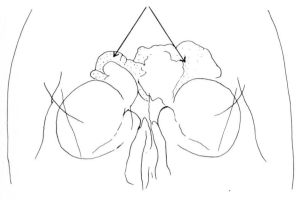

Fig 467.—Caldwell projection showing edematous thickening of mucosa in irregularly compartmented frontal sinus.

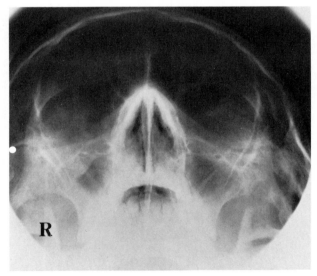

Fig 468.—Boggy thickened mucosa in both maxillary sinuses, more pronounced on the right.

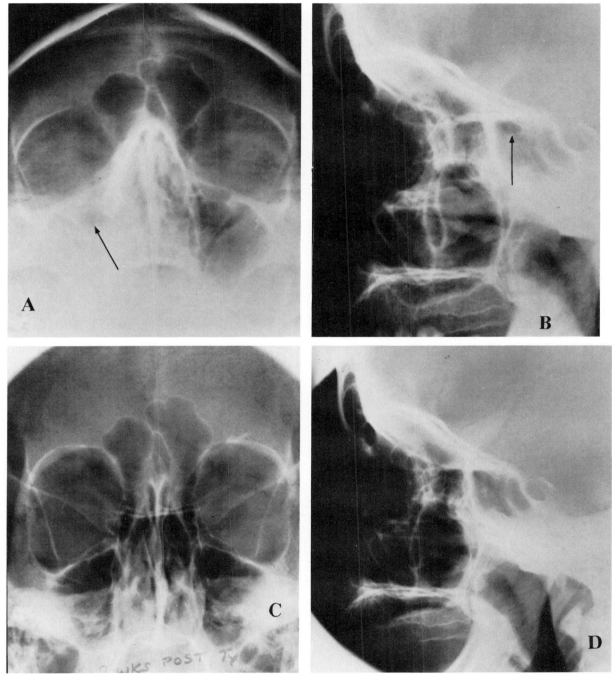

Fig 469.—Upright Waters **(A)** and lateral **(B)** views in a patient with acute right maxillary, ethmoid, and sphenoid sinusitis. Note fluid levels *(arrows)* in maxillary and sphenoid sinuses. After two weeks of anti-biotic therapy, repeat films in Caldwell **(C)** and lateral **(D)** projections show complete clearing.

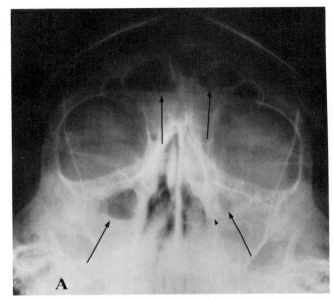

Fig 470.—Upright Waters view **(A)** in a patient with bilateral acute maxillary, ethmoidal, and frontal sinusitis with bilateral air-fluid levels *(arrow)*. Air-fluid level in left maxillary sinus is barely discernible because sinus is almost completely filled with fluid. Re-examination after two weeks of antibiotic therapy shows complete clearing of frontal, ethmoidal, and left maxillary sinuses **(B** and **C)**. The Caldwell projection **(C)** still shows slightly diminished aeration of right maxillary sinus.

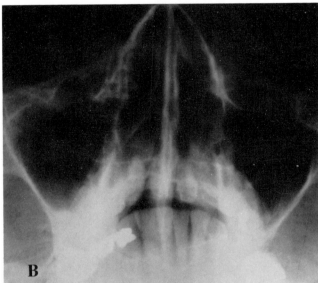

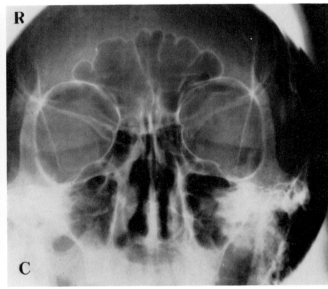

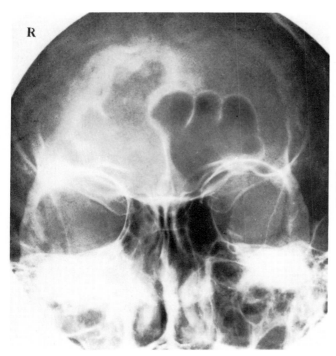

Fig 471.—Chronic right frontal sinusitis of over 15 years duration with sclerotic osteitis of surrounding frontal bone. Slight thickening of left frontal mucosa is also seen, with diminished definition of muco-periosteal border.

Fig 472.—Mucocele of left frontal sinus. There is also clouding of right frontal sinus, but characteristic loss of dense cortical bony outline on the left *(arrowheads)* accompanied by erosion of upper left orbital margin and increased radiopacity of left orbit mark the left-sided lesion a mucocele.

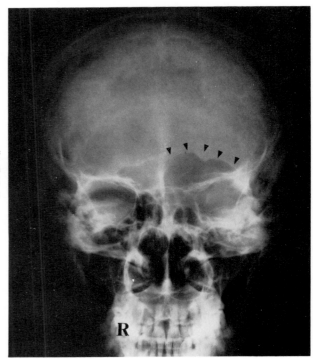

nose in the full-term fetus show considerable development of both the anterior and posterior groups of cells.

The fully developed ethmoidal labyrinths occupy the space between the bony orbits, extending from the frontal sinuses anteriorly to the sphenoid sinuses posteriorly. Of all the paranasal sinuses, the ethmoids vary the most in number (2 to 8 anterior and 1 to 8 posterior cells), size, and location. The ethmoidal cells are arbitrarily divided into anterior and posterior groups. Thus, all cells with ostia below the middle turbinate are termed *anterior cells*, while those having ostia above the middle turbinate are designated *posterior cells*. Since this classification is based upon the location of the ostia, which cannot be visualized on the roentgenogram, it is often impossible to decide whether a cell is anterior or posterior on the basis of position alone. Consequently, there is no sharp dividing line roentgenologically between anterior and posterior ethmoidal cells. In general, the anterior cells represent the upper half of the ethmoidal area in the Caldwell projection, while the posterior cells represent the lower half. Similarly, in the lateral view, there is no sharp demarcation between the frontal sinuses and the anterior ethmoid cells on one hand, and between the sphenoid sinuses and posterior ethmoid cells on the other.

In the adult, the ethmoidal cells are seldom confined to the ethmoid bone. Not infrequently, ethmoidal cells migrate beyond the ethmoidal labyrinth to invade the orbital plate of the frontal bone (Fig 473), the maxilla, the sphenoid (Figs 474 and 475), and the lacrimal, palatine, and nasal bones. These cells, which may occasionally attain considerable size, are termed agger ethmoidal cells (L. *agger*, elevation or mound). Perhaps the most familiar cell in this group is the agger nasi cell anterior to the nasofrontal duct behind the frontal process of the maxilla. Occasionally, a large maxillary agger cell may be mistaken for a supernumerary maxillary sinus.

At birth, the ethmoid cells can be distinguished on a good lateral film. By the end of the first year, the ethmoid cells are sufficiently prominent so that gross pathologic changes can be detected on the roentgenogram. In the well-pneumatized labyrinth, loss of sharp definition of the cell septa can be readily appreciated as the earliest sign of ethmoid disease. This is so significant that the failure to visualize clearly outlined cell walls in a satisfactory lateral roentgenogram indicates ethmoid disease. Later changes include disappearance or thickening of the cell septa and opacification of the cells per se.

MAXILLARY SINUSES

At birth, the maxillary sinus is a narrow slit hugging the lateral wall of the nasal fossa. By the end of the first year the sinus is slightly medial to the infraorbital foramen. The sinus attains a more triangular configuration by the end of the second year. At this time, it extends above the unerupted first molar tooth. There is little room for significant further growth prior to eruption of the teeth and development of the alveolar process. At age 6, therefore, the floor of the sinus is only at the level of the middle meatus. With eruption of the teeth, however (age 8 to 12), gradual expansion occurs, and the floor of the sinus reaches the level of the floor of the nose (Fig 476).

Pneumatization of the alveolar process may begin as early as the sixth year but is usually not demonstrable on the roentgenogram until the 10th or 11th year. Pneumatization of the zygomatic process of the maxilla begins at age 9. Further development of the antrum proceeds more slowly, reaching adult proportions at age 15 to 18, at which time the sinus floor is at the level of the alveolus. With senility, as the teeth are lost, the floor of the sinus once more recedes to the level of the floor of the nose. In children, the unerupted third molar commonly casts a density in Waters' projection that simulates an air-fluid level or a retention cyst. The cause of the density is obvious in the lateral view, however.

The adult maxillary sinus is a pyramidal cavity in the body of the maxilla, bounded above by the floor of the orbit, below by the alveolar process of the maxilla, and medially by the lateral nasal wall. The ostium of the antrum, which communicates with the middle meatus, is located on the medial wall about halfway between the roof and floor. The maxillary sinuses are less subject to variation than are the other paranasal sinuses. In general, they tend to be equal and symmetric, although occasionally one sinus may be smaller due to congenital hypoplasia, severe trauma, or infection early in childhood (Figs 477 and 478).

Occasionally, the antra may be more or less compartmented by complete or incomplete bony septa. A markedly pneumatized pterygoid process should not be mistaken for septation of the maxillary sinus (Fig 479). Likewise, in the presence of extensive lateral pneumatization of the body of the sphenoid, the lateral-lying sphenoid sinus cells are superimposed upon the maxillary sinus in Waters' projection, simulating compartmentation of the maxillary sinus (Fig 480). The cavity of

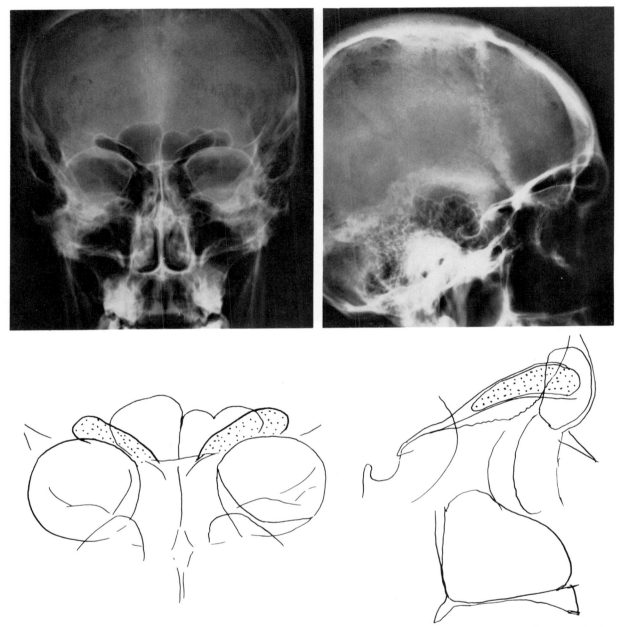

Fig 473.—Extension of ethmoids into orbital roofs ("supraorbital" ethmoids) sometimes gives the appearance of very large frontal sinuses. Ethmoidal extensions shown in Caldwell *(left)* and lateral *(right)* projections are illustrated by stippled shading in the drawing.

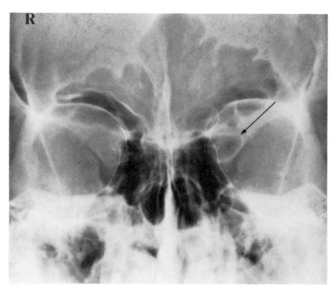

Fig 474.—Agger ethmoid cell in medial end of left lesser sphenoidal wing *(arrow)*.

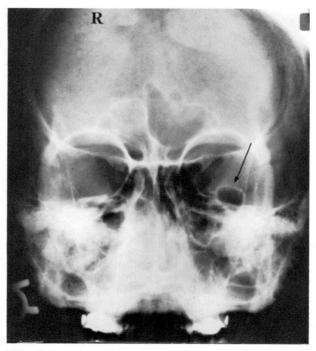

Fig 475.—Large sinus cell in left greater sphenoidal wing *(arrow)*.
Is this an agger ethmoid, or is it sphenoidal in origin?

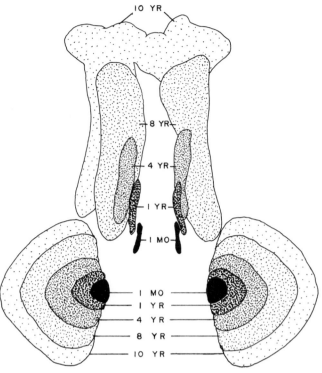

Fig 476.—Schematic diagram of growth of maxillary and frontal sinuses (after Caffey).

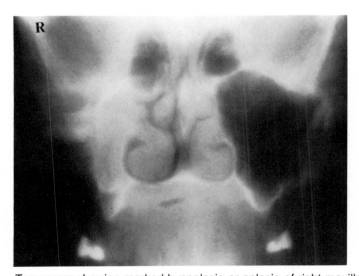

Fig 477.—Tomogram showing marked hypoplasia or aplasia of right maxillary sinus.

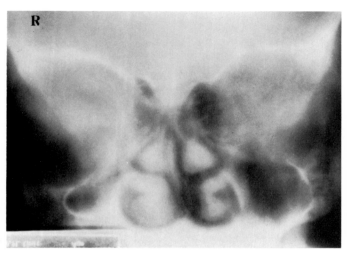

Fig 478.—Neurofibromatosis with orbital and maxillary sinus asymmetry. Tomogram clearly shows enlargement of right orbit and associated hypoplasia of ipsilateral maxillary sinus.

the maxillary sinus consists of the body and four extensions: (1) zygomatic extension (see Fig 480), (2) palatine extension into the floor of the nose, (3) tuberosity extension above the third molar, and (4) alveolar extension projecting into the alveolar process of the maxilla. The degree of pneumatization of all these recesses, and particularly of the alveolar recess, varies considerably. In the edentulous patient with marked alveolar resorption, only a thin layer of bone may separate the antrum from the mouth. This is important in dental extractions of the maxillary molar teeth.

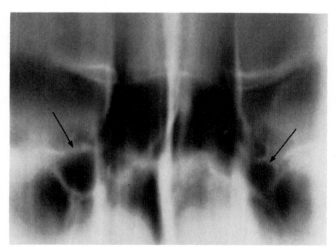

Fig 479.—Anteroposterior tomogram showing asymmetric pneumatization of both pterygoid processes (arrow). In the Waters view, these would be superimposed upon maxillary sinuses, giving erroneous impression of septation of antra.

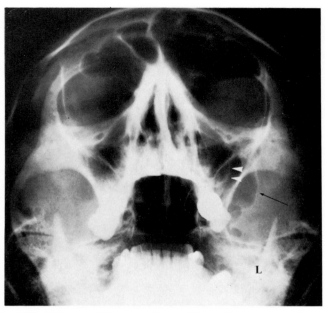

Fig 480.—Asymmetric normal maxillary sinuses due largely to greater pneumatization of zygomatic process of left maxilla (arrow). Note also marked pneumatization of body of sphenoid sinus on the left (arrowheads), mimicking septation of left maxillary sinus.

A few simple caveats concerning the maxillary sinuses may be helpful to the beginner. The soft tissue shadow of the upper lip is commonly superimposed on the floor of the maxillary sinuses in Waters' projection. This should not be confused with localized mucous membrane thickening, because the lip extends beyond the margins of the sinus. Occasionally, prominent flaring alae nasi and soft tissue swelling of the cheek overlie the floor of the sinuses and should not be mistaken for sinus disease. Not uncommonly, the obliquity of the lateral wall of one or both maxillary sinuses results in increased density of this portion of the sinus (Fig 481). A sharp mucoperiosteal line and normal sinus aeration should differentiate this from sinus disease. The vascular groove of the posterior superior alveolar artery midway along the lateral wall of one or both maxillary sinuses should not be confused with a fracture (Fig 482). The infratemporal extension of the innominate line, which projects below the inferior orbital rim in Waters' projection, should not be mistaken for a blow-out fracture of the orbital floor.

In the conventional base view, three lines can be seen in the anterior portion of the skull—one horizontally oriented and two vertically directed (Fig 483). The horizontal line, concave posteriorly, represents the anterior

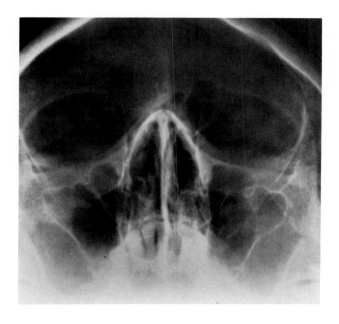

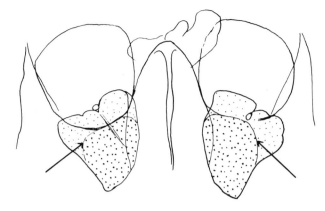

Fig 481.—Waters projection showing normal maxillary sinuses with sloping walls that should not be mistaken for thickened mucosa.

margin of the middle cranial fossa. It is for the most part formed by the greater sphenoidal wing. The more lateral vertical line constitutes the lateral wall of the orbit. Anteriorly, it is formed by the orbital surface of the zygoma; posteriorly, it is formed by the orbital surface of the greater sphenoidal wing. The more medial, S-shaped vertical line represents the lateral wall of the maxillary sinus. The two vertical lines may be superimposed or parallel to each other. The hyperextended base view is occasionally useful to demonstrate both the anterior and posterior walls of the frontal sinuses.

In the Caldwell view, the roof of the maxillary sinus, i.e., the floor of the orbit, is projected below the anterior orbital rim.

In the lateral view, the anterior wall of the maxillary sinus may produce two lines due to its posterior slope as it extends laterally. The most anterior line is more medial than the line just behind it. The roofs of both antra are usually superimposed upon each other. The posterior wall is readily identified, as is the pterygomaxillary fissure and floor.

SPHENOID SINUSES

The sphenoid sinuses develop from mucosal invaginations in the posterior portion of the nares during the fourth month of gestation. At birth, the sphenoid sinuses are still nasal in position. By age 2 to 4, the sinuses begin to pneumatize the sphenoid bone. Pneumatization and resorption of the body of the sphenoid pro-

gress, so that by age 8 to 10 the posterosuperior portion of the sinuses lie beneath the anterior portion of the sella turcica (Fig 484). By the 15th year, the sinuses are usually separated from the hypophysis by a thin lamina of compact bone. As the sphenoid sinuses develop, they tend to pneumatize more rapidly in a posterolateral direction than directly posteriorly. This leads to thinning of the lateral walls of the sinuses and to relatively thick posterior walls.

The adult sphenoid sinuses are usually paired cavities

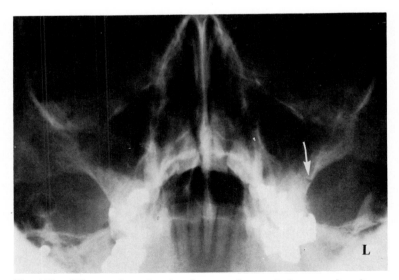

Fig 482.—Waters view showing foramen for posterior superior alveolar artery on the left *(arrow)*. This should not be mistaken for a fracture.

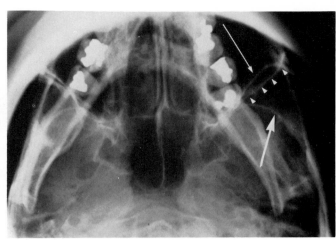

Fig 483.—Base view showing the triple lines important in interpretation of maxillary sinus films. Note orbital surface of greater sphenoidal wing *(arrowheads)*, posterolateral wall of maxillary sinus *(thin arrow)*, and greater sphenoidal wing *(thick arrow).*

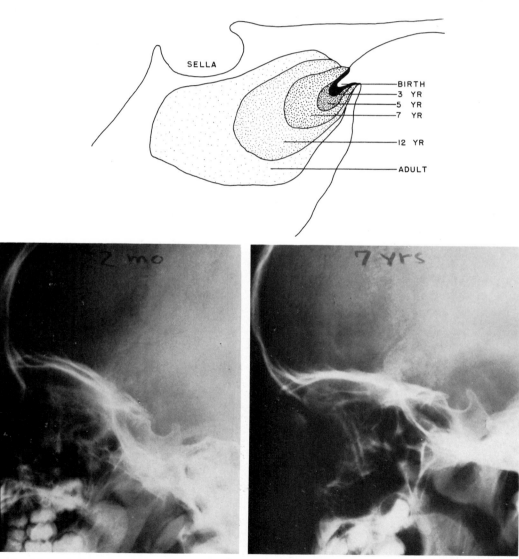

Fig 484.—Diagram *(top)* of lateral view showing progressive development of sphenoid sinuses by invasion of body of sphenoid bone. (According of Caffey.) Lateral radiographs *(bottom)* of 22-month-old boy *(left)* with no pneumatization of sphenoid sinus, and 5 years later *(right)* showing sphenoid sinus pneumatization of juvenile type.

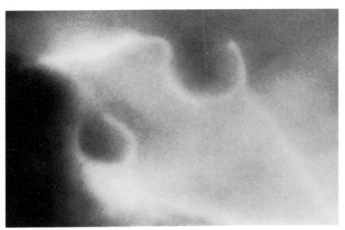

Fig 485.—Lateral tomogram showing conchal type of sphenoid sinus.

occupying a varying portion of the body of the sphenoid. The extent of sphenoid pneumatization, like that of all the other paranasal sinuses, varies widely. The sphenoid sinuses can be divided into three types depending on the degree of pneumatization: (1) the conchal type, with pneumatization limited to the rostral portion of the sphenoid bone (Fig 485); (2) the juvenile type, with pneumatization extending back to the region of the tuberculum sellae or the intersphenoidal synchondrosis (Fig 486); and (3) the adult type, with air cells invading the postsphenoid segment below the sella turcica (Fig 487).

It is important for the radiologist to describe the extent of sphenoid pneumatization in connection with trans-sphenoidal hypophysectomy. With extensive pneumatization into the pterygoid processes and lingula, the vidian canals and the foramen rotundum may become partially or completely incorporated in the sphenoid sinuses. In some patients, the sphenoid sinuses may extend into the clivus, the greater or lesser wings, the pterygoid processes (Fig 488), the rostrum, or the basiocciput. Individual recesses may extend into the superomedial aspect of the orbit, and into the anterior and posterior clinoid processes.

The paired sphenoid sinuses are separated by a septum of variable thickness and location. The septum may be midline in position or, more commonly, deviate to one side, resulting in asymmetric sphenoid sinuses (Fig 489). The midline septum (Fig 490) corresponds to the site of union of the fused presphenoid and postsphenoid centers from each side. Although the septum is usually median in position in the presphenoid segment, it may incline to one side in the postsphenoid segment. The septum is usually intact but may rarely be perforated.

The more common lateral septum originates near the midline and courses posterolaterally to insert near the anterior limb of the carotid groove, adjacent to the internal carotid artery. The least common type of septum is the thick transverse, often incomplete septum that marks the site of the presphenoid and postsphenoid synchondrosis. Occasionally, the septation may be complex (Fig 491). The sphenoid ostium is located in the sphenoethmoidal recess above the most uppermost ethmoid concha, a poor position for efficient drainage.

As a result of their central location, the sphenoid sinuses are intimately related to the hypophysis and optic chiasm above, the cavernous sinus and its contained

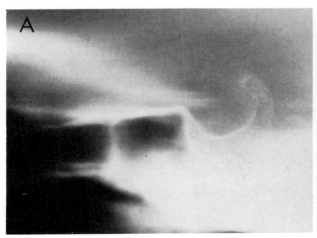
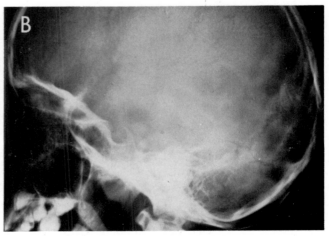

Fig 486.—Two examples (**A** and **B**) of juvenile type of sphenoid sinus pneumatization involving presphenoid, extending back to intersphenoid synchondrosis.

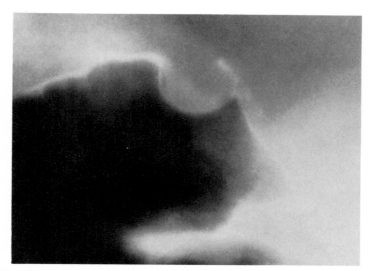

Fig 487.—Adult type of sphenoid sinus pneumatization. In this patient, pneumatization involves almost entire body of sphenoid.

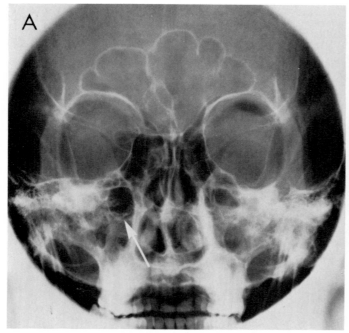

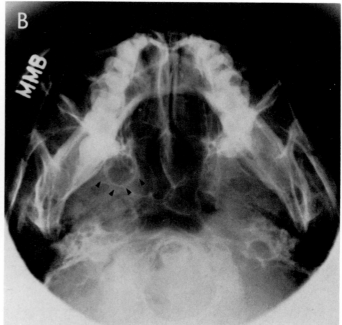

Fig 488.—Caldwell **(A)** and submentovertical **(B)** projections showing pneumatization of right pterygoid process *(arrowheads).* In the Waters projection, this should not be confused with maxillary sinus compartmentation.

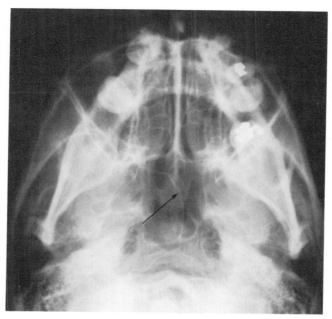

Fig 489.—Asymmetric septum *(arrow)*.

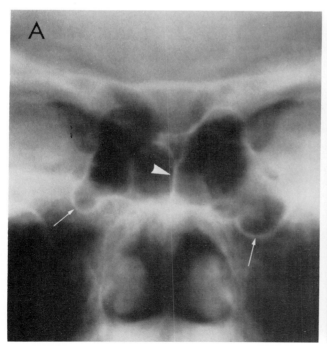

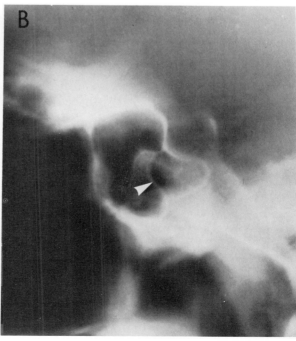

Fig 490.—Anteroposterior **(A)** and lateral **(B)** tomograms with a midline septum *(arrowhead)* corresponding to site of fetal synchon-drosis between presphenoid and postsphenoid centers. Note also asymmetric pneumatization of pterygoid plates *(arrows)*.

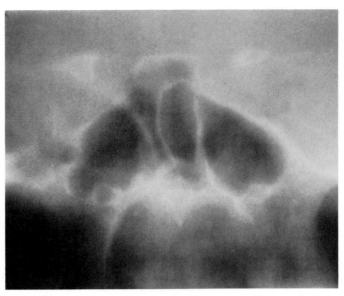

Fig 491.—Anteroposterior tomogram showing complex septation of sphenoid sinuses.

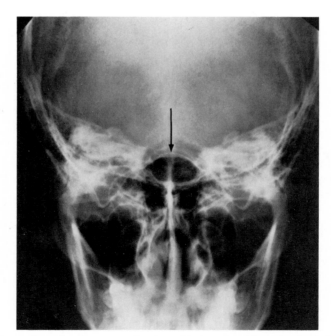

Fig 492.—Granger view showing normal sphenoid sinuses with a clearly defined roof *(arrow)*.

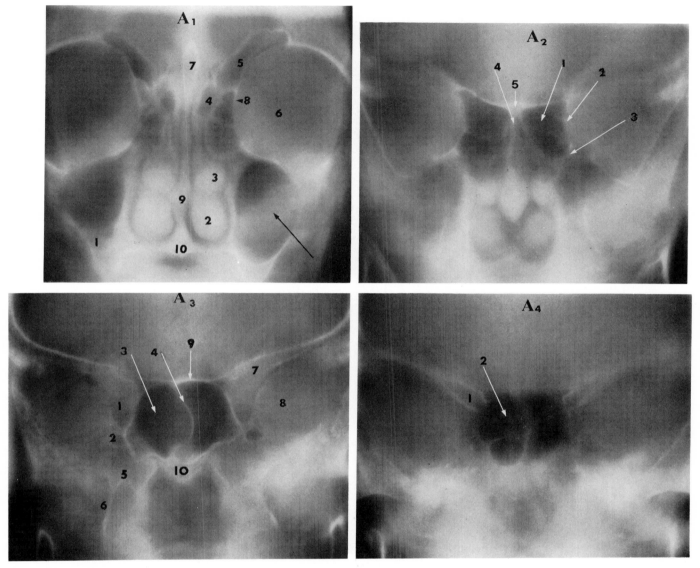

Fig 493.—Anteroposterior tomograms of normal paranasal sinuses—except for benign tumor arising from lateral wall of left maxillary sinus *(arrow)*—in an adult. **A₁,** most anterior section, 17.5 mm cut: maxillary sinus *(1)*, inferior turbinate *(2)*, middle turbinate *(3)*, anterior ethmoid cells *(4)*, supraorbital ethmoids *(5)*, orbit *(6)*, crista galli *(7)*, lacrimal bone *(8)*, nasal septum *(9)*, and roof of hard palate *(10)*. **A₂,** middle section, 15.5 mm cut: posterior ethmoids *(1)*, lamina papyracea *(2)*, ethmoid-maxillary plate *(3)*, perpendicular plate of ethmoid *(4)*, and cribriform plate *(5)*. **A₃,** middle section, 14.5 mm cut: superior orbital fissure *(1)*, foramen rotundum *(2)*, sphenoid sinus *(3)*, septum *(4)*, base of pterygoid processes *(5)*, lateral pterygoid plate *(6)*, lesser sphenoidal wing *(7)*, greater sphenoidal wing *(8)*, planum sphenoidale *(9)*, and sphenoid rostrum *(10)*. **A₄,** posterior section, 13.5 mm cut: anterior clinoid process *(1)* and sphenoid sinus *(2)*.

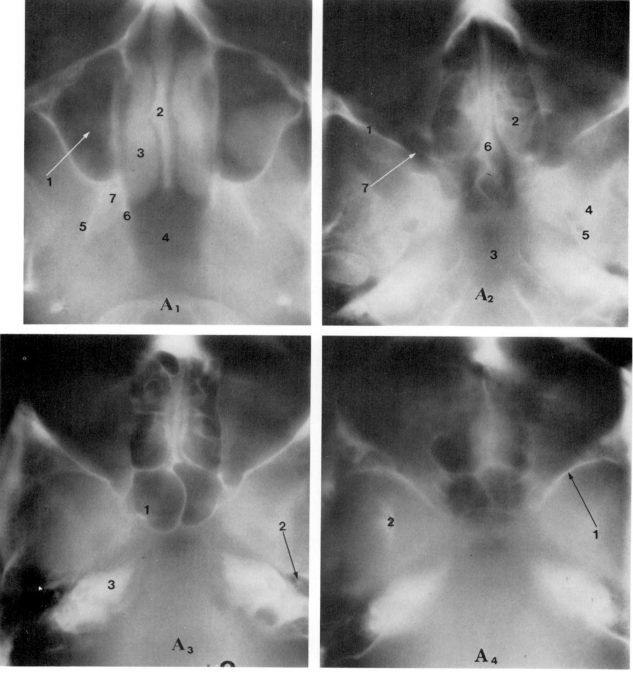

Fig 494.—Submentovertical tomograms. Same patient as in Figure 493. **A₁,** most superior section, 15 mm cut: maxillary sinus *(1)*, nasal septum *(2)*, inferior turbinate *(3)*, nasopharynx *(4)*, lateral pterygoid plate *(5)*, medial pterygoid plate *(6)*, and pterygoid fossa *(7)*. **A₂,** middle section, 13 mm cut: posterolateral wall of orbit *(1)*, ethmoid cells *(2)*, clivus *(3)*, foramen ovale *(4)*, foramen spinosum *(5)*, vomer *(6)*, and inferior orbital fissure *(7)*. **A₃,** middle section, 12 mm cut: sphenoid sinus *(1)*, ossicles *(2)*, and petrous bone *(3)*. **A₄,** inferior section, 11 mm cut: anterior margin of middle cranial fossa *(1)* and middle cranial fossa *(2)*.

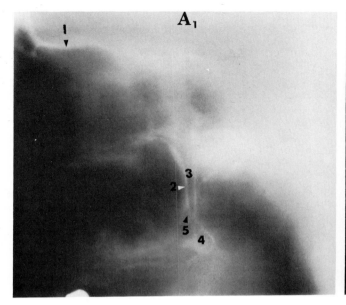

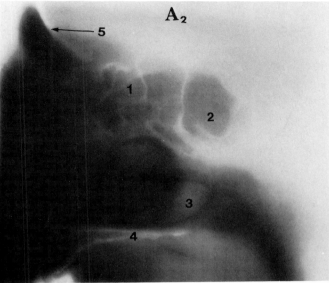

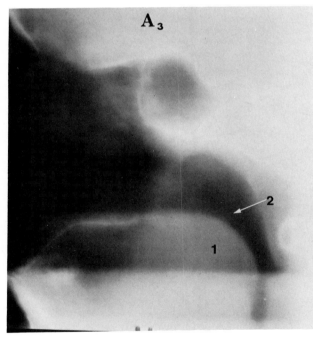

Fig 495.—Lateral tomograms of right paranasal sinuses. Same patient as in Figures 493 and 494. **A₁**, most medial cut, 13 mm: cerebral surface of orbital plate *(1)*, posterior wall of maxillary sinus *(2)*, pterygopalatine fossa *(3)*, pterygoid process *(4)*, and pterygopalatine canal *(5)*. **A₂**, 12 mm cut: posterior ethmoid cells *(1)*, sphenoid sinus *(2)*, posterior end of inferior turbinate bone *(3)*, roof of hard palate *(4)*, and posterior wall of frontal sinus *(5)*. **A₃**, 11 mm cut: tongue *(1)* and nasopharynx *(2)*.

structures laterally, and the vidian nerve and vessels below. Because of secondary involvement of these contiguous structures, sphenoid sinus disease may simulate intracranial lesions, and special studies may be required to establish the correct diagnosis. In this connection, the Granger projection for visualization of the roof of the sphenoid sinus may be helpful. The normal roof is seen as a sharp, white line representing the mucoperiosteal border (Fig 492). On the other hand, the diseased roof shows a poorly defined or thickened outline.

Tomography is extremely helpful in defining the character and extent of a number of disease processes. It exquisitely delineates bone involvement and the extension of invasive tumors, thereby providing more accurate staging and guidelines for surgical treatment (Figs 493 to 495).

REFERENCES

Carmody T. E.: The development of sinuses after birth. *Ann. Otol. Rhinol. Laryngol.* 38:130–134, 1929.

Davis W. B.: *Development and Anatomy of the Nasal Accessory Sinuses in Man.* Philadelphia, W. B. Saunders Co., 1914.

Granger A.: *Radiological Study of the Paranasal Sinuses and Mastoids.* Philadelphia, Lea & Febiger, 1932.

Layton T. B.: *Catalogue of the Onodi Collection.* London, Headley Bros., 1934.

MacMillan A. S.: Personal communication.

Onodi A.: *The Accessory Sinuses of the Nose in Children,* Prausnitz C. (trans). London, John Bale, Sons & Danielsson, 1911.

Samuel E.: *Clinical Radiology of the Ear, Nose and Throat.* London, H. K. Lewis & Co., 1952.

Schaeffer J. P.: *The Nose, Paranasal Sinuses, Nasolacrimal Passageways and Olfactory Organ in Man.* Philadelphia, Blakiston Co., 1920.

Van Alyea O. E.: Sphenoid sinus. *Arch. Otolaryngol.* 34:225–253, 1941.

Vidic B.: The postnatal development of sphenoid sinus and its spread into dorsum sellae and posterior clinoid processes. *Am. J. Roentgenol.* 104:177–183, 1968.

Wasson W. W.: Changes in nasal accessory sinuses after birth. *Arch. Otolaryngol.* 17:197–211, 1933.

Welin S.: The roentgen ray examination of the paranasal sinuses with particular reference to the frontal sinuses. *Br. J. Radiol.* 2:431–437, 1948.

Whalen J. P., Berne A. S.: The roentgen anatomy of the lateral walls of the orbit (orbital line) and the maxillary antrum (antral line) in the submentovertical view. *Am. J. Roentgenol.* 91:1009–1011, 1964.

Yanagisawa E., Smith H. W.: Normal radiographic anatomy of the paranasal sinuses. *Otolaryngol. Clin. North Am.* 6:429–456, 1973.

16

The Ear, Mastoid, and Petrous Pyramid

DEVELOPMENT

At birth, the temporal bone consists of three major components: (1) the squama, forming the roof of the external auditory canal; (2) the tympanic portion, below the squama, forming the floor, anterior wall, and part of the posterior wall of the bony external auditory canal; and (3) the petrous portion, encasing the cochlea, vestibule, and the semicircular canals. The squama and the tympanic portion are derived from membrane, while the petrous portion is derived from cartilage. Although the individual components of the temporal bone are sharply delineated by sutures in the newborn, their boundaries tend to disappear in the adult with sutural closure. The common exceptions are (1) the petrotympanic (glaserian) fissure, separating the posterior wall of the auditory canal from the mastoid process (the chorda tympani nerve traverses this fissure); and (2) the petrosquamosal suture, which persists as a thin, transverse bony septum (Körner's) projecting into the superolateral portion of the mastoid antrum.

At birth, the eustachian tube, tympanic cavity, and antrum are filled with a mucoid, gelatinous material. With the onset of respiration, this substance is gradually discharged into the pharynx through the eustachian tubes. Simultaneously, air enters the tympanic cavity and antrum, which increase in size. According to Bast and Anson, pneumatization of the tympanic and epitympanic cavities is fairly complete at birth. At six months, the pneumatized antrum is clearly demonstrable on the roentgenogram.

ANATOMY

Because the squama is described in detail in chapter 7, dealing with the anatomy of the adult skull, it will not be considered here. Instead, the pertinent anatomy of the isolated temporal bone will be presented in the projections used to study the middle ear and the mastoid process (Figs 496 to 501).

External Ear

The external auditory canal is a short (2 to 2.5 cm) tube running medially and forward from the auricle to the tympanic membrane. Its outer third is cartilaginous, and its inner two-thirds are osseous. Laterally, its vertical diameter is greatest; medially, however, its greatest diameter is in the anteroposterior axis. Because of the slope of the tympanic membrane, the anterior wall and floor of the canal are longer than the posterior wall and roof. The external meatus is clearly demonstrable in the Law projection. Within the shadow of the external meatus, the smaller internal auditory meatus can be recognized. Occasionally, the vertical linear shadow of the handle of the malleus is seen crossing the external auditory meatus. The tympanic membrane is attached superiorly to a bony spur (anterior tympanic spine, scutum, Henle's spine) that separates the external ear from the attic.

Middle Ear

The middle ear (tympanic cavity) lies between the drum membrane and the inner ear (Fig 502). It consists of (1) the epitympanic recess (attic), which lies above the level of the tympanic membrane and contains the head of the malleus and the incus; and (2) the main tympanic cavity, medial to the tympanic membrane.

The tympanic cavity communicates anteromedially with the nasopharynx via the eustachian tube. Posteriorly, the attic communicates with the mastoid antrum by way of the aditus ad antrum. The bony medial wall of the tympanic cavity separates it from the inner ear. In the medial wall is the oval window (fenestra ovalis), which is occluded by the stapes. The roof is formed by the tegmen tympani, a thin plate of bone separating the tympanic cavity from the temporal lobe and its meninges. The floor of the tympanic cavity consists of a thin-walled groove, the hypotympanic recess, which lies below the level of the tympanic membrane. The me-

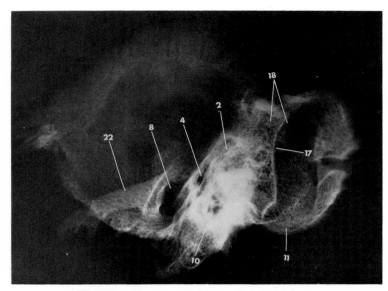

Fig 496.—Dry temporal bone, Law projection.

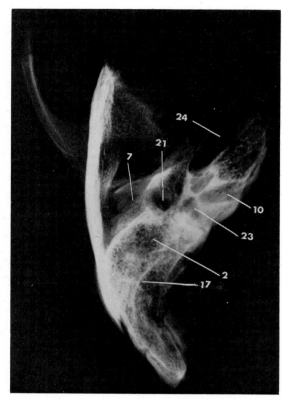

Fig 498.—Dry temporal bone, submentovertical projection.

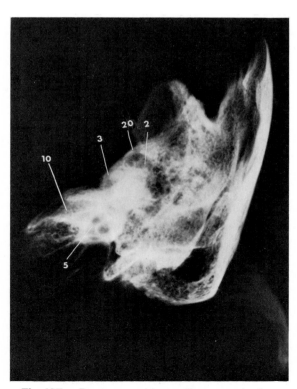

Fig 497.—Dry temporal bone, Towne projection.

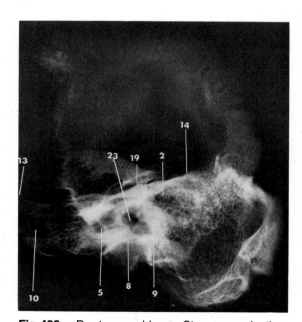

Fig 499.—Dry temporal bone, Stenvers projection.

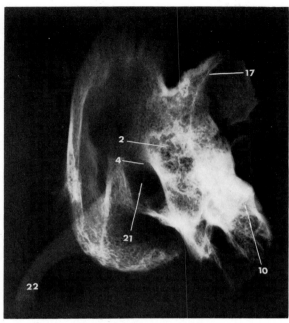

Fig 500.—Dry temporal bone, Mayer projection.

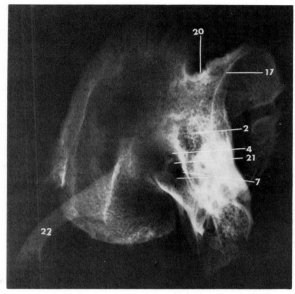

Fig 501.—Dry temporal bone, Owens modification of Mayer projection.

LEGEND FOR FIGURES 496–501

1. aditus ad antrum
2. antrum
3. arcuate eminence
4. attic (epitympanic recess)
5. cochlea
6. eustachian tube
7. external auditory canal
8. glenoid fossa
9. horizontal semicircular canal
10. internal auditory canal
11. mastoid process
12. ossicles

13. petrous apex
14. petrous ridge
15. posterior semicircular canal
16. semicircular canals
17. sigmoid sinus plate
18. sinodural angle
19. superior semicircular canal
20. tegmen tympani
21. tympanic cavity
22. zygomatic process of temporal bone
23. vestibule
24. carotid canal

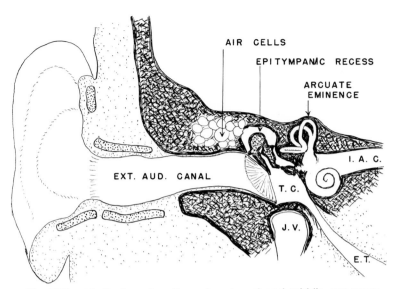

Fig 502.—Vertical section through external and middle ear represented diagrammatically so that parts of internal ear are also shown. Mastoid antrum, although not shown, would be superimposed on epitympanic recess since it lies almost directly posterior to the recess. This view would correspond to a straight anteroposterior roentgenogram. Bone is shown by crosshatching, cartilage by heavy stippling, and other soft tissues by light stippling. Note tympanic cavity (T.C.), eustachian tube (E.T.), jugular vein lying in jugular fossa (J.V.), and internal auditory canal (I.A.C.).

dial wall of the floor is formed by the promontory, the bony capsule of the basal turn of the cochlea. Only a thin plate of bone separates the hypotympanic recess from the jugular bulb inferiorly, and from the internal carotid artery anteriorly.

Rarely, the jugular bulb, which normally lies below the floor of the hypotympanic recess, extends up into the middle ear through a bony dehiscence. The osseous defect and the high position of the jugular bulb are readily demonstrable by tomography in the anteroposterior projection. Similarly, the internal carotid artery may uncommonly buckle laterally in an incomplete bony canal. In both instances, the patient is apt to present with a pulsatile, reddish-blue mass beneath the tympanic membrane.

The three ossicles articulate with one another by synovial-lined joints in a movable chain connecting the tympanic membrane with the oval window. The malleus, the largest most external ossicle, is shaped like a hammer, with the head and handle demarcated by a narrow neck. The head of the malleus lies in the epitympanic recess and articulates with the body of the incus at the incudomalleolar joint. The handle, which

points down in a posteromedial direction, is attached to the superior aspect of the tympanic membrane.

The intermediate ossicle, the incus, lies behind the malleus. It consists of a body and a long and a short process. The long process has a course fairly parallel to that of the handle of the malleus. At its inferior end, the long process bends medially to articulate with the head of the stapes at the incudostapedial joint. The short process is directed posteriorly to its attachment in the posteroinferior portion of the epitympanic recess.

The most medial ossicle, the stapes, is shaped like a stirrup. The base of the stapes occludes the oval window, to which it is attached by the annular ligament. The anterior and posterior limbs of the stirrup are joined to the base. Both limbs arch into a narrow neck and a small head, which articulates with the long process of the incus.

Internal Ear (Figs 503 to 509)

The internal ear, or labyrinth, consists of a series of membrane-lined cavities in the petrous pyramid. This discussion will be limited to the osseous labyrinth, since it is the only portion that can be seen on the roentgenogram. The osseous labyrinth consists of (1) a middle, or vestibular, segment; (2) a posterosuperior, or semicircular canal, segment; (3) an anterior, or cochlear, segment; and (4) the internal auditory canal.

VESTIBULE.—The vestibule is the oval-shaped, central portion of the bony labyrinth behind the cochlea and in front of the semicircular canals. It lies between the tympanic cavity laterally and the internal auditory canal medially. The lateral wall of the vestibule is perforated by the oval and round windows. The oval window is closed by the base of the stapes; the round window is closed by a membrane. The round window connects the middle ear with the basal portion of the cochlea. The vestibule has two small dilatations, the utricle and the saccule. The larger utricle, located in the posterosuperior portion of the vestibule, receives the openings of the semicircular canals. The smaller saccule lies more medially in the anteroinferior portion of the vestibule, and is related to the cochlea. The vestibular aqueduct, arising from the posterior wall of the vestibule, contains the ductus endolymphaticus.

SEMICIRCULAR CANALS.—The three semicircular canals lie above and behind the vestibule, opening into the vestibule by five orifices (one orifice is common to two

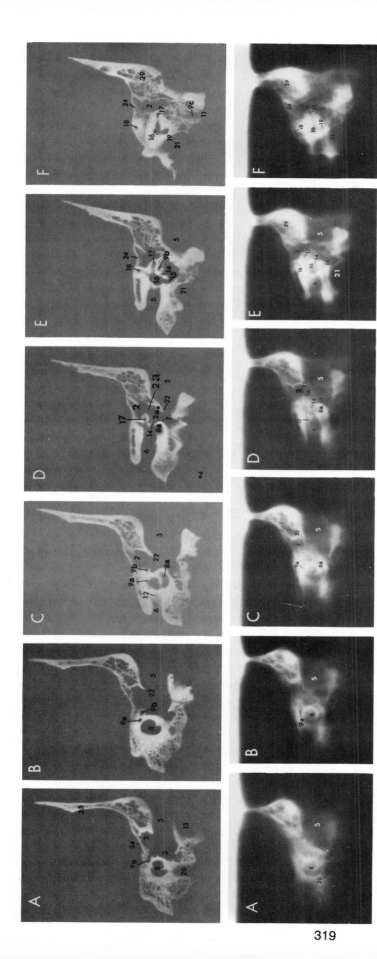

Fig 503.—Anteroposterior projection. Six radiographs *(top)* paired with six tomographic sections *(bottom)* of a dry left temporal bone at varying levels. Progression of levels from **A** to **F** is anterior to posterior at 1.0 to 1.5 mm cuts.

Structures seen particularly well in this projection include the internal auditory canal in its long axis, and the epitympanic recess. (From Schaeffer, R.E.: *Med. Rad. Photog. 48:4–5, 1972.*)

LEGEND FOR FIGURE 503

1. mastoid process
2. mastoid antrum
2a. aditus of antrum
3. middle ear (tympanic cavity)
3a. epitympanic recess (attic)
4. lateral wall of attic
5. external auditory canal
6. internal auditory canal
7. promontory of middle ear
8. cochlea
8a. basal turn of cochlea

9a. facial nerve canal, petrous segment
9b. facial nerve canal, tympanic segment
9c. facial nerve canal, mastoid (descending) segment
10. styloid process
11. stylomastoid foramen
12. crista transversa (crista falciformis)

13. mandibular fossa
14. oval window (fenestra vestibuli)
15. round window (fenestra cochleae)
16. vestibule
17. lateral semicircular canal
18. superior semicircular canal
19. posterior semicircular canal
20. carotid canal
21. jugular fossa

22. scutum (spur)
23. sinus plate
24. tegmen
25. squamous portion of temporal bone
26. crus commune (common limb)
27. arcuate eminence
28. petrous apex
29. mastoid air cells

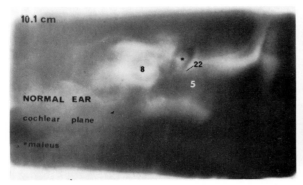
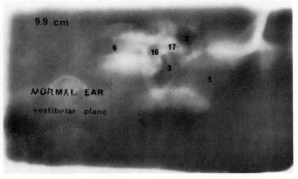
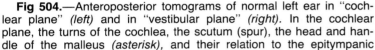

Fig 504.—Anteroposterior tomograms of normal left ear in "cochlear plane" *(left)* and in "vestibular plane" *(right)*. In the cochlear plane, the turns of the cochlea, the scutum (spur), the head and handle of the malleus *(asterisk)*, and their relation to the epitympanic

recess are clearly seen. In the vestibular plane (2 mm more posteriorly), the vestibule, the internal auditory canal, two of the three semicircular canals and the mastoid antrum are well seen. (From Schaeffer, R.E.: *Med. Rad. Photog.* 48:14, 1972.)

canals). The superior semicircular canal, readily recognizable on the plain roentgenogram, lies perpendicular to the long axis of the petrous bone. Its dilated lateral end opens into the upper part of the vestibule. At the other end, it joins the posterior canal to enter the vestibule by a common orifice. Its highest point forms the familiar arcuate eminence near the superior margin of the petrous bone.

The posterior semicircular canal, also vertical in position, runs fairly parallel to the posterior surface of the petrous bone. It opens into the lower part of the vestibule at one end and into the superior semicircular canal at the other.

The short lateral (horizontal) semicircular canal arches posteriorly and laterally at right angles to the other two canals. Both ends of the lateral canal open into the upper outer part of the vestibule. The lateral wall of this canal forms the medial wall of the aditus ad antrum.

THE COCHLEA.—The cochlea, which constitutes the anterior portion of the bony labyrinth, lies between the vestibule and the internal carotid artery. The first, or basal, coil of the cochlea forms the promontory on the medial wall of the tympanic cavity. The anteroinferior aspect of the cochlea is directly behind the posterior wall of the carotid canal as it bends anteromedially. The cochlea is arranged around a bony central core (the modiolus) in a spiral of two and a half turns, with the apex of the spiral pointing anterolaterally. The base of the modiolus is related to the lateral aspect of the internal auditory canal. Only the modiolus and the bony capsule can be visualized on the plain roentgenogram.

There are two orifices in the first portion of the basal turn of the cochlea: (1) the round window (fenestra

cochlea), opening into the medial wall of the tympanic cavity; and (2) an opening into the vestibule. The tiny cochlear aqueduct is more medial in position than the vestibular aqueduct. It extends from the basal cochlear turn posteromedially to a notch directly below the internal auditory canal.

Tomography of the Internal Ear

The ideal technique for studying the detailed anatomy of the internal ear is pluridirectional tomography with 1-mm cuts. It is important to use low kV, small fields, a 0.3-mm focal spot, and no grid. A diaphragm with a hole close to the tube and another hole at the end of the cone helps reduce secondary radiation. The most useful tomographic projections are the anteroposterior, the lateral, and the submentovertical. All of these views are not necessary in every case. In order to avoid unnecessary radiation, I take only the views which are required to solve the problem at hand. In most cases, tomograms in the anteroposterior (AP) and lateral projections are adequate. According to Littleton, a single AP tomogram of the skull made with hypocycloidal motion using the Polytome (74 kV(p), 220 mas, no grid, no additional filter, 2.5 × 3.5-inch field measured on the film) produces the following radiation: 1,500 mR to the skin, less than 1 mR to the gonads and thyroid gland, and 800 to 1,600 mR (average, 1,300 mR) to the ipsilateral lens and 16 to 20 mR to the opposite lens. Because of this, Berger et al. have suggested posteroanterior tomography to reduce the radiation to the lens. The measured dose to the lens for six cuts in the posteroanterior projection is 50 to 340 mR.

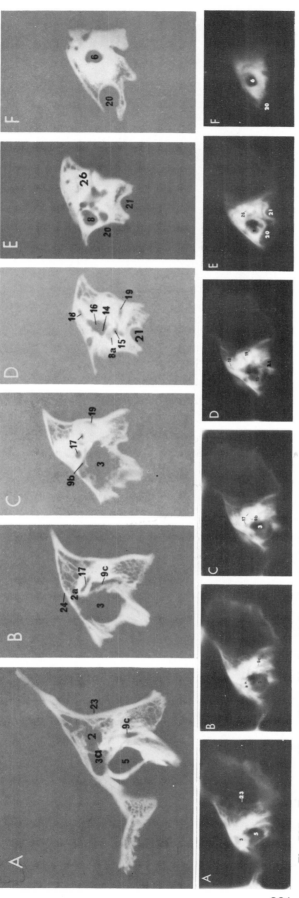

Fig 505.—Tomographic sections of isolated left temporal bone in lateral projection. Six radiographs (top) paired with six tomographic sections (bottom) of dry left temporal bone at varying levels. Progression of levels from **A** to **F** is from lateral surface toward medial surface of bone. Posterior aspect of bone is on the reader's right. Lateral projection shows relation between epitympanic recess and mastoid antrum, as well as descending portion of facial canal. The bottom section **B** shows the handle of the malleus (anterior) and the long process of the incus (posterior) (asterisks). (From Schaeffer, R.E.: Med. Rad. Photog. 48:6–7, 1972.)

LEGEND FOR FIGURE 505

1. mastoid process
2. mastoid antrum
2a. aditus of antrum
3. middle ear (tympanic cavity)
3a. epitympanic recess (attic)
4. lateral wall of attic
5. external auditory canal
6. internal auditory canal
7. promontory of middle ear
8. cochlea
8a. basal turn of cochlea

9a. facial nerve canal, petrous segment
9b. facial nerve canal, tympanic segment
9c. facial nerve canal, mastoid (descending) segment
10. styloid process
11. stylomastoid foramen
12. crista transversa (crista falciformis)

13. mandibular fossa
14. oval window (fenestra vestibuli)
15. round window (fenestra cochlear)
16. vestibule
17. lateral semicircular canal
18. superior semicircular canal
19. posterior semicircular canal
20. carotid canal
21. jugular fossa

22. scutum (spur)
23. sinus plate
24. tegmen
25. squamous portion of temporal bone
26. crus commune (common limb)
27. arcuate eminence
28. petrous apex
29. mastoid air cells

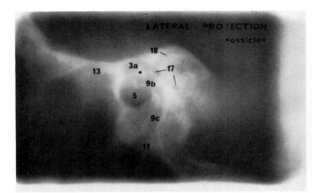

Fig 506.—Lateral tomograms of a normal left ear made at two levels. At the more superficial of the two levels *(left),* the facial nerve canal is visible down to its point of exit at stylomastoid foramen, and ossicular mass *(asterisk)* can be seen in epitympanic recess. Two limbs of lateral semicircular canal are also visible. At the second level *(right),* 8 mm deeper than the first level, a deep jugular fossa is visible, but carotid canal is not shown to good advantage. Internal auditory canal is clearly visible. Thin, bony band that stretches across diameter of internal auditory canal is edge-on view of crista falciformis. (From Schaeffer, R.E.: *Med. Rad. Photog.* 48:15, 1972.)

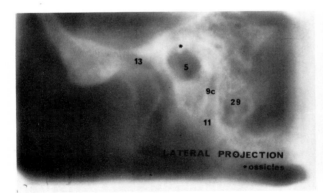
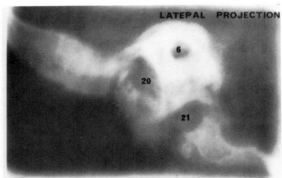

Fig 507.—Lateral tomograms of normal left ear made at two levels. Comparison with Figure 506 shows that appearance of same structures can vary from one person to another. At the more superficial of the two levels *(left),* the facial nerve canal, ossicular mass *(asterisk),* and the relation of external auditory canal to mandibular fossa are clearly shown. Visualization of this relation is helpful in orienting structures from front to back. At the deeper of the two levels *(right),* 1.2 cm medial to the first level, relation between carotid canal and jugular fossa is seen to good advantage. Spur of bone that divides carotid canal from jugular fossa is shown clearly, and cross-sectional aspect of internal auditory canal is visible. (From Schaeffer, R.E.: *Med. Rad. Photog.* 48:15, 1972.)

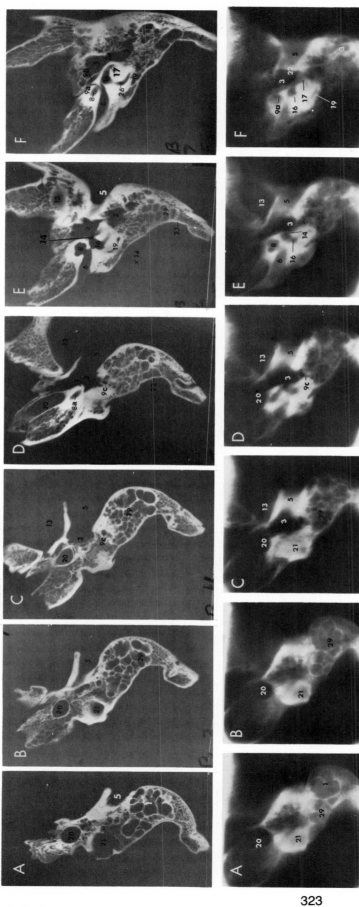

Fig 508.—Submentovertical projection. Six radiographs *(top)* paired with tomographic sections *(bottom)* of a dry left temporal bone at varying levels. Progression of levels from **A** to **F** is caudad to cephalad. Lateral aspect of skull is on the reader's right, anterior aspect at the top, and posterior aspect at the

bottom. Base view provides information on internal auditory canal and shows relation between carotid canal and jugular fossa. (From Schaeffer, R.E.: *Med. Rad. Photog.* 48:10–11, 1972.)

LEGEND FOR FIGURE 508

1. mastoid process
2. mastoid antrum
2a. aditus of antrum
3. middle ear (tympanic cavity)
3a. epitympanic recess (attic)
4. lateral wall of attic
5. external auditory canal
6. internal auditory canal
7. promontory of middle ear
8. cochlea
8a. basal turn of cochlea

9a. facial nerve canal, petrous segment
9b. facial nerve canal, tympanic segment
9c. facial nerve canal, mastoid (descending) segment
10. styloid process
11. stylomastoid foramen
12. crista transversa (crista falciformis)

13. mandibular fossa
14. oval window (fenestra vestibuli)
15. round window (fenestra cochleae)
16. vestibule
17. lateral semicircular canal
18. superior semicircular canal
19. posterior semicircular canal
20. carotid canal
21. jugular fossa

22. scutum (spur)
23. sinus plate
24. tegmen
25. squamous portion of temporal bone
26. crus commune (common limb)
27. arcuate eminence
28. petrous apex
29. mastoid air cells

323

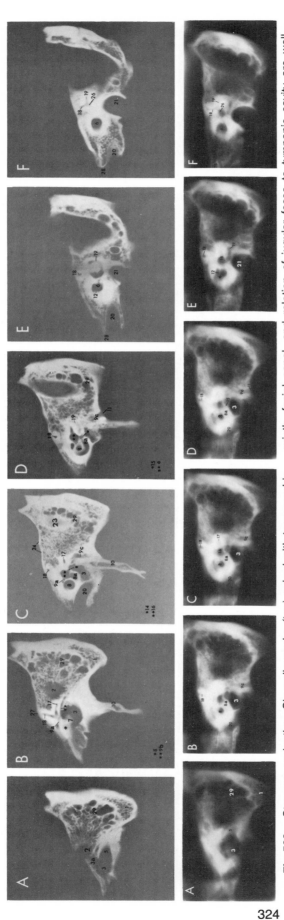

Fig 509.—Stenvers projection. Six radiographs (top) paired with tomographic sections (bottom) of a dry left temporal bone at varying levels. Progression of levels from **A** to **F** is anterior to posterior. Anteromedial aspect of bone is on the reader's left, and posterolateral aspect on the reader's right. Jugular fossa, lab-

yrinth, facial canal, and relation of jugular fossa to tympanic cavity are well shown in this projection. (From Schaeffer, R.E.: *Med. Rad. Photog.* 48:8–9, 1972.)

LEGEND FOR FIGURE 509

1. mastoid process
2. mastoid antrum
2a. aditus of antrum
3. middle ear (tympanic cavity)
3a. epitympanic recess (attic)
4. lateral wall of attic
5. external auditory canal
6. internal auditory canal
7. promontory of middle ear
8. cochlea
8a. basal turn of cochlea

9a. facial nerve canal, petrous segment
9b. facial nerve canal, tympanic segment
9c. facial nerve canal, mastoid (descending) segment
10. styloid process
11. stylomastoid foramen
12. crista transversa (crista falciformis)

13. mandibular fossa
14. oval window (fenestra vestibuli)
15. round window (fenestra cochleae)
16. vestibule
17. lateral semicircular canal
18. superior semicircular canal
19. posterior semicircular canal
20. carotid canal
21. jugular fossa

22. scutum (spur)
23. sinus plate
24. tegmen
25. squamous portion of temporal bone
26. crus commune (common limb)
27. arcuate eminence
28. petrous apex
29. mastoid air cells

ANTEROPOSTERIOR PROJECTION

Most of the important osseous structures can be visualized at two levels: the anterior, or cochlear, plane, and a more posterior vestibular plane (see Figs 503 and 504). The cochlear plane lies approximately 1 mm behind the anterior wall of the external auditory canal near the root of the tragus. Among the structures demonstrated in the cochlear plane are the external auditory canal, the spur, the lateral wall of the attic, the ossicles, the tympanic cavity and epitympanic recess, the cochlea, and the carotid canal. The malleus and incus have the appearance of an obliquely oriented club in the epitympanic recess. The bulbous part of the club represents the head of the malleus, while the tapered part corresponds to the superimposed handle of the malleus and long arm of the incus.

The vestibular plane is approximately 4 mm posterior to the plane of the cochlea. The structures visualized at this level include the external auditory canal, the spur and mastoid antrum, the vestibule and oval window, the superior and lateral semicircular canals, the internal auditory canal, the jugular fossa and tubercle, the hypoglossal canal, and the occipital condyle. Although the ossicles are not ideally demonstrated in the vestibular plane, the incus can usually be seen.

Among the structures not seen in the anteroposterior projection are the posterior semicircular canal, the stapes, the cochlear (round) window, and the third portion of the facial canal.

LATERAL PROJECTION

Multiple sections are necessary to visualize the bony external canal, the middle ear and ossicles, the round window, the descending portion of the facial canal, the cochlea, vestibule, and semicircular canals, and the internal auditory canal and carotid ridge (see Figs 505 to 507). The three most important levels to study are those through the ossicles, the round window, and the internal auditory canal.

Potter pointed out the resemblance to a molar tooth of the combined shadow of the malleus and incus in the lateral view. The crown of the tooth consists of the head of the malleus and body of the incus; its parallel roots are formed by the handle of the malleus and the long process of the incus. The stapes is not seen because of its obliquity.

The V-shaped, ridgelike inferior margin of the petrous pyramid is clearly visualized when the internal auditory canal is in sharp focus. The anterior wall of the V is formed by the carotid canal, and the posterior wall by the jugular fossa.

The lateral view is inadequate to evaluate the cochlea, the vestibule, the labyrinthine windows, and the first portion of the facial canal.

SUBMENTOVERTICAL PROJECTION

Several sections must be cut from cephalad to caudad in order to visualize all of the structures (see Fig 508). The more anterior sections include the mastoid air cells, the epitympanic recess, and the semicircular canals. Slightly more posteriorly, the internal auditory canal, part of the horizontal portion of the facial canal, the ossicular mass, and lateral wall of the epitympanic recess are visible. Still more posteriorly, the basal turn of the cochlea and its termination in the vestibule and the oval window are visualized. The most posterior section demonstrates the hypotympanium and the internal orifice of the cochlear aqueduct below the internal auditory canal.

SEMIAXIAL AND STENVERS PROJECTIONS

In the semiaxial projection (see Fig 509), the head of the supine patient is rotated 20 degrees toward the involved side. The central ray enters close to the medial canthus of the eye. Because the principal direction of the medial (labyrinthine) wall of the middle ear cavity is in a plane 20 to 25 degrees from the sagittal plane of the skull, the semiaxial projection is ideal for visualization of the oval window, the promontory, the horizontal semicircular canal, and the horizontal segment of the facial nerve canal.

I rarely use the Stenvers view, except for fractures of the petrous bone. It is excellent for a detailed assessment of the posterior semicircular canal, because the canal is parallel to the axis of the petrous pyramid in this projection.

INTERNAL AUDITORY CANAL—The long axis of the internal auditory canal makes a right angle with the sagittal plane of the skull. The petrous pyramid forms the hypotenuse of the right angle, since its long axis is oriented at a 45-degree angle to the sagittal plane. The porus, or medial end, of the canal enters the posterior fossa, approximately 1.0 to 1.5 cm posterior to the tip of the petrous pyramid. The closed lateral end of the canal is demarcated by the bony lamina cribrosa, abutting the vestibule. The lateral half of the canal is divided by the thin transverse falciform crest into two unequal segments. The smaller superior segment contains the facial nerve and nervus intermedius anteriorly, and the superior vestibular nerve posteriorly. The larger inferior segment houses the cochlear nerve anteriorly, and the inferior vestibular nerve posteriorly. The internal auditory canal also transmits the internal auditory artery and a few small veins.

The canal may be straight, oval-shaped, or slightly tapered at its medial end. The height or vertical diameter varies from 3 to 8 mm (average, 4 mm). The length of the posterior wall of the canal varies from 4 to 11 mm (average, 8 mm). These measurements are easy to make because the posterior wall and the superior and inferior tips of the porus are well defined. On the other hand, the anterior lip is less well demarcated from the posteromedial aspect of the petrous apex.

The following criteria are helpful in differentiating the normal from the abnormal canal: (1) the normal crista falciformis lies at, or above, the center of the canal (a crista below the center of the canal is abnormal); (2) the concave medial end of the normal posterior wall is well defined bilaterally; (3) a difference of 3 mm or more in length of the posterior wall of the two canals is abnormal; (4) a difference of more than 2 mm in vertical height from side to side is abnormal; and (5) significant differences in the shape of the canal compared with the opposite side should be viewed with suspicion (Figs 510 and 511).

Patients with neurofibromatosis may exhibit considerable enlargement of the internal auditory canal due to dural ectasia, without having an intracanalicular eighth nerve tumor. The latter can only be excluded by posterior fossa myelography (Fig 512). Rarely, a normal patient may present with unilateral enlargement of the internal auditory canal as a congenital variant (Figs 513 and 514). This diagnosis, too, can only be established by posterior fossa myelography.

Occasionally, there is a small, rounded bony knob present unilaterally or bilaterally on the superior margin of the petrous bone. This is a normal variant that should not be confused with a petrosal meningioma (see Fig 121).

FACIAL (FALLOPIAN) CANAL—The seventh cranial, or facial, nerve arises from the lower border of the pons and passes anteromedially to enter the internal auditory canal. The nerve lies anteriorly in the lateral half of the internal auditory canal above the falciform crest. It exits from the lateral end of the internal auditory canal to enter its own canal, the facial canal.

The entire canal, approximately 5 cm long, is divided into three segments: The first, or petrous, segment (genu), about 1.5 cm in length, extends from the lateral end of the internal auditory canal to the geniculate ganglion, coursing anterolaterally between the cochlea and the vestibule. The second, or tympanic, portion doubles back posteriorly and runs horizontally immediately below the lateral semicircular canal. The third, or descending, segment, about 1.5 cm in length, has a vertical course just behind the external auditory canal; it exits at the stylomastoid foramen. The chorda tympani arises from the facial nerve in the mid-descending portion and courses anteriorly between the handle of the malleus and the long process of the incus.

PNEUMATIZATION OF THE MASTOID

The mastoid process does not exist at birth. As it develops in the early years of life, the cells on the lateral

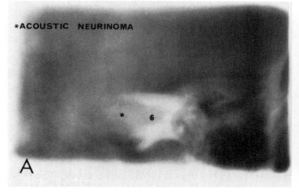
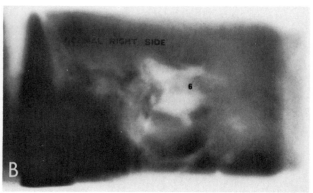

Fig 510.—Anteroposterior tomography in a patient with left acoustic neurinoma. **A,** left ear. Medial portion of internal auditory canal (6) is enlarged by acoustic neurinoma (asterisk). **B,** normal right ear. (From Schaeffer, R.E.: Med. Rad. Photog. 48:18–19, 1972.)

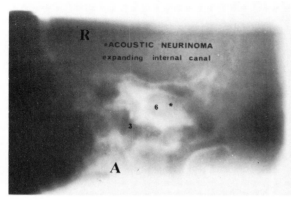
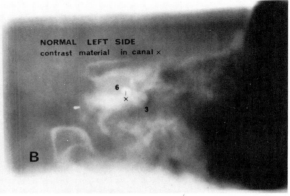

Fig 511.—Anteroposterior tomography in a patient with right acoustic neurinoma. **A,** right ear. Medial portion of internal auditory canal (6) is enlarged by the tumor *(asterisk).* **B,** normal left ear contains a drop of residual Pantopaque in the canal from a previous posterior fossa myelogram. (From Schaeffer, R.E.: *Med. Rad. Photog.* 48:20, 1972.)

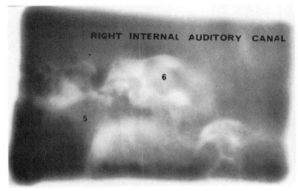
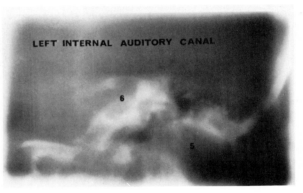

Fig 512.—Anteroposterior tomography of both ears in a patient with neurofibromatosis showing bilateral striking enlargement of internal auditory canals. Note external auditory canal *(5)* and internal auditory canal *(6).* (From Schaeffer, R.E.: *Med. Rad. Photog.* 48:20, 1972.)

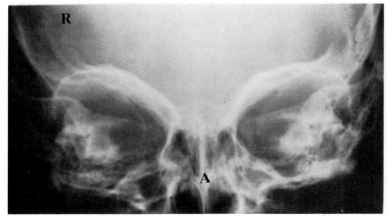
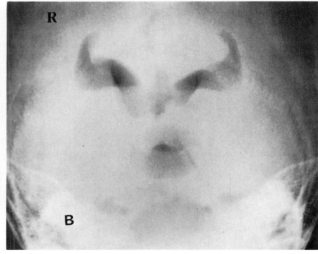

Fig 513.—**A,** bilateral symmetric enlargement of internal auditory canals in a patient with no overt evidence of neurofibromatosis. **B,** upright pneumoencephalogram showing normal configuration of both cerebellopontine cisterns. Posterior fossa myelography demonstrated no evidence of intracanalicular defect. This must, therefore, be considered a normal variant.

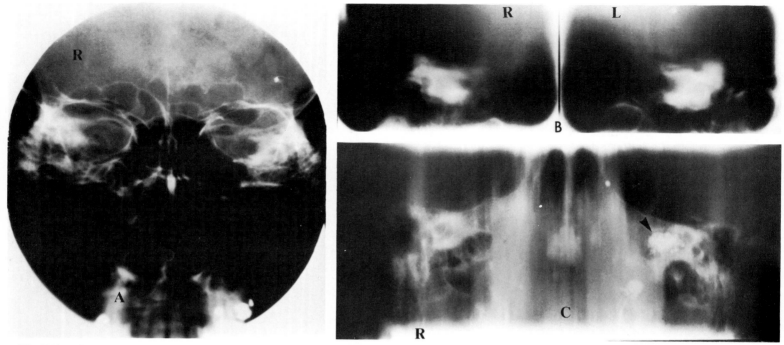

Fig 514.—A, posteroanterior radiograph showing flaring of medial aspect of left internal auditory canal. **B,** anteroposterior tomography demonstrating some generalized enlargement of left canal. **C,** poste-rior fossa myelogram with Pantopaque filling the canal, and no intra-canicular defect *(arrowhead).* This represents a normal variation.

aspect of the antrum fan laterally and posteriorly. The entire normal mastoid process is pneumatized by the fifth year of life (Figs 515 to 518).

Normal Variations

In some persons, normal epithelial growth is retarded and pneumatization diminished to varying degrees. Consequently, there are three relatively distinct types of "normal" mastoids (Figs 519 to 522): (1) pneumatic, characterized by large, thin-walled, intercommunicating cells lined with a delicate mucous membrane continuous with that of the tympanic cavity (see Fig 519); (2) diploic, made up of spongy bone containing marrow (see Fig 520); and (3) mixed, consisting of varying degrees of pneumatized and diploic bone (see Fig 521). The sclerotic, eburnated mastoid with no cellular development is an abnormal finding due to old disease.

Pneumatization

A number of theories have been advanced to explain the marked variation in pneumatization of the mastoid. The most widely accepted view is that of Wittmaack, who demonstrated that pneumatization depends upon a sound, intact mucous membrane in the tympanic cav-ity. According to this theory, the pneumatic cellular mastoid is indicative of a normal mucosa, whereas cellular development other than pneumatic is the result of otitis media in infancy with alteration of the mucosa of the middle ear and antrum.

Although the mastoid process assumes its adult form by the fifth year, the cells continue to develop up to puberty, and possibly for some time thereafter. The size and the shape of the cells in normal pneumatic mastoids vary considerably. In general, however, the cells tend to be smaller centrally and become progressively larger as they fan out peripherally. The terminal cell at the tip of the mastoid is often rather large.

Genetically, all the cells in the temporal bone are derived from the mucous membrane of the primary cavities of the eustachian tube, tympanic cavity, and antrum. However, there is a remarkable variability in location of various cell groups. Meltzer believes that the position of the lateral sinus influences the topographic localization of mastoid cell groups. Neumann has described the following possible locations of cells (Fig 523):
1. Zygomatic cells
2. Cells along the floor of the middle fossa
3. Marginal cells (behind the lateral sinus)
4. Cells overlying the lateral sinus

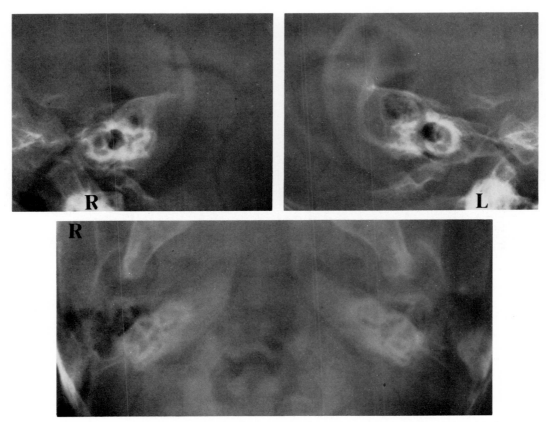

Fig 515.—Normal left mastoid at age 6 months. Right mastoid was involved in acute mastoiditis that was completely controlled by anti- biotics. The contrast of the right with the normal left mastoid empha- sizes the normalcy of the latter.

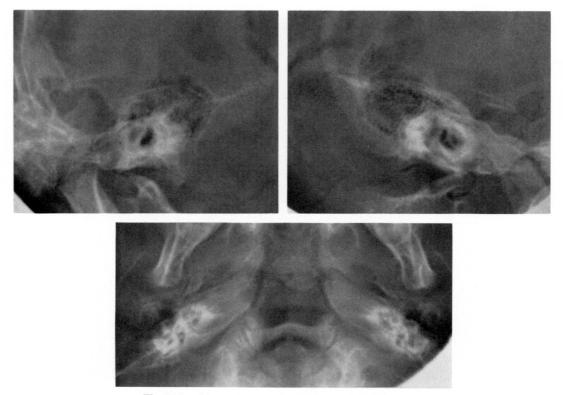

Fig 516.—Normal mastoids bilaterally at age 1 year.

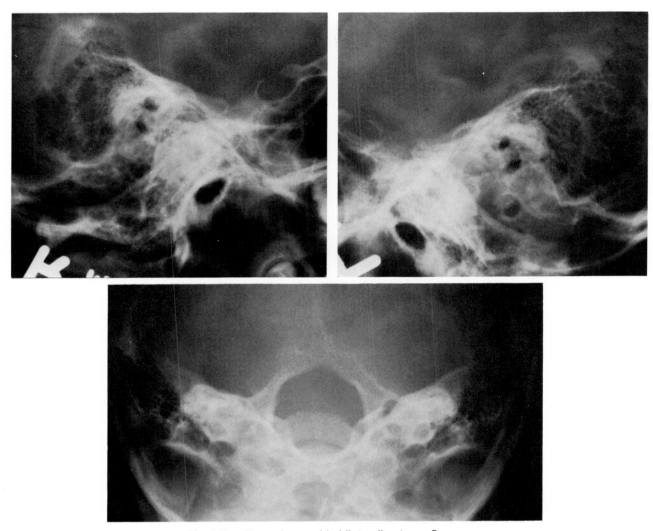

Fig 517.—Normal mastoids bilaterally at age 5 years.

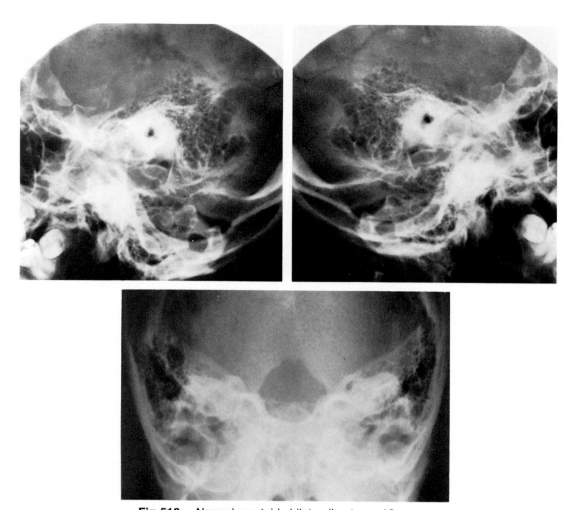

Fig 518.—Normal mastoids bilaterally at age 16 years.

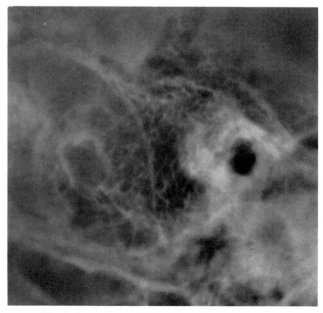

Fig 519.—Pneumatic type of normal mastoid.

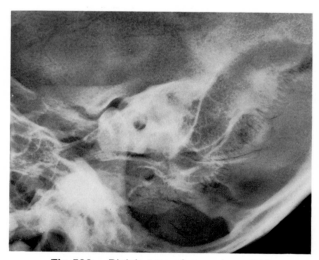

Fig 520.—Diploic type of normal mastoid.

332

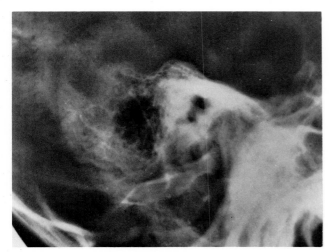

Fig 521.—Mixed type of normal mastoid, showing some pneumatization along with diploic spongy bone.

5. Retrofacial cells
6. Cells extending under the labyrinth
7. Cells in the mastoid tip
8. Cells around the bony portion of the eustachian tube
9. Cells in the squama
10. Petrosal, or "angle," cells

The degree of pneumatization of the petrous bone varies considerably; occasionally, the entire petrous apex may be pneumatized (Fig 524). In general, pneumatization of any area in one petrous pyramid is usually accompanied by some degree of pneumatization on the

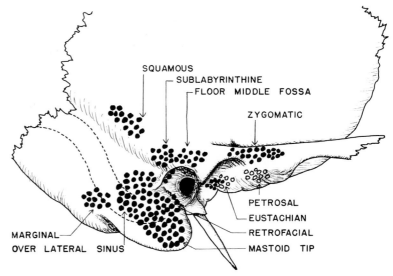

Fig 523.—Distribution of possible locations of mastoid cells. Actually, the peripheral groups of cells are not isolated, but are represented as such in the diagram for the purpose of clarity. (After Tremble.)

opposite side. Although some asymmetry in pneumatization is frequent, marked asymmetry is usually the result of mastoid disease in infancy (Fig 525) or previous surgery (Fig 526).

In the well-pneumatized petrous bone, acute petrositis may be recognized either by loss of sharp definition of the bony cortex, or by clouding of the cells with slightly increased radiopacity (Fig 527). As the infection progresses, there may be actual destruction of bone. In

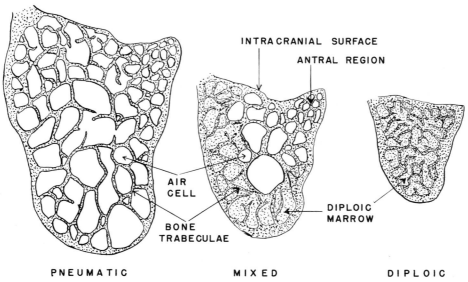

Fig 522.—Diagram of mastoid types (after Lederer).

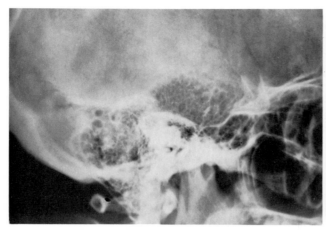
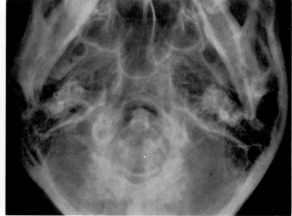

Fig 524.—Extensive pneumatization of petrous bone. Mastoid processes are large, and mastoid cells extend to tips of petrous pyramids and far into zygomatic processes anteriorly.

chronic petrositis, the usual roentgenologic finding is dense sclerosis (Fig 528).

The variable location of the lateral sinus and its relationship to the posterior wall of the external auditory meatus are important to the surgeon. In the extremely well-pneumatized mastoid, it is not always possible to visualize the entire lateral sinus. However, its anterior wall is usually seen as a sharp, linear density curving toward the external auditory canal. In the sclerotic or poorly pneumatized mastoid, both walls of the sinus are usually clearly demonstrable.

Recognition of Departure from the Normal

In studying roentgenograms of the mastoids, one must consider the type and extent of cellular development, the presence or absence of cellular opacity, the sharpness of definition of the cell walls, the appearance of the petrous apex, and the position of the lateral sinus and emissary vessel.

The earliest roentgenologic evidence of mastoiditis is an overall haziness and clouding of the mastoid cells. This change may be produced by (1) edema of the mas-

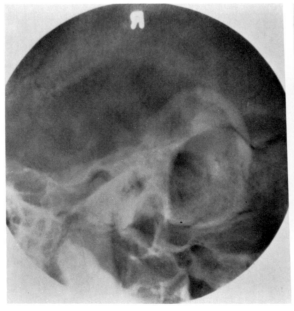
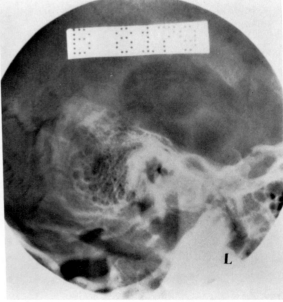

Fig 525.—Asymmetric development of mastoid process due to old infection during childhood. Normal left mastoid contrasts sharply with sclerotic right mastoid, which exhibits no pneumatization beyond the periantral triangle.

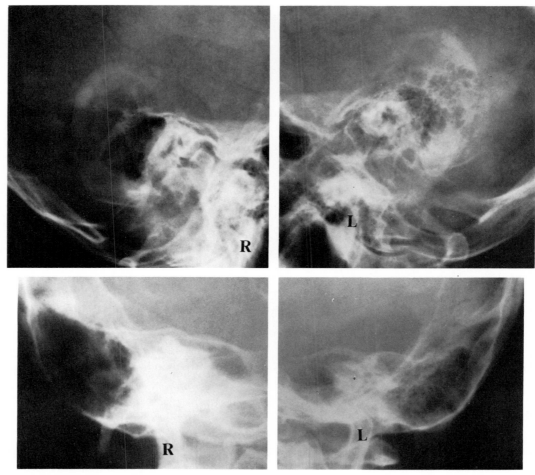

Fig 526.—Asymmetric pneumatization of mastoids due to previous right mastoidectomy in childhood. Law projection *(top)*; Stenvers projection *(bottom)*.

toid mucosa and exudation into the cells without bone destruction (Fig 529), (2) exudation into the cells with bone destruction (Fig 530), and (3) swelling of the external soft tissues overlying the mastoid process (Fig 531). The demonstration of faint haziness overlying the mastoid does not necessarily mean that the patient has, or will develop, clinical mastoiditis. On the other hand, this may well be the first roentgenologic manifestation of mastoiditis.

Although haziness and clouding are not too difficult to recognize in the well-pneumatized mastoid, they may not be readily appreciated in the diploic mastoid. It is impossible, roentgenologically, to differentiate simple edema of the mastoid mucosa from early mastoiditis. It is perhaps more important to differentiate early mastoid disease from simple swelling of the external soft tissues. In this regard, clinical examination, in con-

junction with films of the mastoid tips, usually leads to the correct diagnosis.

The infection may be arrested at the stage of exudation or may progress from the mucosa to involve bone. The latter stage is characterized by actual destruction of the intercellular septa (Fig 532). A comparison with the normal side is helpful in the detection of mastoid disease and early cell necrosis. In the final analysis, accurate diagnosis depends upon close correlation of the clinical and roentgenologic findings.

In evaluating patients for the presence of a cholesteatoma, it is important to pay attention to several key structures: the spur, Körner's septum, and the mastoid antrum (Figs 531 to 533). The spur is a sharply defined bony projection at the junction of the superior medial margin of the external auditory canal and the lateral attic wall. If the spur is ill-defined, eroded, or destroyed,

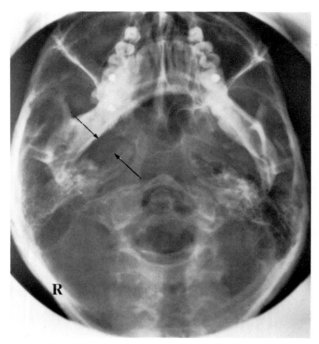

Fig 527.—Submentovertical radiograph showing acute petrositis of right petrous apex with bone destruction *(arrows)*. (From Young, B.R.: *The Skull, Sinuses and Mastoids* [Chicago, Year Book Medical Publishers, 1948].)

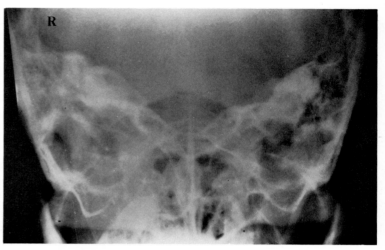

Fig 528.—Chronic right mastoiditis and petrositis.

a middle ear infection or cholesteatoma is likely to be present. Körner's septum is another seminal landmark, which is normally represented by a thin, transverse sliver of bone projecting into the mastoid antrum from its superior lateral margin. An absent septum is usually indicative of a cholesteatoma or a previous mastoidectomy.

Tomography cannot always differentiate cholesteatoma from chronic otitis media, since both conditions can produce bone destruction of the ossicles, lateral wall of the attic, tympanic cavity, and mastoid antrum. However, a cholesteatoma is more likely in the pres-

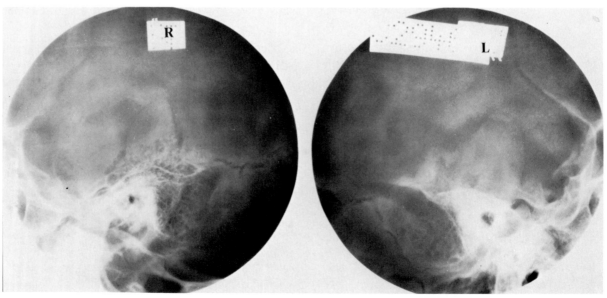

Fig 529.—Clouding of left mastoid cells due to edema associated with otitis media. Normal right mastoid is shown for comparison.

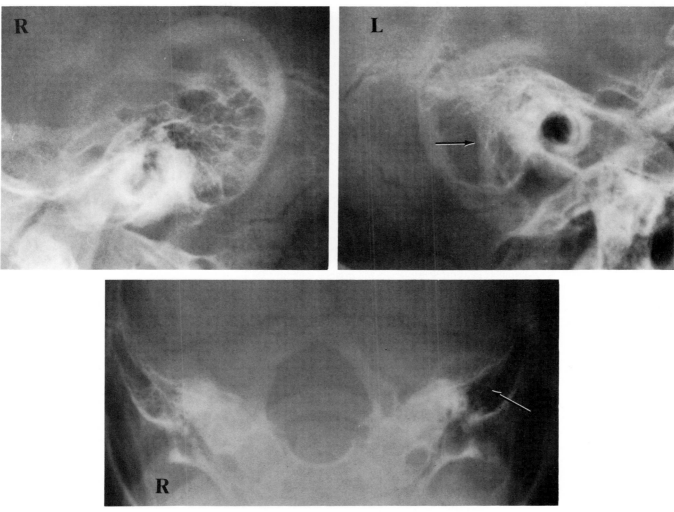

Fig 530.—Acute left mastoiditis with exudation into cells
and early bone destruction *(arrows).*

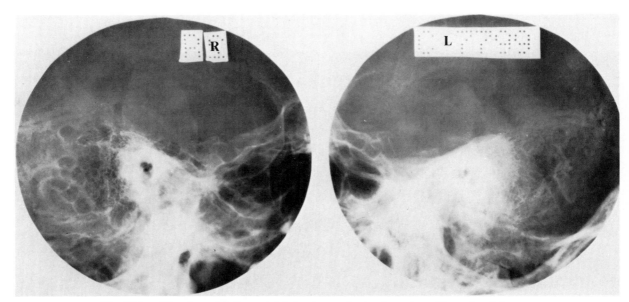

Fig 531.—Clouding of left mastoid due to marked external swelling of soft tissues resulting in overall increased radiopacity without loss of cellular outlines.

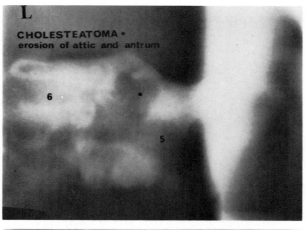

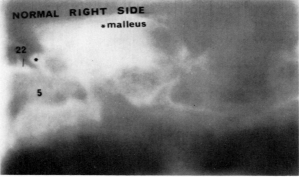

Fig 532.—Anteroposterior tomograms in a patient with large cholesteatoma of the left ear. Left ear *(top):* Entire lateral wall of attic and much of external auditory canal are eroded *(asterisk).* There is also extensive erosion of the antrum and complete destruction of the ossicles. Bony density in superior portion of eroded attic may represent an ossicular fragment. Lateral semicircular canal is truncated due to fistula proven at surgery. Right ear *(bottom):* Scutum is normal and malleus *(asterisk)* fits nicely into relatively small normal attic. External auditory canal *(5);* internal auditory canal *(6);* and scutum *(22).* (From Schaeffer, R.E.: *Med. Rad. Photog.* 48:17, 1972.)

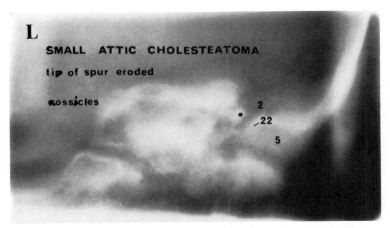

Fig 533.—Anteroposterior tomogram of left ear showing small cholesteatoma. The important feature is the rounding and blunting of the scutum. Ossicular mass *(asterisk)* is also farther from lateral wall of attic than normal due to bone erosion. Mastoid antrum *(2)*; external auditory canal *(5)*; scutum *(22)*. (From Schaeffer, R.E.: *Med. Rad. Photog.* 48:18, 1972.)

ence of a large aditus ad antrum or antrum, ossicular erosion, and displacement. In this connection, it is important to remember that the normal mastoid antrum may vary considerably in size. Uncommonly, a very large normal antrum, i.e., 15 mm, can simulate a cholesteatoma. The important differential diagnostic criterion is the presence or absence of focal bone destruction.

The normal antrum is visualized as a radiolucency lateral to the superior semicircular canal. In the newborn, the antrum lies at a higher level than in the adult; it drifts posteriorly and inferiorly with progressive pneumatization and development of the mastoid bone. In general, the antra tend to be symmetric from side to side and usually do not exceed 6 mm (transverse) × 10 mm (vertical) in size. The anterior wall of the antrum opens into the tympanic cavity through the aditus. The posterior wall opens into the mastoid air cells separating the antrum from the somewhat more inferior and posterior lateral sinus. The superior wall or roof lies below the temporal lobe in the middle cranial fossa. The medial wall, which is usually quite anterior to the lateral sinus, is indented by the lateral semicircular canal and the canal for the facial nerve.

REFERENCES

Bast T., Anson B. J.: *The Temporal Bone and the Ear.* Springfield, Ill., Charles C Thomas, Publisher, 1949.

Brunner S.: Radiological examination of temporal bone in infants and children. *Radiology* 82:401–405, 1964.

Buckingham R. A., Valvassori G. E.: Tomographic anatomy of the temporal bone. *Otolaryngol. Clin. North Am.* 6:337–362, 1973.

Camp J. D., Allen E. P.: Microtia and congenital atresia of the external auditory canal. *Am. J. Roentgenol.* 43:201–203, 1940.

Farrell F. W. Jr., Hantz O.: Protruding jugular bulb presenting as a middle ear mass: Case report and brief review. *Am. J. Roentgenol.* 128:685–687, 1977.

Fowler E. P. Jr.: Certain fundamentals in regard to suppuration of the petrosal pyramid: Normal and pathological anatomy of the petrous pyramid. *Ann. Otol. Rhinol. Laryngol.* 44:1056–1068, 1935.

Fowler E. P. Jr., Swenson P. C.: Petrositis. *Am. J. Roentgenol.* 41:317–342, 1939.

Guinto F. C., Jr., Himadi G. M.: Tomographic anatomy of the ear. *Radiol. Clin. North Am.* 12:405–417, 1974.

Glasgold A. I., Horrigan W. D.: The internal carotid artery presenting as a middle ear tumor. *Laryngoscope* 82:2217–2221, 1972.

Hanafee W. N., Gussen R.: Correlation of basal projection tomography in clinical problems. *Radiol. Clin. North Am.* 12:419–430, 1974.

Jensen J., Rovsing H.: *Fundamentals of Ear Tomography.* Springfield, Ill., Charles C Thomas, Publisher, 1971.

Juster M., Fischgold H.: *Etude radioanatomique de l'os temporal.* Paris, Masson & Cie, 1955.

Lapayowker M. S., Liebman E. P., Ronis M. L., et al.: Presentation of the internal carotid artery as a tumor of the middle ear. *Radiology* 98:293–297, 1971.

Lindsay J. R.: Petrous pyramid of the temporal bone. *Arch. Otolaryngol.* 31:231–255, 1940.

Lloyd T. V., Van Aman M., Johnson J. C.: Aberrant jugular bulb presenting as a middle ear mass. *Radiology* 131:139–141, 1979.

Meltzer P. E.: Mastoid cells: Their arrangement in relation to the sigmoid portion of the transverse sinus. *Arch. Otolaryngol.* 19:326–335, 1934.

Overton S. B., Ritter F. N.: A high placed jugular bulb in the middle ear: A clinical and temporal bone study. *Laryngoscope* 83:1986–1991, 1973.

Potter G. D.: The lateral projection in tomography of the petrous pyramid. *Am. J. Roentgenol.* 104:194–200, 1968.

Potter G. D.: *Sectional Anatomy and Tomography of the Head.* New York, Grune & Stratton, 1971.

Samuel E.: *Clinical Radiology of the Ear, Nose and Throat.* London, H. K. Lewis & Co., 1952.

Schillinger R.: Pneumatization of the mastoid. *Radiology* 33:54–67, 1939.

Steffen T. N.: Vascular anomalies of the middle ear. *Laryngoscope* 78:171–197, 1968.

Taylor H. K.: Roentgen findings in suppuration of the petrous apex (petrositis). *Am. J. Roentgenol.* 30:156–162, 1933.

Taylor H. K.: Suppuration of the petrosal pyramid: Roentgenologic problems. *Arch. Otolaryngol.* 18:458–463, 1933.

Tremble G. E.: Pneumatization of the temporal bone. *Arch. Otolaryngol.* 19:172–182, 1934.

Valvassori G. E.: The radiological diagnosis of acoustic neuromas. *Arch. Otolaryngol.* 83:582–587, 1966.

Valvassori G. E.: The abnormal internal auditory canal: The diagnosis of acoustic neuroma. *Radiology* 92:449–459, 1969.

Valvassori G. E., Buckingham R. A.: *Tomography and Cross Section of the Ear.* Toronto, W. B. Saunders Co., 1975.

Valvassori G. E., Pierce R. H.: The normal internal auditory canal. *Am. J. Roentgenol.* 92:1232–1241, 1964.

Waltner J. G.: Anatomic variations of the lateral and sigmoid sinuses. *Arch. Otolaryngol.* 39:307–312, 1944.

Welin S.: On the roentgen diagnosis of cholesteatoma in the temporal bone. *Acta Radiol.* 25:227–239, 1944.

Welin S.: Beiträge zur Röntgendiagnostik der Otitis med. acuta und ihrer Komplikationen im Schläfenbein. *Acta Radiol.*, suppl. 42, 1951.

Winderen L., Zimmer J.: Cholesteatoma of the middle ear. *Acta Radiol.*, suppl. 111, 1954.

Wittmaack K.: Über die normale und die pathologische Pneumatisation des Schläfenbeines, Jena. Fischer, 1918.

Wittmaack K.: Zur Frage der Bedeutung der Mittelohrenzundungen des frühesten Kindesalters für später. *Arch. Ohren-Nasen Kehlkophfh.* 129:207–250, 1931.

17

Computed Tomography of the Skull

STEPHEN G. ROTHMAN *and* EDWARD N. RAUSCHKOLB

With increasing availability of computed tomography (CT) scanners and recognition of their role in the evaluation and management of neurologic problems, the standard radiographic skull series may become superfluous in many cases. Much of the information obtained from routine skull films and even from tomography can be acquired by utilizing the variable mean and window capabilities of current CT scanners. However, the skull cannot be adequately studied from images that are primarily designed for optimal portrayal of the brain. The images must be replayed for bone detail.

While the spatial resolution of current scanners is inferior to that of film-screen techniques, the contrast resolution is significantly better. In addition, the axial projection is ideal for evaluating the facial bones, sinuses, orbits, and basal foramina without the need to place a possibly unstable patient in an awkward or potentially dangerous position. Reconstruction or coronal tomography can play an adjunctive role. The ability to precisely localize abnormalities such as tumor calcifications, as well as evaluate the cerebral ventricles, is a great advantage over plain films.

FACIAL BONES AND PARANASAL SINUSES

The most inferior cut through the maxilla (Fig 534) demonstrates the relationship between the alveolar ridge and the rami of the mandible. This view is useful for the evaluation of tumors of the oral cavity and their extension into the alveolar ridge.

Slightly superior to this section, the nasal cavity and septum, and inferior portions of the maxillary antrum are clearly displayed (Fig 535). The soft tissue mass immediately behind the nasal cavity is the tongue. Moving superiorly, the nasal cavity is visualized communicating with the nasopharynx. At this level the nasolacrimal duct is seen anterior to the medial wall of the maxillary sinus. The medial and lateral pterygoid plates are also noted (Fig 536). The condylar process of the mandible abutting the temporomandibular joint comes into focus at the next higher level, along with the posterosuperior extension of the maxillary sinus below the orbit (Fig 537). This relationship is important in planning radiation therapy for maxillary sinus tumors, since failure to recognize the superior extent of a tumor may result in inadequate treatment.

It is important to realize that the scan is essentially a horizontal beam image because the patient is supine. Hence, air-fluid levels are well visualized (Fig 538).

As we ascend further into the orbits, the lamina papyracea (the lateral wall of the ethmoid sinus) and the delicate ethmoid intercellular septae come into view (Fig 539). The sphenoid sinus with its variable septa is noted more posteriorly. The axial plane is ideally suited for evaluation of the orbital surface of the sphenoid bone which constitutes the posterolateral orbital wall (Fig 540). The scan in Figure 541, A demonstrates facial dislocation in a severely injured patient who also had a conventional brain CT scan at the same time.

Many scanners permit tilting of the gantry to produce scans with varying degrees of angulation from the canthomeatal line. The ability to angulate the gantry makes it possible to view complex structures in different planes (Fig 542).

As in other radiographic techniques, it may be usful to visualize the patient in two right-angle projections. Patients can, therefore, be repositioned to obtain coronal scans (Fig 543, A to D).

CT in the axial and coronal planes is useful in the localization of intraocular foreign bodies (Fig 544, A and B). Unlike routine radiographs, CT visualizes nonmetallic foreign material so long as its attenuation coefficient differs from that of water. Similarly, tumors involving the orbit can be studied to evaluate extension of tumor and destruction of bone (Fig 545).

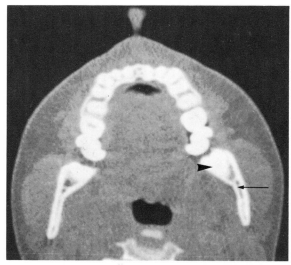

Fig 534.—Scan through alveolar ridge. Note part of mandible (←) and last mandibular molar behind the maxillary teeth (▶).

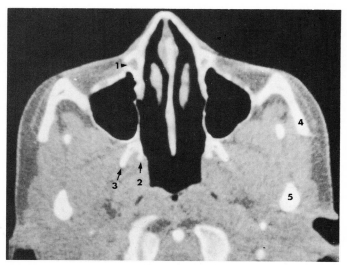

Fig 536.—Next higher scan through pterygoid plates. Nasolacrimal duct *(1)*, medial pterygoid process *(2)*, lateral pterygoid process *(3)*, zygoma *(4)*, and condylar process of mandible *(5)*.

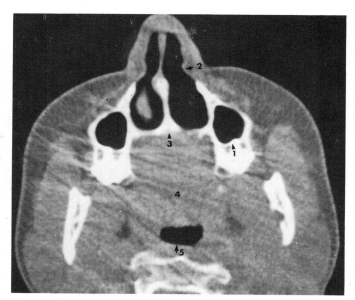

Fig 535.—Next higher scan through inferior portion of maxillary sinuses. Maxillary sinus *(1)*, nasal cavity *(2)*, nasal septum *(3)*, tongue *(4)*, and pharynx *(5)*.

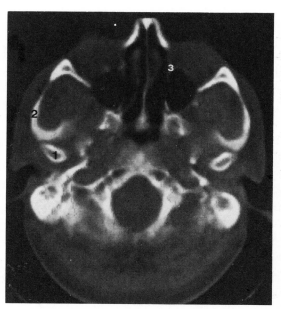

Fig 537.—Scan at level of mandibular condyle. Mandibular condyle *(1)*, zygomatic arch *(2)*, and posterior-superior extension of maxillary sinus *(3)*.

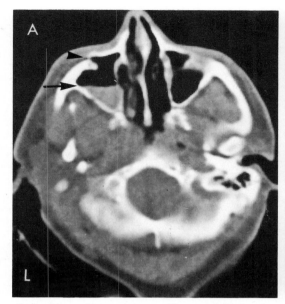

Fig 538.—A, scan through maxillary sinuses. Note airfluid level (→) and displaced fracture of anterior maxillary wall (▶) on the left side. **B,** scan 1 cm higher showing indentation of anterior half of zygomatic arch (▶) and fracture of orbital surface of the left sphenoid bone (→).

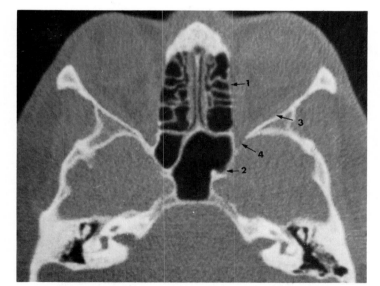

Fig 539.—Scan through ethmoid sinuses. Ethmoid sinus *(1),* sphenoid sinus *(2),* orbital surface of greater sphenoid wing *(3),* and superior orbital fissure *(4).*

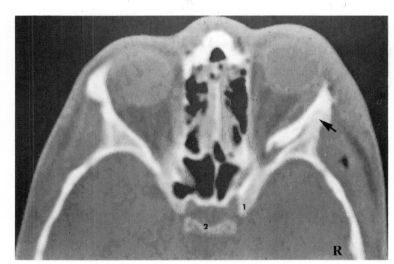

Fig 540.—Fracture of right orbit. Zygomatic portion of orbit is displaced posteromedially (←). Anterior clinoid process *(1)* and dorsum sellae *(2).*

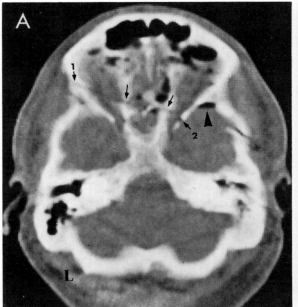

Fig 541.—A, craniofacial dislocation. Complex fracture line extends obliquely across skull base from left greater sphenoid wing *(1)* through the ethmoids (↓) and contralateral optic canal *(2)*. Ethmoids and sphenoid sinuses are opacified. Air is seen within the orbit and intracranially anterior to temporal lobe (▲). **B,** a second patient with similar fracture without craniofacial dislocation. Optic canal fracture *(1)* and posterior orbital wall fracture *(2)*.

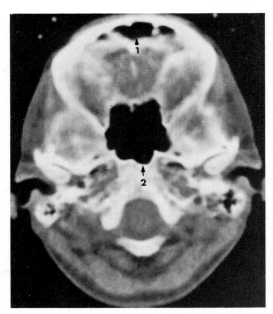

Fig 542.—Scan produced with central ray angled 20 degrees to canthomeatal line. Note that frontal sinuses *(1)* are in same plane as sphenoid sinuses *(2)*.

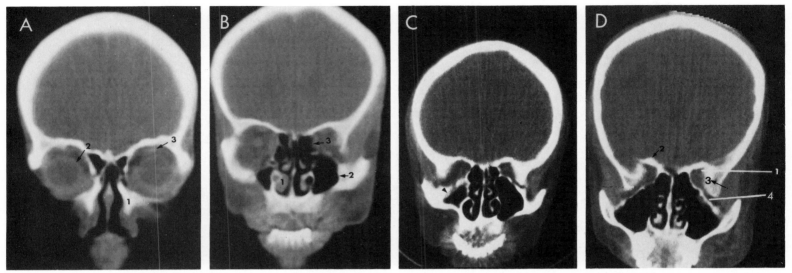

Fig 543.—A, coronal CT scan through most anterior portion of maxilla *(1)*. Note density of choroidal layer of eye *(2)* compared to rest of globe. Both superior rectus muscles *(3)* can be identified. **B,** a scan 1 cm more posterior demonstrates nasal turbinates *(1)*, maxillary sinuses *(2)*, and ethmoid sinuses *(3)*. **C,** midmaxillary scan showing mucosal thickening in right maxillary sinus (▼). **D,** somewhat oblique coronal scan through superior orbital fissures *(1)*. Note the lesser sphenoidal wing *(2)*, greater sphenoidal wing *(3)*, and inferior orbital fissure *(4)*.

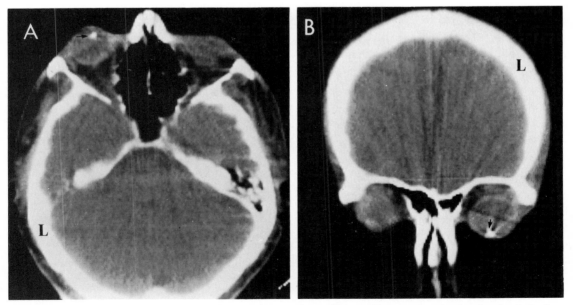

Fig 544.—A and **B,** axial and coronal scans in a patient with a radiopaque ocular foreign body (→). The two right-angle projections allow precise localization prior to surgical removal.

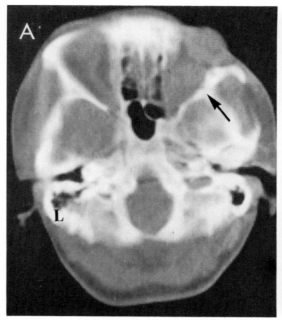
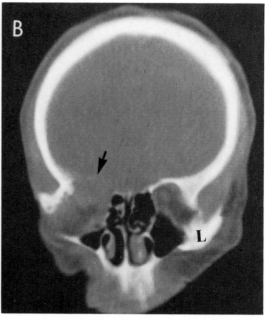

Fig 545.—A and **B,** axial and coronal scans in a patient with a malignant lacrimal gland tumor. Note thickening and irregularity of posterior orbital wall (↖) on axial scan. Orbital roof is destroyed and absent on the coronal scan (↓).

Tumors of the paranasal sinuses are well demonstrated by CT. A nasopharyngeal soft tissue mass in a young male displacing but not destroying the nasal septum and medial wall of the maxillary sinus is virtually diagnostic of angiofibroma (Fig 546). Malignancies involving the paranasal sinuses can also be studied with benefit prior to radiation treatment planning (Fig 547). CT is more sensitive than conventional tomography in the evaluation of the paranasal sinuses because it can identify thin spicules of bone that are difficult to see even on pluridirectional tomography.

BASAL FORAMINA

CT provides an ideal method for studying the skull base. No awkward positioning is required—merely minimal angulation of the gantry to obtain scans horizontal to the orbitomeatal line.

A single scan (Fig 548) through the base of the skull demonstrates most of the significant anatomy. Traversing the floor of the middle cranial fossa are the foramina ovale and spinosum. The foramen lacerum paralleling the carotid canal is seen medially behind the foramen ovale. The scan in Figure 549 was performed with the central ray angled 20 degrees to the canthomeatal line, centered slightly lower than in Figure 548. This angulation provides a single view of the entire clivus and the important posterior structures.

Many of the congenital variations at the craniocervical junction can be visualized quite readily by CT (Fig 550, *A* and *B*). The extent of the bony deformity and the neural compression in basilar invagination are ideally studied by this technique (Fig 551). Occasionally, tumors destroy portions of the skull base (Fig 552).

Tumors of the temporal bone and mastoid, while

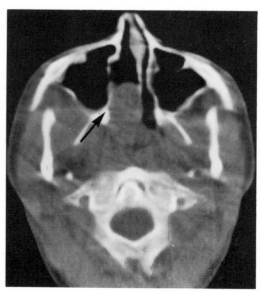

Fig 546.—Young adult male with a soft tissue nasal and nasopharyngeal mass that bows the nasal septum and medial maxillary wall (↑). Diagnosis: angiofibroma.

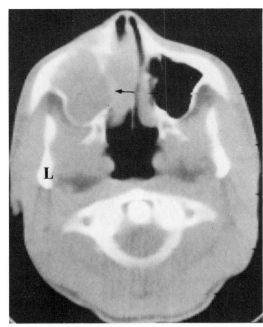

Fig 547.—Scan in a patient with maxillary carcinoma. Left maxillary sinus is filled with mass that has destroyed medial sinus wall and extends into nasal cavity (←).

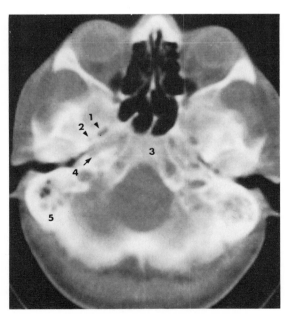

Fig 548.—Scan through floor of middle cranial fossa. Foramen ovale (1), foramen spinosum (2), clivus (3), carotid canal (4), and mastoid process (5).

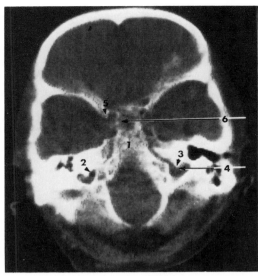

Fig 549.—Scan performed with central ray angled 20 degrees to canthomeatal line provides visualization of entire clivus on one view. Clivus (1), pars nervosa of jugular foramen (2), jugular spine (3), and pars vascularis of jugular foramen (4). The more superior and anterior structures are also seen because of the angulation. Anterior clinoid process (5) and sella turcica (6).

fairly uncommon lesions, present a challenge because the extent of bone destruction and brain invasion dictate the mode of therapy. Glomus jugulare tumors characteristically exhibit marked contrast enhancement (Fig 553, A and B). On the other hand, carcinoma of the ear rarely enhances significantly following contrast infusion (Fig 553, C). Hence, these two lesions can usually be distinguished by CT without resorting to angiography.

Cerebrospinal fluid otorrhea and basilar skull fractures in areas traditionally difficult to evaluate by standard radiography are probably also best studied by CT (Fig 554, A and B).

CALVARIA

The bony calvaria is more difficult to study with CT since, for the most part, the plane of the skull is perpendicular to the plane of the image. In addition, as one proceeds superiorly toward the vertex, the apparent thickness of the skull increases because the calvaria becomes more tangential to the plane of the image (Fig 555). This spurious thickening can readily be distinguished from the thickening and disorganization which occurs in Paget's disease (Fig 556). Focal thickening can also occur normally, as a normal variant in the frontal region in hyperostosis frontalis interna (Fig 557), or abnormally, as in fibrous dysplasia (Fig 558).

Vascular channels produce normal lucencies within

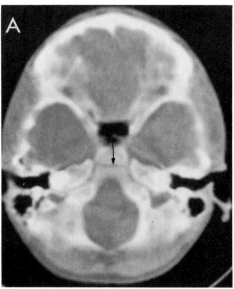 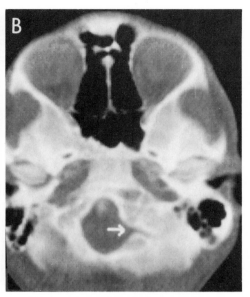

Fig 550.—A, axial scan in adult patient with persistent spheno-occipital synchondrosis (↓). **B,** axial scan in another patient with congenital cleft in occipital bone (→). This most likely represents failure of fusion of synchondrosis between exoccipital and supraoccipital portions of bone.

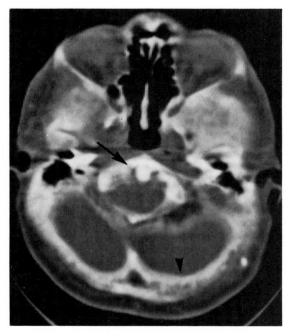 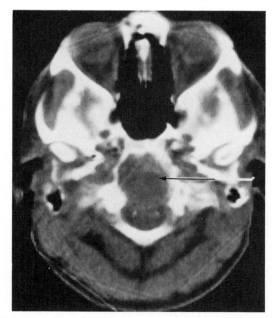

Fig 551.—Patient with acquired basilar invagination. Note disorganization of petrous and occipital bones characteristic of Paget's disease (▲). Entire ring of C-1 and tip of the dens lie within posterior fossa (↑).

Fig 552.—Slightly oblique axial scan showing irregular destruction of anterior rim of foramen magnum and clivus (←) due to large clivus chordoma.

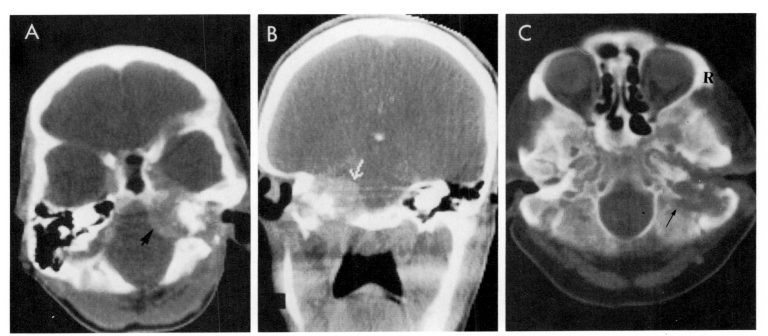

Fig 553.—A and **B,** axial and coronal scans in a patient with glomus jugulare tumor, which destroys most of petrous bone (↙). Unlike the carcinoma shown in **C,** this tumor enhances prominently following intravenous contrast infusion. This is the hallmark of a glomus jugulare tumor. **C,** scan through external auditory canals in patient with carcinoma. Note soft tissue mass replacing air in the right external canal. Mass extends posteriorly and medially to destroy mastoid and petrous bones (↗) but does not enhance following intravenous contrast injection.

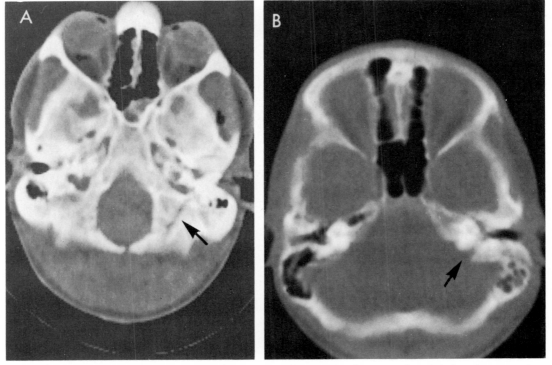

Fig 554.—A and **B,** two axial scans in a patient with complex fracture of occipital and temporal bones (↑). Note extension of fracture into middle ear with opacification of mastoid.

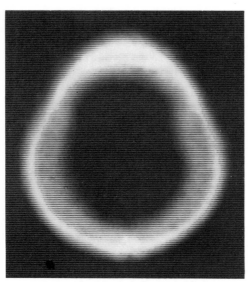

Fig 555.—Axial scan performed just below the vertex. There is artifactual expansion of calvaria due to parallelism of bony calvaria with beam of scanner at this level.

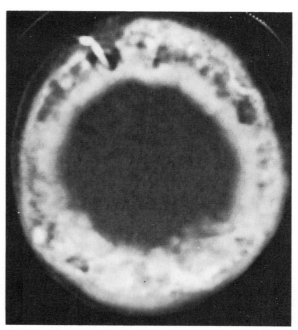

Fig 556.—Axial scan in a patient with Paget's disease. Calvaria is thickened and disorganized. Note characteristic alternating areas of hyperostosis and bone destruction.

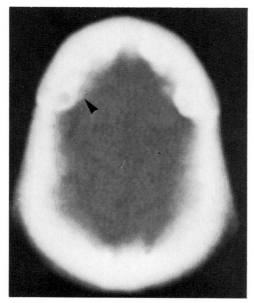

Fig 557.—Hyperostosis frontalis interna. Note irregularity of inner table of skull (▲).

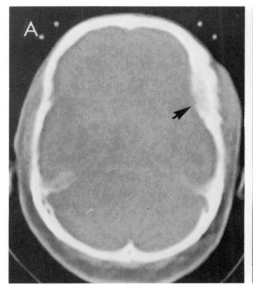 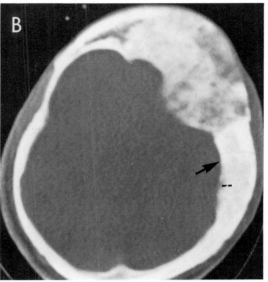

Fig 558.—**A,** axial scan in a patient with small area of fibrous dysplasia (↑). Cortical bone of outer table of skull is not seen in area of lesion; inner table is thickened and homogeneous. **B,** similar scan on another patient with much more extensive fibrous dysplasia. Tables of skull are indistinguishable posteriorly (↑) and anteriorly. In frontal region there is large area of inhomogeneity that represents osteogenic sarcomatous degeneration.

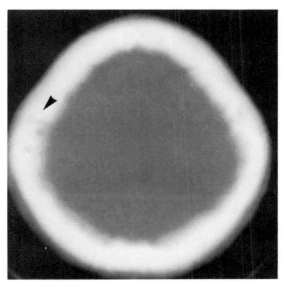

Fig 559.—Axial scan in a normal patient. Lucencies in calvaria represent normal diploic venous channels (▲).

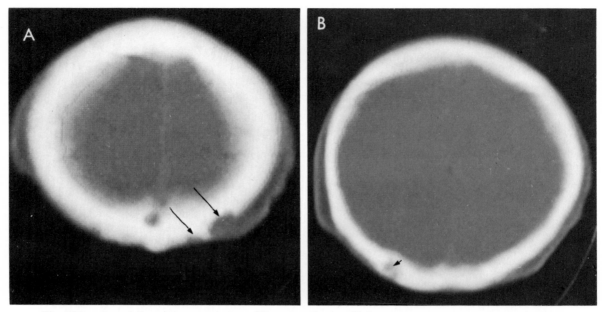

Fig 560.—**A** and **B,** axial scans in two different patients with bony metastases to calvaria. Lesions cause irregular destruction of the skull as well as expansion of inner and outer tables (↘).

the bone (Fig 559). These must be distinguished from metastatic disease, which can produce similar, yet more irregular, asymmetric lucencies (Fig 560, *A* and *B*). The nature of soft tissue masses of the head can frequently be elucidated (Fig 561). Virtually all of these lesions would be entirely invisible on the CT image without specifically displaying the attenuation levels for bone. In this regard, some clarification is in order. CT of the calvaria need rarely be performed as a primary procedure because the routine skull films answer most clinical questions. However, since brain CT is commonly done, it is worthwhile making two sets of images (one for the brain and one for bone) when the clinical situation warrants it. Head trauma best illustrates this point. Nearly all patients with significant head trauma have a CT study of the brain. Delineating the site of a linear fracture by plain films is not as significant as demonstrating the underlying epidural hematoma. In cases of depressed skull fracture, however, it is important to evaluate the degree of bone depression and fragmentation (Fig 562).

One of the exciting areas where CT has proved advantageous is the evaluation of the petrous bone. High-resolution scanning algorithms are available on many scanners, which permit resolution of 11 line pairs per centimeter. These scans differ from conventional brain CT scans in several important ways. Because high-resolution scans are by nature very thin sections, the vol-

ume averaging effect is reduced. The pixel size (as small as 0.15 mm) is also reduced, which results in magnification and higher geometric resolution. Finally, the sampling rate over the anatomical area scanned is increased, thereby producing more measurements of lin-

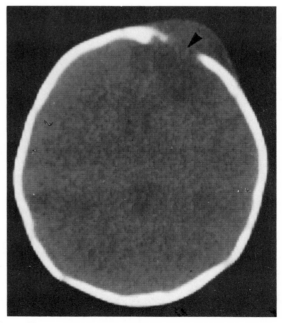

Fig 561.—Traumatic leptomeningeal cyst. Note large cyst extending through obvious bone defect (▲)—child with history of previous cranial trauma.

Index